# Treatment of esophageal varices

# Treatment of esophageal varices

Proceedings of the Tokyo Symposium
on the Treatment of Esophageal Varices,
Tokyo, Japan, 21 – 22 January 1988

*Editor:*

**YASUO IDEZUKI**

Second Department of Surgery,
The University of Tokyo, Faculty of Medicine, Tokyo, Japan

 1988

EXCERPTA MEDICA, AMSTERDAM - NEW YORK - OXFORD

International Congress Series 794
ISBN 0-444-80999-6

*Published by:*
Elsevier Science Publishers B.V.
  (Biomedical Division)
P.O. Box 211
1000 AE Amsterdam
The Netherlands

*Sole distributors for the USA and Canada:*
Elsevier Science Publishing Company, Inc.
52 Vanderbilt Avenue
New York, NY 10017
USA

**Library of Congress Cataloging in Publication Data**

Tokyo Symposium on the Treatment of Espohageal
    Varices (1988)
    Treatment of esophageal varices.

    (International congress series ; 794)
    Includes bibliographies and index.
    1. Esophageal varices--Endoscopic surgery--Congresses.
2. Portal hypertension--Surgery--Congresses.
3. Hemodynamics--Congresses.  4. Esophageal varices--
Surgery--Japan--Congresses.  I. Idezuki, Yasuo,
1934-     .  II. Title.  III. Series: International
congress series ; no. 794.  [DNLM: 1. Esophageal and
Gastric Varices--surgery--congresses.  2. Hemodynamics--
congresses.  3. Sclerosing Solutions--therapeutic use--
congresses.  W3 EX89 no.794 / WI 720 T646t 1988]
RD539.5.T65  1988      617'.5480592      88-31095
ISBN 0-444-80999-6 (U.S.)

Printed in The Netherlands

# Preface

Methods of control of bleeding from ruptured esophagogastric varices have been a target of interest of many physicians and surgeons since establishment of the concept of portal hypertension in the 1930s. However, treatment of esophagogastric varices has always been one of the most controversial issues in surgery and this seems still to be so since the new development of endoscopic sclerotherapy in recent years.

Many surgical procedures have been proposed and performed in patients in the past; however, the most logical and appropriate method of treatment for varices has not been uniformly agreed. One important reason for this is probably because the treatment of varices in most cases is a symptomatic one and does not improve the eventual course of the original diseases of the liver causing portal hypertension and varices. When portal decompression operations were introduced in the 1940s, it was considered that the final sulution had been found; however, after 20 years of experience with these decompression procedures, they were abandoned by many surgeons because the mortality and morbidity associated with these operations were intolerably high and the results of controlled trials reported from many institutions had revealed that the patients' life expectancy was not improved by these shunt operations. In the late 1960s, selective shunt operations were introduced by Dr. Warren and by Dr. Inokuchi, and also the reappraisal and modification of direct operations on the esophagogastric varices were started and gradually became popular in Japan. Again 20 years have elapsed since the introduction of these new procedures, and now the long-term integrity of selective shunts is being questioned and the procedures are being modified again. Discrepancies in the results of direct operations reported from Japan and those reported from the United States and European countries have been significant, and non-shunting operations have not become popular in most of the Western countries.

Although controversies over the issue during the last four decades have mostly been over the methods of operation used by surgeons, since the recent development of endoscopic sclerotherapy controversy now exists between surgeons and physicians over surgery versus endoscopic sclerotherapy. In many institutions the recent development of sclerotherapy has had a great impact on surgeons as well as physicians. It seems that even selection of patients for surgery has been transferred to the hands of physicians from those of surgeons in many of the institutions in many countries.

Each doctor by nature, whether he is a physician or a surgeon, believes in his own treatment, which seems quite natural and is understandable, but often tends to become dogmatic in his selection of patients for a particular treatment. However, it is important to be thoroughly aware of up-to-date results with each method of treatment and to analyse the data from other institutions critically but fairly in order to clarify and to solve the problems facing us. Only a scientific attitude and a critical mind will lead to the right conclusions.

We have invited almost all the prominent physicians and surgeons in Japan who have been engaged in this area so that the current trends in the treatment of varices in Japan will be dealt with comprehensively. We have also invited the most important physicians and surgeons from around the world who have been pioneers in the treatment of varices and have been actively engaged in this field, so that the current trends in other countries will also be well represented.

It is important that in solving this complicated and controversial issue that physicians and surgeons get together and exchange their results and ideas. Most of the practical problems in treating patients with varices have been brought up and discussed among the participants during the two-day symposium. I believe that the most recent results and solid data on treatment of esophagogastric varices from around the world are included in this volume. I sincerely hope that this information will be utilized in the future development of the treatment of varices and portal hypertension.

In the United States and in some of the European countries, liver transplantation is being performed as an ultimate form of treatment of bleeding varices in cirrhotic patients. Certainly, this may be a form of radical treatment for these patients, but liver transplantation still has its own problems and the number of patients to benefit from this radical approach will be limited.

**Yasuo Idezuki**

*A note from the editor:* The original manuscript by Dr. W. Dean Warren covering his talk at the symposium could not be included in this volume because of his severe condition due to the advance of his unrelenting illness. Those who attended the symposium should recall his invaluable endeavours and contributions to the symposium despite his severe illness. It is greatly appreciated that the authors, J.B. Lippincott Company and The Emory University Journal of Medicine have kindly permitted us to use the article by Henderson, Millikan and Warren which appeared in the Emory University Journal of Medicine as a substitute in this volume (Chapter 20).

# The Tokyo Symposium on the Treatment of Esophageal Varices (Tokyo, Japan, 21 – 22 January 1988)

**PRESIDENT**
Yasuo Idezuki              (The University of Tokyo)

**ADVISORY BOARD TO EXECUTIVE COMMITTEE**

| | |
|---|---|
| Fumihiro Ichida | (Niigata University) |
| Kiyoshi Inokuchi | (Saga Prefectural Hospital) |
| Kunio Okuda | (Chiba University) |
| Toshitsugu Oda | (National Medical Center of Hospital) |
| Takao Sakita | (Showa General Hospital) |
| Tatsuo Wada | (Kanagawa Cancer Center) |

**EXECUTIVE COMMITTEE**

| | |
|---|---|
| Haruo Aoki | (Fujita-Gakuen Health University) |
| Toshio Isomatsu | (Sapporo Teishin Hospital) |
| Kaoru Umeyama | (Osaka City University) |
| Hiroshi Oka | (The University of Tokyo) |
| Eizo Okamoto | (Hyogo College of Medicine) |
| Keiichi Ono | (Hirosaki University) |
| Reiji Kasukawa | (Fukushima Medical College) |
| Haruo Kameda | (The Jikei University) |
| Seiichiro Kobayashi | (Tokyo Women's Medical College) |
| Michio Kobayashi | (Medical College of Oita) |
| Kenji Koyama | (Akita University) |
| Toshio Sato | (Tohoku University) |
| Mitsuo Sugiura | (Juntendo University) |
| Keizo Sugimachi | (Kyusyu University) |
| Tadayoshi Takemoto | (Yamaguchi University) |
| Takayoshi Tobe | (Kyoto University) |
| Fusahiro Nagao | (The Jikei University) |
| Masayoshi Namiki | (Asahikawa Medical College) |
| Terukazu Mutoh | (Niigata University) |
| Sadahiro Yamamoto | (Aichi Medical University) |

**ORGANIZING COMMITTEE**

| | |
|---|---|
| Yoshiya Kumagai | (Mitsukoshi Health and Ware Foundation) |
| Hiroaki Suzuki | (The Jikei University) |
| Yasuhiro Takase | (The University of Tsukuba) |
| Yusuke Tada | (The University of Tokyo) |
| Shunji Futagawa | (Juntendo University) |

**EXECUTIVE SECRETARY**
Kensho Sanjo              (The University of Tokyo)

# Acknowledgements

The Committee of The Tokyo Symposium on the Treatment of Esophageal Varices wishes
to thank the following for their valuable contributions:

**Supporter's organization:**
  Ministry of Education, Science and Culture of Japan
  Second Department of Surgery,
    University of Tokyo, Faculty of Medicine

**Main sponsors:**
  Shionogi & Co., Ltd.
  Eisai Co., Ltd.
  Yamanouchi Pharmaceutical Co., Ltd.
  Sankyo Co., Ltd.
  Tsumura Juntendo Inc.
  Taiho Pharmaceutical Co., Ltd.
  Morishita Pharmaceutical Co., Ltd.
  Warner-Lambert K.K.
  Ajinomoto Co., Ltd.
  Toshiba Medical System Co., Ltd.

**Sponsors:**
  Green Cross Corporation
  Kaigen Co., Ltd.
  Lederle (Japan) Ltd.

**Publication coordinator**
  Jeff International Project Inc., Tokyo

# Contents

**Preface**
*Y. Idezuki* .................................................................... v
**The Tokyo Symposium on the Treatment of Esophageal Varices** ........................ vii
**Acknowledgements** .................................................... ix

## INDICATIONS AND RESULTS OF ENDOSCOPIC SCLEROTHERAPY

**Chairpersons:** *Tadayoshi Takemoto and Haruo Kameda*

**Chapter 1**
Indications and early and long-term results of paravariceal immediate, elective and prophylactic injection sclerotherapy
*K.-J. Paquet* .................................................................... 1
**Chapter 2**
Results of endoscopic sclerotherapy: influence of hepatic reserve and cause of varices
*E.P. DiMagno* .................................................................... 23
**Chapter 3**
Indication and results of injection sclerotherapy
*E. Okamoto, A. Shu and Y. Nakai* .................................................... 37
**Chapter 4**
Endoscopic sclerotherapy for esophageal varices by combined injection technique with 1% Polidocanol
*Y. Watanabe, M. Kohyama, R. Ohmasa, K. Masuda, H. Suzuki and O. Miho* ............. 45
**Chapter 5**
Endoscopic injection sclerotherapy: application, results and prediction of recurrence after the treatment
*Y. Yazaki, H. Maguchi, S. Okano, Y. Tominaga, T. Suzuki, M. Mizuno, C. Sekiya, A. Uehara and M. Namiki* .................................................................... 53
**Chapter 6**
Clinical evaluation of endoscopic injection sclerotherapy for esophageal varices
*K. Tanikawa and A. Toyonaga* ........................................................ 67
**Chapter 7**
A combination method for endoscopic injection sclerotherapy with ethanolamine oleate and polidocanol on esophageal varices
*R. Kasukawa, M. Masaki, K. Obara and H. Mitsuhashi* ............................... 75
**Chapter 8**
Indication and technique of endoscopic injection sclerotherapy
*K. Sugimachi, S. Kitano, M. Hashizume and H. Yamaga* ............................... 85
**Chapter 9**
Elective treatment of esophageal varices by injection sclerotherapy
*Y. Takase, Y. Kobayashi and S. Shibuya* ............................................. 95
**Chapter 10**
Indications of injection sclerotherapy for varices of the cardia
*Y. Kumagai and H. Makuuchi* ........................................................ 105
**Chapter 11**
Pathological findings after endoscopical injection sclerotherapy for esophageal varices
*M. Arakawa and M. Kage* ............................................................ 111

# INDICATIONS AND RESULTS OF NON-SHUNTING OPERATIONS

**Chairpersons:** *Toshio Sato and Hiroshi Takagi*

**Chapter 12**
Oesophageal transection for varices: rationale, indications, technique and results
*R.A.J. Spence* ................................................................... 123
**Chapter 13**
Indications and results of portal-azygos disconnection surgeries (terminal esophago-proximal gastrectomy, proximal gastric transection and autosuture proximal gastrectomy) under endoscope assistance
*S. Yamamoto* ................................................................... 141
**Chapter 14**
Experience with non-shunting operation for esophageal varices, 1980 – 87
*M. Sugiura, S. Futagawa, M. Fukasawa, Eiichi Kinoshita, R. Nakanishi and Y. Nishimura* . 149
**Chapter 15**
Late results of 224 cases of esophageal transection for esophageal varices
*S. Kobayashi and K. Takasaki* ................................................... 161
**Chapter 16**
Indications and results of transabdominal esophageal transection for esophageal varices
*K. Umeyama, T. Yamashita, K. Yoshikawa and T. Ishikawa* ......................... 167
**Chapter 17**
Indications and results of non-shunting operations for esophageal varices
*Y. Idezuki, K. Sanjo, H. Koyama, H. Sakamoto and N. Kokudo* ...................... 175
**Chapter 18**
Indications and results of non-shunting operations: experience in 190 cases
*K. Ouchi, T. Sato and K. Koyama* ............................................... 187
**Chapter 19**
The role of non-shunting surgery in the treatment of esophageal varices in comparison to injection sclerotherapy
*K. Yoshida, K. Tsukada and T. Muto* ............................................. 195

# INDICATIONS AND RESULTS OF SELECTIVE SHUNTS

**Chairpersons:** *Sadahiro Yamamoto and Tatsuzo Tanabe*

**Chapter 20**
Selective variceal decompression by the distal splenorenal shunt: an Emory perspective 20 years later
*J.M. Henderson, W.J. Millikan, Jr. and W.D. Warren* ............................... 205
**Chapter 21**
The importance of hepatic functional reserve as a determinant of prognosis after portal decompression
*F.E. Eckhauser, J.G. Turcotte and G.D. Zuidema* ................................. 239
**Chapter 22**
Evaluation of shunting operation for the treatment of portal hypertension
*Yan-Ting Huang* ................................................................ 247
**Chapter 23**
Mesocaval shunts
*K.G. Swan, J.J. Flanagan and J.M. Rocko* ....................................... 257
**Chapter 24**
Indication, results and prognosis of distal splenorenal shunt
*K.-J. Paquet* ................................................................... 271
**Chapter 25**
Selective shunts for esophageal varices via trans-left gastric venous and trans-splenic routes — their rationale and clinical results
*M. Kobayashi, K. Inokuchi and K. Sugimachi* ..................................... 277

**Chapter 26**
Indication and results of distal splenorenal shunt
*T. Isomatsu* ................................................................. 287
**Chapter 27**
Long-term results of superselective distal splenorenal shunt
*H. Katoh and T. Tanabe* ....................................................... 299

## HEMODYNAMICS OF ESOPHAGEAL VARICES

**Chairpersons:** *Hiroshi Oka and Takayoshi Tobe*

**Chapter 28**
Experimental and clinical effects of vasopressin
*K.G. Swan, J.J. Flanagan and D.M. Rosa* ....................................... 303
**Chapter 29**
The hemodynamics of esophago-gastric varices: significance of esophago-gastric arterial inflow
in their formation
*H. Aoki, A. Hasumi and M. Shimazu* ........................................... 315
**Chapter 30**
Continuous intravenous infusion of pitressin for esophageal variceal bleeding and combined
therapy for esophageal varices
*J. Ono and T. Katsuki* ........................................................ 329
**Chapter 31**
The effect of an amino acid solution granule-enriched with branched chain amino acids, and
arginine, in patients with portal systemic encephalopathy
*K. Sanjo, Y. Idezuki and H. Oka* .............................................. 339
**Chapter 32**
Emergency control of bleeding esophageal varices using a transparent tamponade tube (Idezuki's
tube)
*M. Hagiwara, Y. Sato, M. Sakai and H. Watanabe* ............................... 347
**Chapter 33**
Angiographic study of hemodynamics in portal hypertension
*S. Futagawa, R. Nakanishi, Y. Hishimura and M. Sugiura* ........................ 355

## TREATMENT OF ESOPHAGEAL VARICES IN JAPAN

**Chairperson:** *Taketo Katsuki*

**Chapter 34**
Study on portal hypertension in Japan: activities of the Japanese Research Society for Portal
Hypertension during a period of 20 years
*K. Inokuchi* .................................................................. 361

**Chairperson:** *Tatsuo Wada*

**Chapter 35**
Current status of treatment of esophageal varices in Japan: endoscopic sclerotherapy in Japan
*Y. Idezuki* ................................................................... 367

## Summary of general discussion on the treatment of esophageal varices

**Chairpersons:** *W.D. Warren and Yasuo Idezuki* ........................................ 375

*K.-J. Paquet*                    *Kiyoshi Inokuchi*
*Roy A.J. Spence*                 *Mitsuo Sugiura*
*Kenneth G. Swan*                 *Sadahiro Yamomoto*
*Frederic E. Eckhauser*           *Kyuichi Tanikawa*
*Eugene P. DiMagno*               *Yasuhiro Takase*
*Huang Yan-Ting*                  *Hiroshi Ashida*

**Closing remarks** ................................................................. 379

**Author index** ................................................................... 381

**Subject index** .................................................................. 383

© 1988 Elsevier Science Publishers B.V. (Biomedical Division)
*Treatment of esophageal varices*
*Y. Idezuki, editor*

Chapter 1

# Indications and early and long-term results of paravariceal immediate, elective and prophylactic injection sclerotherapy

K.-J Paquet

*Department of Surgery and Vascular Surgery, Heinz-Kalk Hospital, Am Gradierbau, D-8730 Bad Kissingen, FRG*

As so often happens, interest in an old technique has been renewed. Injection sclerotherapy was introduced in 1939 by Crawfoord and Frenckner [1] and in 1955 Macbeth [2] reported good results in 30 patients. A few other reports followed in ear, nose and throat journals but then shunt procedures became popular and have been an elective standard treatment for the past 20 years. Lately, however, surgeons have become disillusioned with shunt surgery, particularly for emergency bleeding. While Orloff et al. [3] still recommend emergency portacaval shunts, despite a mortality of 49% in the first 138 patients, shunting is an elective procedure in most centers. Even then the late encephalopathy has been found to be significant, and not only in those with very poor liver function. Against this background, Johnston and Rodgers and our group in 1973 [4, 5] published remarkably good results from sclerotherapy, controlling bleeding in 93 (92%) out of 117 patients with a total admission mortality of 18 (19%). Several other centers in Europe, South Africa and the United States then adapted the technique. However, around this time Warren and Inokuchi [6, 7] were starting their selective shunts, aimed at reducing the incidence of encephalopathy, so now is an opportune time in the treatment of this difficult disease to assess the role of injection sclerotherapy.

Stelzner and Lierse [8] noted that at the esophagogastric junction in rhesus monkeys (Fig. 1) the gastric subglandular veins pierce the muscularis mucosa to become subepithelial in position for the lowest few centimetres of the esophagus. Varices are useful collateral channels bypassing a venous block. It is only the few that happen to impinge on the esophageal mucosa that are dangerous and it is only these that need treatment [9]. Experiences in more than 1000 emergency endoscopies of the upper gastrointestinal tract in patients with liver cirrhosis and variceal hemorrhage have demonstrated that the source of bleeding can be found in the lower part of the esophagus in more than 90% of cases. This is the rationale for local sclerotherapy rather than larger operations to bypass or ligate all the collateral chan-

2

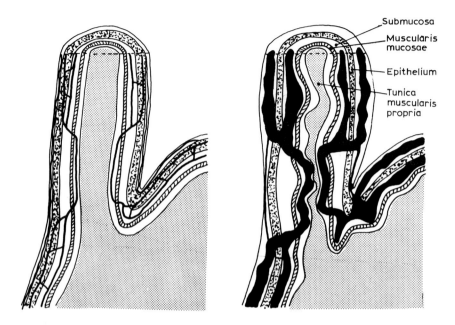

Submucosa

Muscularis
mucosae

Epithelium

Tunica
muscularis
propria

FIG. 1  Anatomical localization of esophageal varices in the lower part of the esophagus in rhesus monkeys; they are localized subepithelially.

TABLE 1  Different groups treated by paravariceal endoscopic sclerotherapy (01.01.1969 – 01.09.1987; $n$ = 1761) at the Department of Surgery, University of Bonn, and the Heinz-Kalk Hospital, Bad Kissingen, FRG

| Group I | : | Acute and uncontrollable variceal hemorrhage ($n$ = 540 – 232 (group Ia) = 308) |
|---|---|---|
| Group Ia | : | Prospective evaluation ($n$ = 232; 01.01.1982 – 01.01.1987) |
| Group II | : | Acute variceal hemorrhage – prospective controlled randomized trial ($n$ = 22 (43); 01.01.80 – 01.01.81) |
| Group III | : | Elective treatment of variceal hemorrhage ($n$ = 1016) |
| Group IVa | : | Prophylactic treatment of esophageal varices 1. Prospective controlled randomized trial ($n$ = 36; 01.01.78 – 01.01.80) |
| Group IVb | : | 2. Prospective evaluation ($n$ = 82; 01.01.80 – 01.09.86) |
| Group V | : | Acute and elective treatment of variceal hemorrhage in childhood ($n$ = 65; 01.01.72 – 01.09.87) |

nels. Our group has performed the method of paravariceal injection for more than 17 years and collected experience on more than 1750 patients, divided into 5 different groups (Table 1). The classification according to Child-Pugh [10, 11] is shown in Table 2.

Endoscopic sclerotherapy of esophageal varices is a therapeutic procedure to treat bleeding esophageal varices and to prevent further variceal bleeding. This procedure involves the passage of an esophagoscope, visualization of the esophageal varices and injection of a sclerosing agent into the varices or into the area surrounding the varices – paravariceally. The mechanism of injection sclerosis to control variceal hemorrhage is not understood completely, and involves a series of pathological events. The sclerosing agents are thought to damage the intima of varix and to cause intraluminal thrombosis followed by necrosis, polymorphonuclear leucocyte in-

TABLE 2   Sclerotherapy of the esophageal wall in esophageal varices: total number and classification after Child-Pugh ($n$ = 1761; 01.01.1969 – 01.09.1987 Department of Surgery, University of Bonn, and Heinz-Kalk Hospital, Bad Kissingen)

|  | Classification | | |
|---|---|---|---|
|  | Child A | Child B | Child C |
| Number | 317 | 370 | 1074 |
| Percent | 18 | 21 | 61 |

TABLE 3   Indications for injection sclerotherapy of esophageal varices

1. Acute, particularly uncontrollable bleeding esophageal varices
2. Prevention of recurrent hemorrhage from esophageal varices
3. Complete thrombosis of the portal venous system
4. Shunt thrombosis in patients with intrahepatic block
5. Bleeding esophageal varices in babies and children
6. Varices III – IV with teleangiectasias and IVP over 30 cmH$_2$O

TABLE 4   Additional devices for endoscopic sclerotherapy of bleeding esophageal varices

Flexible tube
Balloons for tamponade
X-ray monitoring

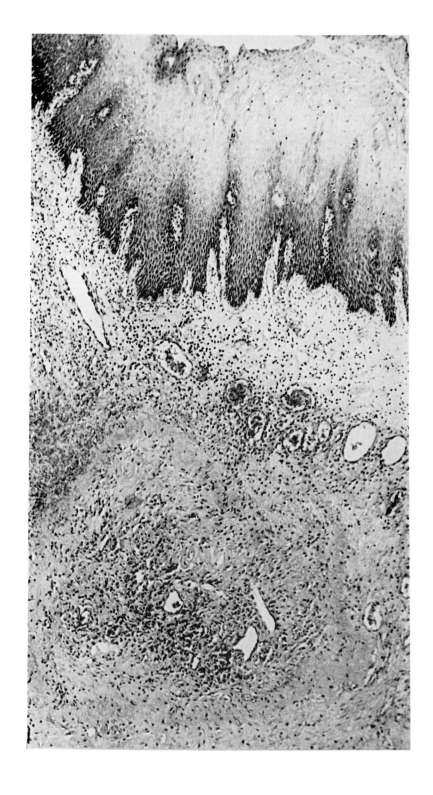

filtration, and localized inflammation. This, in turn, is thought to progress to intravascular fibrous organization, intimal thickening and perivenous fibrosis. By using the paravariceal approach the varices as collaterals are protected by scar tissue and thickening of the epithelium and mucosa and still perfused (Fig. 2).

The technique to perform endoscopic sclerotherapy is not standardized. Physicians differ in the indications for treatment. Our main indications are listed in Table 3. We must consider several different points. Will injection sclerotherapy be performed during the acute hemorrhage as emergency treatment or will it be performed after conservative management with vaso- or glycylpressin or balloon tamponade or only if this conservative management is not effective? Will it be applied as long-term management to prevent recurrent bleeding or are there indications for its prophylactic use (Table 4)? Is it suitable for all patients without respect to their liver function or should it only be chosen for patients with decompensated liver function, especial-

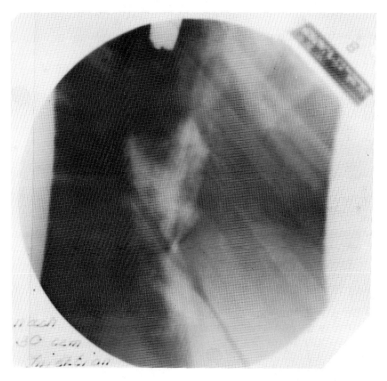

FIG. 3  X-ray control of paravariceal or submucosal injection of sclerosant diluted by contrast medium; the X-ray picture is taken three minutes after injection; all injected substance is still localized in the injection areas and has not entered the systemic circulation.

---

FIG. 2  Histological specimen of the terminal esophagus after paravariceal endoscopic injection sclerotherapy and resection of 3 cm terminal esophagus; esophageal varices are still perfused.

ly Child C patients? Can the results of endoscopic sclerotherapy be improved if this type of treatment is combined with other methods such as drugs, laser or shunt operation and performed as acute or long-term management? Are additional devices necessary for endoscopic sclerotherapy of esophageal varices such as an additional tube, which is recommended by the King's College Hospital in London, or different types of balloon or is X-ray monitoring during injection necessary or advisable? We prefer to do it by free-hand technique without special devices. We only sometimes check the localization of injection if it is para- or intravariceal by X-ray monitoring (Fig. 3). The schedule of our method of paravariceal endoscopic sclerotherapy is shown in Table 5.

Furthermore, physicians and surgeons differ (Table 6) with regard to volume of sclerosing agent, the type, number, place, depth and frequency of injections, the type of endoscope and anaesthetic and attractive supportive measures.

TABLE 5   Schedule of paravariceal endoscopic sclerotherapy

| | |
|---|---|
| 1. Acute: | 5 – 15 ml 0.5% polidocanol in portions of 1 ml up to the stop of hemorrhage. |
| 2. Elective: | (a) 40 ml 0.5% polidocanol in 40 portions in the terminal esophagus. |
| | (b) After 7 days the same; if there are no ulcerations, take 1% polidocanol; in the case of ulcerations wait or inject only 20 ml. |
| | (c) Usually 1 – 6 sessions using the same schedule till teleangiectasias disappeared and epithelium and mucosa are completely covered by fibrous tissue. |
| | (d) Simultaneous selection of the patients for elective and selective shunt operation. |
| | (e) Endoscopic control after 4 months and resclerosis if necessary 90%. Inject per session 0.5 or 1% polidocanol in 40 portions of 0.75 ml. |
| | (f) Thereafter endoscopic control every 4 – 12 months. |
| 3. Prophylactic: | Same schedule as in 2. |

TABLE 6   Differences in the techniques of endoscopic sclerotherapy of esophageal varices

1. Different substances for injection, e.g. polidocanol, ethanolamine, etc.
2. Volume per injection
3. Place and depth of injection: intra-, para- and combined injection
4. Schedule of sclerotherapy, e.g. injection once per week, etc.; control after 3 – 4 months
5. Type of endoscope, rigid or flexible
6. Methods of compression during injection

TABLE 7  Results of main uncontrolled studies of emergency injection sclerotherapy using a rigid esophagoscope (on general anaesthesia) in patients with acute variceal bleeding

| References | No. of patients | Emergency injection sclerotherapy | | Hemostasis (immediate) (%) | Inpatient mortality (%) |
|---|---|---|---|---|---|
| | | Method | Timing | | |
| Johnston and Rogers (1973) | 117 | Ethanolamine 5% i.v. | After tamponade | 93 | 18 |
| Paquet et al. (1978) | 51 (211) | Polidocanol 1% p.v. | Uncontrollable hemorrhage | 91 | 20 |
| Palani et al. (1981) | 22 | Sodium morrhuate 5% i.v. | After tamponade and/or vasopressin | 79 | 29 |
| Terblanche et al. (1981) | 66 (93 admissions) | Ethanolamine 5% i.v. | After tamponade | 92 | 28 |
| Alwmark et al. (1982) | 50 | Polidocanol 1% p.v. | After vasopressin and tamponade | 89 | 14 |
| Barsoum et al. (1982) | 100 | Ethanolamine 5% i. + p.v. | Within 12 – 24 h of admission | 72 | 21 |
| Fleig et al. (1983) | 25 | Polidocanol 1% p.v. | After ineffective tamponade | 92 | 40 |
| Total | 600 | | | 87 | 24 |

TABLE 8 Results of the main uncontrolled studies of emergency injection sclerotherapy using a flexible endoscope in patients with acute variceal bleeding

| References | No. of patients | Emergency injection sclerotherapy | | Hemostasis (immediate) (%) | Inpatient mortality rate (%) |
| | | Method | Timing | | |
|---|---|---|---|---|---|
| Lewis et al. (1981) | 19 | Simultaneous gastric balloon tamponade and sodium morrhuate, 5%, intravariceal | Immediate | 93 | 42 |
| Kjaergaard et al. (1982) | 61 | Polidocanol, 3%, paravariceal | After tamponade in 29 patients (bleeding stopped in the 32 others) | 92 | 31 |
| Stray et al. (1982) | 8 | Polidocanol, 1%, paravariceal | Immediate or after tamponade | 85 | 37 |
| Takase et al. (1982) | 30 | Simultaneous oesophageal balloon tamponade and ethanolamine oleate, 5%, in-intravariceal | After tamponade | 96 | 37 |
| Soehendra et al. (1983) | 120 | Polidocanol, 1%, submucosal and travariceal | Immediate or after tamponade | 84 | 36 |
| Paquet (1983) | 386 | Polidocanol, 1%, paravariceal | Immediate | 92 | 22 |
| Nilsson (1984) | 43 | Polidocanol, 1%, submucosal and intravariceal | Immediate or after tamponade and vasopressin | 100 | 19 |
| Total | 812 | | | 92 | 32 |

## Results

Endoscopic sclerotherapy has been used to control acute variceal hemorrhage which persists despite maximal medical therapy, to prevent recurrent variceal hemorrhage in patients with a history of esophageal hemorrhage, and to prevent a hemorrhage even in patients with esophageal varices who never bled.

*Emergency injection sclerotherapy*
The aim of emergency sclerotherapy of esophageal varices is to stop the variceal bleeding by either thrombosis of the bleeding varices secondary to an intravariceal injection of the sclerosant or acute thickening of the bleeding varix wall secondary to a submucosal injection of the sclerosant close to this varix. Since the method was brought up to date by Johnston, Rodgers and our group in 1973 [4, 5], a myriad of technical innovations have appeared. A rigid as well as a flexible endoscope was used, the former requiring general anaesthesia. The results of 15 uncontrolled studies, applying rigid (Table 7) and flexible endoscopes are demonstrated here [4, 12 – 24]: 600 patients were managed by ethanolamine, polidocanol and sodium morrhuate by injection sclerotherapy during uncontrollable hemorrhage, after treatment with tamponade or vasopressin or within 12 – 24 hours of the admission or after ineffective tamponade. Immediate hemostasis was achieved in 72 – 93% (median 87%) and inpatient mortality varies from 14 – 40% (median 24%) in patients treated with the rigid endoscope. If patients were treated with a flexible endoscope the numbers were quite similar (Table 8) in 812 patients treated with sodium morrhuate, polidocanol and ethanolamine immediately after tamponade or after tamponade and vasopressin. The median value of immediate hemostasis was 92% and inpatient mortality 32%.

In two controlled trials (Table 9) it could be demonstrated that emergency injection sclerotherapy (i.e. immediate para- or intravariceal injection during emergency endoscopy because of acute variceal hemorrhage) can significantly improve hemostasis and survival in comparison with other conservative measures [25, 26].

Our group compared in a controlled randomized trial the effect of the Sengstaken-Blakemore tube (SBT) with paravariceal endoscopic sclerosis (IES) in 22

TABLE 9   Results of two controlled trials of emergency injection sclerotherapy of bleeding esophageal varices using flexible endoscopes

| References | No. of patients | Method of emergency injection sclerotherapy i.v., p.v. | Hemostasis (immediate) (%) (sc/c) | Survival rate after 1 year (%) |
|---|---|---|---|---|
| Paquet and Feussner (1985) | 21 | Polidocanol 0.5 + 1% p.v. | 90 (55) | 79 (38) |
| Larson et al. (1986) | 44 | Tetradecylsulfate 3% i.v. | 85 (47) | 62 (54) |

TABLE 10   Results of a randomized controlled trial comparing Sengstaken-Blakemore
tube (SBT) to emergency endoscopic sclerotherapy (ES) during emergency

|  | | SBT | ES | Statistical significance |
|---|---|---|---|---|
| 1. | No. of patients | 22 | 21 | NS |
| 2. | Primary control of hemorrhage | 16 (73%) | 20 (95%) | NS |
| 3. | Recurrence of hemorrhage | 7[a] (44%) | 4[a] (20%) | NS |
| 4. | Control of recurrent hemorrhage | 3[b] (43%) | 3[b] (75%) | NS |
| 5. | Definite control of hemorrhage per patient | 12/22 (55%) | 19/21 (90%) | $P < 0.01$ |
| 6. | Definite control of hemorrhage per bleeding episode | 19/29 (66%) | 23/25 (92%) | $P < 0.01$ |
| 7. | No. of acute complications | 2 (10%) | 2 (10%) | NS |
| 8. | No. of transfusions required | 5 (23%) | 3 (14%) | NS |
| 9. | Mortality at 30 days | 6/22 (27%) | 2/21 (10%) | $P < 0.01$ |
| 10. | Mortality at 6 months | 11/22 (50%) | 3/21 (14%) | $P < 0.01$ |
| 11. | Late total mortality | 17/22 (77%) | 7/21 (33%) | $P < 0.001$ |

The probabilities were calculated using Fisher's exact probability test. NS = > 0.05. Data in rows 1 – 10
are calculated for the first six months of the trial.
[a] 7/16 = 44%; 4/20 = 20%.
[b] 3/7 = 43%; 3/4 = 75%.

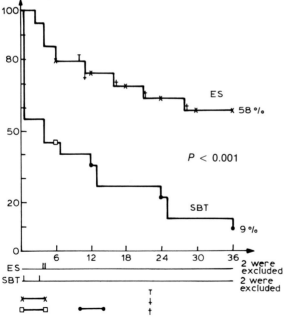

FIG. 4   Cumulative survival curve using the method of Kaplan-Meier for the controlled randomized trial comparing the Sengstaken-Blakemore tube (SBT) with emergency endoscopic
sclerotherapy (ES) during emergency endoscopy.

and 21 patients, respectively. Bleeding was controlled in 16 of 22 patients (73%) with SBT and in 20 of 21 with IES (95%) (Table 10). Recurrences of hemorrhage occurred in 7 of 16 patients controlled by SBT (44%) and 4 of 20 controlled by IES (20%). These differences are statistically not significant. Rebleeding was controlled again in 3 of 7 by SBT (43%) and by IES in 3 of 4 patients (75%) (Table 10). Thus, definitive control of hemorrhage was accomplished in 12 of 22 patients (55%) and in 19 of 29 bleeding episodes (66%) with SBT, and in 19 of 21 patients (90%) and in 23 of 25 bleeding episodes (92%) with IES, which is statistically significantly more than with SBT ($P < 0.01$). Six of the 22 SBT patients (27%) died within 30 days of admission, compared to 2 of the 21 IES patients (10%). This difference is statistically significant ($P < 0.01$), too. The cumulative survival curve using the method of Kaplan-Meier (Fig. 4) [27, 28] demonstrates a statistically significant difference in favour of IES after 6 months ($P < 0.01$) and a higher significance after 36 months ($P < 0.001$).

On the basis of these results since January 1982 we performed in our hospital immediate endoscopic injection sclerosis (IEIS) of bleeding esophageal varices during emergency endoscopy. We have prospectively treated 232 patients up to the first of

TABLE 11   Etiology of the intra- and prehepatic block and Child-Pugh classification of a prospective evaluation of immediate endoscopic injection sclerosis (IEIS) ($n$ = 232; 01.01.1982 – 01.01.1987)

|   |   | Number | Percent |
|---|---|---|---|
| **A.** | **Underlying disease** | | |
| | Alcoholic cirrhosis | 138 | 59.5 |
| | Posthepatic cirrhosis | 47 | 20.3 |
| | Cirrhosis of unknown etiology | 17 | 7.3 |
| | Primary biliary cirrhosis | 11 | 4.7 |
| | Extrahepatic bile duct atresia | 2 | 0.9 |
| | Secondary biliar cirrhosis | 1 | 0.4 |
| | Liver cirrhosis (total) | 216 | 93.1 |
| | Prehepatic block | 9 | 3.9 |
| | Liver fibrosis | 5 | 2.2 |
| | Schistosomiasis | 1 | 0.4 |
| | Mucoviscidosis | 1 | 0.4 |
| | Non-cirrhotic patients (total) | 16 | 6.9 |
| **B.** | **Classification** | | |
| | Child-Pugh A[a] | 53 | 23 |
| | Child-Pugh B | 70 | 30 |
| | Child-Pugh C | 109 | 47 |
| | Total | 232 | 100 |

[a] Non-cirrhotic patients are classified as Child-Pugh A.

January 1987 with the following Child-Pugh criteria [29]: 53 (23%) A, 70 (30%) B and 109 (47%) C. More than 93% had liver cirrhosis, with 60% being of alcoholic origin (Table 11). If IEIS by the free technique was not successful after 15 minutes a Linton-Nachlas tube was inserted for 6 – 12 hours. In cases of recurrences of hemorrhage a second emergency endoscopy and IEIS and, if this was not successful, a gastroesophageal disconnection was performed directly. During the bleeding-free interval Child-Pugh A and B patients were selected using special criteria for shunt operation. All sclerotherapy patients were checked after 4 months and thereafter every 6, 9 and 12 months and reinjected if necessary. Bleeding was controlled in 93% with IEIS and in 97% with the combination of IEIS and Linton-Nachlas tube. Definite control of hemorrhage was accomplished in 94%. Thirty-five patients died during the first days of admission (15.1%). The main causes of death were liver failure and variceal hemorrhage. Only 2 patients were lost to follow up. The main causes of 39 late deaths (29.8%) were liver failure, hepatocellular cancer and hemorrhage. The calculated cumulative survival curve using the method of Kaplan-Meier demonstrates a five-year life expectancy of about 45% (Fig. 5). Thus IEIS during emergency endoscopy is established as a primary therapeutic mode to successfully control bleeding esophageal varices. It seems to be superior to elective sclerotherapy. In spite of that we recommend this strategy only for a very experienced operator and endoscopist who must be available day and night and who has an experienced endoscopy team with at least two additional persons at hand.

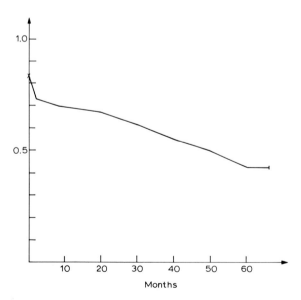

FIG. 5  Survival curve using the method of Kaplan-Meier in the prospective evaluation of IEIS.

TABLE 12  Long-term results of controlled trials of elective endoscopic sclerotherapy of bleeding esophageal varices using a flexible endoscope

| Reference | No. of patients (sc/c) | Rebleeding reduced | Survival prolonged (therapy/control) |
|---|---|---|---|
| Westaby et al. (1983) | 56/60 | Significant | 78/43 |
| Terblanche et al. (1983) | 38/37 | Significant | Not significant |
| Copenhagen ES Trial (1984) | 93/94 | Significant (beginning at 40th day) | 57/27 (after 40 days) |
| Söderlund (1985) | 54/53 | Significant | Not significant |
| Korula et al. (1985) | 56/60 | Significant | 51/35 (significant if urgent shunts are excluded) |
| | 297/309 | Significant | |

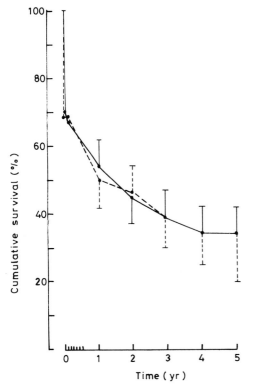

FIG. 6  Cumulative survival in the controlled trial of Terblanche et al. [31] comparing elective endoscopic sclerotherapy (———) and controls (– – –); bleeding and controls were managed by endoscopic sclerotherapy.

14

*Elective endoscopic sclerotherapy*
Several controlled trials (Table 12) have shown that endoscopic sclerotherapy of esophageal varices significantly reduces the incidence of recurrent bleeding [30 – 34]. The uniformly positive outcome of these trials (with some exceptions; for example the trial of Terblanche (Fig. 6 [31]) has firmly established the efficacy of endoscopic sclerotherapy. This efficacy is, as found by most investigators, quite variable in the reported trials. In most of the studies it decreases more and more when more phases of injection sclerotherapy were performed. Only Terblanche et al. could not demonstrate a difference in the incidence of recurrent variceal bleeding between the sclerotherapy and the control groups in the first 3 months of the trial.

Effective sclerotherapy not only lowers the incidence of rebleeding but also increases life expectancy. It is to be expected that only those trials which show a marked reduction in the bleeding risk of the sclerotherapy group have documented an improvement in the survival rate. The difference in the percentage of recurrent hemorrhage in the Cape Town study [31] precluded a significant effect on survival. Cumulative survival in the London study (Fig. 7) [30], however, showed a one-year survival of 75% in the sclerotherapy and 58% in the control group ($P < 0.01$). In the final report of this trial [35], after a follow-up of 6 years, an even better survival in the sclerotherapy group was reported ($P < 0.001$). In the sclerotherapy group 18 deaths occurred (5 from variceal bleeding), in marked contrast with the 32 deaths (25 from hemorrhage) in the control group. These findings are confirmed by our own results of a retrospective analysis of more than 1000 patients over a period of nearly 18 years (Table 13): hospital mortality is now under 10% and the complication rate estimated by control endoscopy and resclerosis in weekly intervals during treatment is now about 10%. The estimated natural history of variceal bleeding in

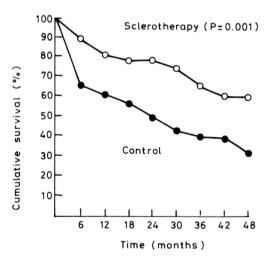

FIG. 7 Cumulative survival curve of the controlled trial at King's College Hospital in London comparing elective endoscopic sclerotherapy and control; bleeding in the control group was not usually managed by endoscopic sclerotherapy.

patients with cirrhosis [36, 37] is shown in Table 14 according to Child-Pugh classification. After 2 years it varies between 65% (Child-Pugh A) and 23% (Child-Pugh C). By sclerotherapy it can be prolonged in A patients to 95, in B patients to 78 and in C patients to 53%, mainly by prevention of rebleeding (Table 15). This is readily apparent in our personal cumulative survival curve (Fig. 8) [38].

TABLE 13   Indications for sclerotherapy of the esophageal wall after acute bleeding of esophageal varices in the non-bleeding interval (01.01.1969 – 01.09.1987, n = 1016; Group III; Department of Surgery, University of Bonn, and Heinz-Kalk Hospital, Bad Kissingen)

| Number | Percent | Disease |
|--------|---------|---------|
| 752 | 74.0 | Decompensated liver cirrhosis |
| 193 | 19.0 | Compensated liver cirrhosis (a shunt was refused or not recommended) |
| 51 | 5.0 | Prehepatic block |
| 15 | 1.5 | Osteomyelosclerosis |
| 5 | 0.5 | Others |

TABLE 14   Estimated natural history of variceal bleeding in patients with liver cirrhosis, according to Child's classification (from Graham and Lacey-Smith [36] and Burroughs et al. [37])

| Child classification | Survival rate after 1 month | 1 year | 2 years |
|----------------------|-----------------------------|--------|---------|
| A | 85 | 76 | 65 |
| B | 75 | 52 | 39 |
| C | 65 | 35 | 23 |

TABLE 15   Survival following prospective paravariceal elective injection sclerotherapy of 200 consecutive patients according to Child classification (personal unpublished data)

| Classification | No. of patients | Survival | |
|----------------|-----------------|----------|--------|
| | | 1 year | 2 years |
| Child A | 45 | 99 | 95 |
| Child B | 60 | 79 | 78 |
| Child C | 95 | 62 | 53 |

16

*Prophylactic endoscopic sclerotherapy*
The findings of our controlled trial of prophylactic endoscopic sclerotherapy, published 1982 [39], are impressive. Between January 1978 and January 1980, 65 of 71 patients entered the study under the indications shown in Table 16. When entry was closed 14 of 33 (40%) control patients had died, in contrast with 2 of 32 (6%) of those (Table 17) having received prophylactic paravariceal injection sclerotherapy ($P < 0.01$) One year later the study was terminated when 94% of the control group had died versus only 19% of the sclerotherapy group ($P < 0.001$) (Fig. 9). The cause of death in the control group was predominantly variceal hemorrhage, whereas the majority of patients in the sclerotherapy group succumbed because of liver failure without bleeding. These results are well confirmed by the study by Witzel et al. [40] (Fig. 10). On the other hand, Sauerbruch and some other groups [41 – 44] found that the mortality rate in multicenter controlled trials from a few months to seven years was 28% in the sclerotherapy group and 35% in the control. This is not statistically significant. None of the other preliminary studies

TABLE 16   Indications for prophylactic sclerotherapy of esophageal varices during a prospective controlled randomized trial ($n$ = 71, 01.01.1978 – 01.01.1980)

| Diagnosis | Number | Percent |
|---|---|---|
| 1.  Varices (III) – IV with so called erosions or angiectases on the cupula | 25 | 35 |
| 2.  Varices II – III with a clotting factor below 30% | 15 | 21 |
| 1 + 2 | 31 | 44 |
| Total | 71 | 100 |

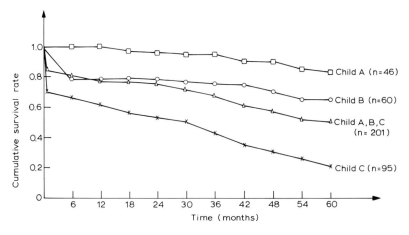

FIG. 8   Cumulative survival curve using the method of Kaplan-Meier for 200 consecutive patients treated by paravariceal elective injection sclerotherapy prospectively.

TABLE 17   Late results of a prospective controlled randomized trial of the value of paravasal sclerotherapy of esophageal varices in liver cirrhosis prior to hemorrhage ($n$ = 71 (63); 01.01.1978 – 01.01.1981)

| | Group Ia ($n$ = 32): conservative treatment | | Group 1b ($n$ = 31): sclerosing procedure | |
|---|---|---|---|---|
| | Number | Percent | Number | Percent |
| Hemorrhage | 29 | 90 | 3 | 9.6 |
| Complication | 2 | 7 | 6 | 19.3 |
| Death | 30 | **94** | 6 | **19.3** |

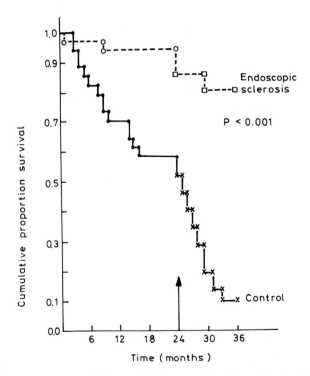

FIG. 9   Cumulative survival curve according to Kaplan-Meier in our prospective controlled randomized trial on paravariceal prophylactic endoscopic sclerotherapy.

18

found a statistically significant improved survival and only some studies showed a significantly reduced bleeding rate after sclerotherapy. Therefore in the final discussion of an international symposium on prophylaxis of variceal hemorrhage in Munich in January 1986 the panel agreed that prophylactic sclerotherapy should only be carried out within controlled trials.

Our group started a new controlled trial one year ago and has included up to the 1st of January 1988 18 patients under the following indications: varices degree III to IV with teleangiectasias on top and an intravariceal esophageal pressure measured by fine needle puncture of over 30 cmH₂O. Preliminary results show that in these patients there is a high risk of bleeding and consequently death from variceal hemorrhage. Furthermore these results demonstrate a statistically reduced bleeding rate by prophylactic sclerotherapy and a tendency to prolonged survival. Unfortunately the numbers are too small to draw any conclusion.

**Conclusion**

The grade of severity of liver failure is a decisive factor in the early course and survival of patients with acute variceal hemorrhage. In these cirrhotic patients early rebleeding is a major ominous event. Thus, preventing early recurrences of acute variceal bleeding should be the major goal of treatment. This can be achieved from our point of view best by emergency or early injection sclerotherapy of esophageal varices. Endoscopic sclerotherapy has thus emerged as an effective treatment with a low incidence of serious side-effects. This modern mode of treatment can arrest acute bleeding with a success rate of over 90% and with regular control and resclerosis often eradicates varices by an intravariceal approach or protects them with scar tissue by the paravariceal injection technique. An 'avariceal or protected stage' can be maintained by further injection if required.

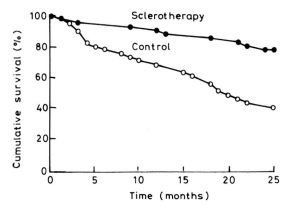

FIG. 10   Cumulative survival curve of the prospective controlled randomized trial of Witzel et al. [40].

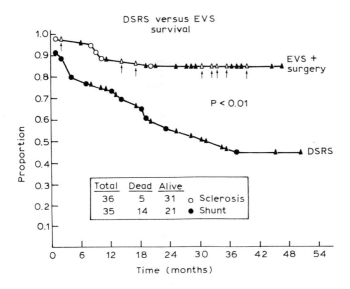

FIG. 11  Preliminary results of the controlled trial of the Warren group comparing elective endoscopic sclerotherapy to elective distal splenorenal shunt operation; about 30% of the sclerotherapy group moved to the shunt group because of recurrences of hemorrhage and were declared as 'failure'.

On the other hand, the data strongly suggest that recurrences of variceal bleeding can only be prevented with an acceptable degree of safety. This has been clearly shown in two controlled trials comparing sclerotherapy to shunt operation by Cello et al. [45] and the Warren group [46]. Therefore additional measures such as shunt or devascularization operations are necessary in about 30% of the patients to provide optimal prevention of recurrent bleeding and improve survival. This has been demonstrated (Fig. 11) in the controlled trial carried out by the Warren group. The two-year survival rate in the failure group of sclerotherapy in which distal spleno-renal shunt was performed was over 80%. Never before in the past have such impressive results been published. However, this has been our policy for 15 years to treat recurrences of hemorrhage by shunt operation if they are Child-Pugh A or B and by the devascularization procedure if they are Child-Pugh C. The results using mesocaval interposition shunt with special selection criteria have recently been published [47] and the results of distal splenorenal shunts are presented in Chapter 26 of this volume.

### References

1   Crawfoord C, Frenckner T, New surgical treatment of varicous veins of the esophagus. Act Otolaryngol 1939; 27: 422 – 429.
2   Macbeth RG. Treatment of esophageal varices in portal hypertension by means of sclerosing injections. Br Med J 1955; 2: 877 – 880.

3   Orloff MJ, Charters AC, Chandler JG, et al. Portocaval shunt as emergency procedure in unselected patients with alcoholic cirrhosis. Surg Gynecol Obstet 1975; 141: 59 – 68.

4   Johnston GW, Rodgers HW. A review of 15 years experiences in the use of sclerotherapy in the control of acute hemorrhage from esophageal varices. Br J Surg 1973; 60: 797 – 800.

5   Raschke E, Paquet K-J. Management of hemorrhage from esophageal varices using endoscopic method. Ann Surg 1973; 99: 177 – 181.

6   Warren WD, Zeppa R, Fomon JJ. Selective transsplenic decompression of gastroesophageal varices by distal splenorenal shunt. Ann Surg 1967; 166: 437 – 455.

7   Inokuchi K, Kobayashi M, Ogawa Y, Saku M, Nagusue N. Results of left gastric vena caval shunt for esophageal varices: analysis of 100 clinical cases. Surgery 1975; 78: 628 – 639.

8   Stelzner S, Lierse W. Der angiomuskuläre Verschluß der Speiseröhre. Langenbecks Arch Klin Chir 1981; 321: 35 – 42.

9   Spence RAJ. Pathogenesis of variceal bleeding – the role of esophageal mucosal changes: International Symposium on Prophylaxis of Variceal Bleeding, Munich, January 1986, p. 35 – 39.

10   Child CG. Surgery and portal hypertension. In: Engelbert J, Dunfield H, eds. Major problems in clinical surgery, Vol. I. Philadelphia: WB Saunders, 1964.

11   Pugh PNH, Murray-Lyon IM, Dawson JL, Pietroni MC, Williams R. Transsection of the esophagus for bleeding esophageal varices. Br J Surg 1973; 60: 646 – 652.

12   Paquet K-J, Oberhammer E. Sclerotherapy of bleeding esophageal varices by means of endoscopy. Endoscopy 1978; 10: 7 – 12.

13   Palani CK, Abuabara S, Krafft AR, Jonasson O. Endoscopic sclerotherapy in acute variceal hemorrhage. Am J Surg 1981; 141: 164 – 168.

14   Terblanche J, Nordhover JMA, Bornman P, et al. A prospective evaluation of injection sclerotherapy in the treatment of acute bleeding from esophageal varices. Surgery 1979; 85: 239 – 245.

15   Alwmark A, Bengmark S, Börjesson B, et al. Emergency and long term endoscopic esophageal sclerotherapy of bleeding esophageal varices. A prospective study of 50 consecutive cases. Scand J Gastroenterol 1982; 17: 409 – 412.

16   Barsoum MS, Boulus FI, ElRobby AA, et al. Tamponade and injection sclerotherapy in the management of bleeding esophageal varices. Br J Surg 1982; 69: 76 – 78.

17   Fleig WE, Stange EF, Rüttenauer K, Ditschuneit H. Emergency endoscopic sclerotherapy for bleeding esophageal varices: a prospective study in patients not responding to balloon tamponade. Gastrointest Endosc 1983; 29: 8 – 14.

18   Paquet K-J. Endoscopic paravariceal injection sclerotherapy of the esophagus – indications, technique, complications: results of a period of 14 years. Gastrointest Endosc 1983; 29: 310 – 317.

19   Kjaergaard J, Fischer A, Miskowiak J, et al. Sclerotherapy of bleeding esophageal varices. Longterm results. Scand J Gastroenterol 1982; 17: 363 – 367.

21   Stray N, Jacobsen CD, Rosserland A. Injection sclerotherapy of bleeding esophageal and gastric varices using a flexible endoscope. Acta Med Scand 1982; 211: 125 – 129.

22   Takase Y, Osaki A, Orirj K, et al. Injection sclerotherapy of esophageal varices for patients undergoing emergency and elective surgery. Surgery 1982; 92: 474 – 479.

23   Soehendra N, deHeer K, Kempeneers I, Runge M. Sclerotherapy of esophageal varices: acute arrest of gastrointestinal hemorrhage or long-term therapy? Endoscopy 1983; 15: 136 – 140.

24   Nilsson F. Management of active bleeding from esophageal varices by sclerotherapy. 5th International Symposium in Gastrointestinal Emergencies. Modena, April 1984.

25    Paquet K-J, Feussner H. Endoscopic sclerosis and esophageal balloon tamponade in acute hemorrhage from esophagogastric varices: a prospective controlled randomized trail. Hepatology 1985; 5: 580 – 583.

26    Larson AW, Cohen H, Zweiban B, Chapman D, Gourdji M, Korula J, Weiner J. Acute esophageal variceal sclerotherapy. Results of a prospective randomized controlled trial. JAMA 1986; 255: 497 – 500.

27    Kaplan EL, Meier P. Nonparametric estimation from incomplete observation. J Am Stat Assoc 1958; 53: 457 – 481.

28    Peto R, Pike MC, Armitage P, et al. Design and analysis of randomized clinical trials requiring prolonged observation of each patient. Br J Cancer 1977; 35: 1 – 40.

29    Paquet K-J, Kalk J-Fr, Koussouris P. Immediate endoscopic sclerosis of bleeding esophageal varices – a prospective evaluation over five years. Surg Endosc 1988; 2: 18 – 23.

30    MacDougall BRD, Westaby D, Theodossi A, et al. Increased long-term survival in variceal hemorrhage using injection sclerotherapy. Results of a controlled trial. Lancet 1982; i: 124 – 127.

31    Terblanche J, Bornman TC, Kahn D, et al. Failure of repeated injection sclerotherapy to improve long-term survival after esophageal variceal bleeding. A five year prospective controlled clinical trial. Lancet 1983; ii: 1328 – 1332.

32    Soederlund C. Endoscopic sclerotherapy of esophageal varices, a clinical study. Acta Chir Scand Suppl 1985; 151: 1 – 23.

33    The Copenhagen variceal sclerotherapy project. Sclerotherapy after first variceal hemorrhage in cirrhosis, a randomized multicenter trial. N Engl J Med 1984; 311: 1594 – 1600.

34    Korula J, Balart LA, Radvan G, Zweiban BE, Larson AW, Kao HW, Yamada S. A prospective randomized controlled trial of chronic esophageal variceal sclerotherapy. Hepatology 1985; 5: 584 – 589.

35    Westaby D, MacDougall BRD, Williams R. Improved survival following injection sclerotherapy for esophageal varices: final analysis of a controlled trial. Hepatology 1985; 5: 827 – 830.

36    Graham DY, Lacey-Smith J. The course of patients after variceal hemorrhage. Gastroenterology 1981; 80: 800 – 809.

37    Burroughs AK, Sanchez A, Bass NM, et al. Can endoscopic sclerotherapy influence significantly the course of cirrhotic patients who survive variceal bleeding? Gut 1983; 24: 972 – 977.

38    Paquet K-J. Unpublished data.

39    Paquet K-J. Prophylactic endoscopic sclerosant treatment of the esophageal wall in varices – a prospective controlled randomized trial. Endoscopy 1982; 14: 4 – 7.

40    Witzel L, Wolbergs G, Merki H. Prophylactic endoscopic sclerotherapy of esophageal varices. A prospective controlled study. Lancet 1985; i: 773 – 778.

41    Sauerbruch T, Weinzierl M, Ansari H, Paumgartner G. Injection sclerotherapy of esophageal variceal hemorrhage. A prospective long-term follow-up study. Endoscopy 1987; 19: 181 – 184.

42    Fleig WE, Stange EG, Wördehoff D, Rainer K, Ditschuneit H. Endoscopic sclerotherapy for the primary prophylaxis of variceal bleeding in cirrhotic patients. Preliminary results of a randomized controlled trial. International Symposium on Prophylaxis of Variceal Bleeding, Munich, 1986; p. 133.

43    Koch H, Henning H, Grimm H, et al. Prophylactic sclerosing of esophageal varices – Results of a prospective controlled study. Endoscopy 1986; 18: 40 – 43.

44    Gregory P, Hartigan P, Amodeo D, et al. Multicenter study – Prophylactic sclerotherapy for esophageal varices in alcoholic liver disease. Results of a cooperative

randomized trial. Gastroenterology 1986; 92: 1414.

45   Cello JP, Grendell JH, Crass RA, et al. Endoscopic sclerotherapy versus portacaval shunt in patients with severe cirrhosis and acute variceal hemorrhage. N Engl J Med 1984; 311: 589 – 594.

46   Warren WD, Henderson JM, Millikan WJ, et al. Distal splenorenal shunt vs. endoscopic sclerotherapy for long-term management of variceal bleeding: a report of a prospective randomized trial. Ann Surg 1986; 203: 454 – 462.

47   Paquet K-J, Kalk J-Fr, Koussouris P. A prospective evaluation and long-term results of mesocaval interposition shunts. Acta Chir Scand 1987; 153: 423 – 429.

© 1988 Elsevier Science Publishers B.V. (Biomedical Division)
*Treatment of esophageal varices*
*Y. Idezuki, editor*

Chapter 2

# Results of endoscopic sclerotherapy: influence of hepatic reserve and cause of varices

Eugene P. DiMagno

*Department of Medicine, Mayo Foundation, Rochester, MN 55905, USA*

In the United States, esophageal sclerotherapy has been enthusiastically accepted as the best method to treat patients with variceal hemorrhage [1, 2]. This opinion has gained popularity because 1) mortality of patients with esophageal varices who are acutely bleeding is unacceptably high even when vasopressin and esophageal tamponade are used and 2) even though elective surgical shunts reduce rebleeding, survival is unaffected [3 – 6].

In several control trials endoscopic sclerotherapy has been reported to reduce rebleeding rates [7 – 9] and to decrease mortality [9, 10], but in other trials this conclusion was not reached [11]. A major problem in evaluating sclerotherapy trials is that they have not taken into consideration variables other than treatment that might affect rebleeding and mortality. In some surgical series, survival has been associated with the degree of hepatic reserve (Child's classification [3 – 6]). In sclerotherapy trials, however, the relationships among liver function, cause of varices, survival and rebleeding rates have not been considered adequately.

Recently, to investigate these relationships we performed a retrospective study to estimate the probabilities of survival and bleeding-free intervals and to relate them to the cause of esophageal varices and underlying liver function in patients who had and patients who had not received sclerotherapy. This analysis considered patients who were admitted to hospitals affiliated with our institution for well-documented bleeding esophageal varices between 1978 and 1980 (before the routine use of esophageal sclerotherapy) and between 1980 and 1982 (when esophageal sclerotherapy was used).

The purpose of this paper is to summarize this published work [12] and to comment on the role of esophageal variceal sclerotherapy in the treatment of esophageal varices. The following methods and results sections are essentially reprinted from reference 12 without any substantial change.

**Methods**

*Patients*

All patients who were admitted to the Mayo Clinic affiliated hospitals with a history of bleeding varices were identified for the time intervals between June 1, 1978, to June 30, 1980, and July 1, 1980, to December 31, 1982. We selected these two time periods because fiberoptic endoscopic esophageal variceal sclerosis was not routinely used prior to June 1980. Thereafter, all patients with bleeding varices have been treated with this procedure.

Eighty patients who did not receive sclerotherapy and 162 patients who were sclerosed were seen during the first and second intervals respectively. All patients had acute endoscopically proven variceal hemorrhage defined as 1) bleeding from varices or 2) blood in the upper gastrointestinal tract in the presence of varices without any other lesion to explain bleeding at the time of endoscopy. None of the 80 patients comprising the non-sclerotherapy group seen between 1978 and 1980 received or have received sclerotherapy, whereas each of the 162 patients seen from 1980 to 1982 have been sclerosed (sclerotherapy group).

In each patient the severity of liver function was assessed by a modified [11, 13] Child's classification [14] (Table 1), and the etiology of esophageal varices categorized (Table 2). Standard published criteria were used to make the diagnoses of chronic active hepatitis [15], primary biliary cirrhosis [16] and primary sclerosing cholangitis [17]. A diagnosis of alcoholic liver disease was accepted if criteria for other liver diseases were not present and a history of alcohol abuse was obtained from the patient or family members. A liver biopsy was performed if the prothrombin time was less than 14 s (45% of non-sclerotherapy and 43% of sclerotherapy patients).

TABLE 1   Modified Child's risk grading

| | Score | | |
|---|---|---|---|
| | 1 | 2 | 3 |
| Encephalopathy | Nil | Slight-Moderate | Moderate-Severe |
| Ascites | Nil | Slight | Moderate-Severe |
| Bilirubin[a] (mg/100 ml) | < 2 | 2 – 3 | > 3 |
| Albumin (g/100 ml) | ≥ 3.5 | 2.8 – 3.4 | < 2.8 |
| Prothrombin index | > 70% | 40 – 70% | < 40% |
| Prothrombin time in our modification | (≤ 14 s) | (15 – 17 s) | (≥ 18 s) |

[a] For primary biliary cirrhosis the bilirubin score is adjusted: 1 = < 4; 2 = 4 – 10, 3 = > 10 mg/100 ml. To determine Child's class, scores are summed: Class A = 5 – 7; Class B = 8 – 10, Class C = 11 – 15. Reprinted with permission, from Ref. 12.

TABLE 2 Numbers and percentages ( ) of patients in each Child's class (upper panel) and by etiology of esophageal varices (lower panel) for the non-sclerotherapy and sclerotherapy groups (reprinted with permission, from Ref. 12)

| Child's class | Non-sclerotherapy | | Sclerotherapy | |
|---|---|---|---|---|
| | $n$ | (%) | $n$ | (%) |
| A | 29 | (36) | 75 | (46) |
| B | 33 | (41) | 65 | (40) |
| C | 18 | (23) | 22 | (14) |
| Totals | 80 | | 162 | |
| Alcoholic liver disease | 28 | (35) | 63 | (39) |
| Non-alcoholic causes for esophageal varices | 52 | (65) | 99 | (61) |
| Cryptogenic cirrhosis | 20 | (25) | 23 | (14) |
| Chronic active liver disease | 10 | (13) | 23 | (14) |
| Primary biliary cirrhosis | 12 | (15) | 20 | (12) |
| Primary sclerosing cholangitis | 2 | (3) | 8 | (5) |
| Extrahepatic portal vein thrombosis | 5 | (6) | 16 | (10) |
| Other | 3 | (4) | 9 | (6) |

*Follow-up and statistical methods*

Death certificates were obtained in all deceased patients. Of patients alive at last follow-up, 72% of the non-sclerotherapy and 100% of the sclerotherapy patients were re-examined at our institution. Every live patient of the sclerotherapy group returned for follow-up sclerotherapies. In addition, at the time of the latest accrual of data, all live patients in both groups were contacted by letter and/or phone call to verify survival and frequency of rebleeding episodes.

The Kaplan-Meier method was used to estimate survival and bleeding free interval probabilities [18], but statistical comparisons between the non-sclerotherapy and sclerotherapy groups were not made because of the retrospective nature of this study. The entry point for these analyses was either date of sclerotherapy for bleeding varices, or the date of bleed (non-sclerotherapy group). Within study groups the association of severity and etiology of liver disease with survival and with duration of time to rebleeding was assessed using the log rank test [18]. Criteria for obliteration of esophageal varices included non-visualization of previously present varices and/or no bleeding when varices punctured with the sclerosing needle.

Acutely bleeding patients were routinely sclerosed after 24 h treatment with esophageal balloon tamponade and intravenous vasopressin. We used a two channel Olympus TGF-2D endoscope (Olympus Corp of America, New Hyde Park, NY 11042) which had a balloon (Knight-Grimm-Sanders cuff; outside diameter 14 mm, Foregger Hospital Equipment, Allentown, PA 18105) tied to it with silk suture so the distal end of the balloon was 7 cm from the tip of the endoscope [19]. A nylon catheter with a 21 gauge Woods point needle incorporated into its tip was used to inject ethanolamine oleate (Allen & Hambury's a Glaxo Canada Limited Company, Toronto, Canada) into varices. Two to 4 ml of ethanolamine were used per injection and 17–20 ml were used per procedure. Intravariceal injection followed by balloon tamponade was employed. Sclerotherapy was repeated at 4 to 6 week intervals until the varices were obliterated. The median time between the first and second sclerotherapy was 28 days.

TABLE 3   Mean values (± SE) or percent of patients for each factor in non-sclerotherapy (*n* = 80) and sclerotherapy (*n* = 162) groups

| Factor | Non-sclerotherapy | Sclerotherapy |
|---|---|---|
| Time between bleed and entry into study[a] | '0' | 8 days (2–24 inner quartile range) |
| Number of variceal bleeds prior to entry into study including index hemorrhage | | |
| 1 | 51% | 21% |
| 2 | 30% | 37% |
| 3–4 | 19% | 42% |
| Characterization of index bleeding episode | | |
| Major[b] | 74% | 92% |
| Minor | 26% | 8% |
| Ascites | | |
| None | 35% | 44% |
| Moderate | 15% | 19% |
| Severe | 50% | 37% |
| Encephalopathy | | |
| None | 71% | 81% |
| Moderate | 13% | 12% |
| Severe | 16% | 7% |
| Bilirubin (mg%) | | |
| Conjugated | 2.5 ± 0.5 | 1.4 ± 0.2 |
| Total | 4.1 ± 0.7 | 2.8 ± 0.3 |
| SGOT (u/dl)[c] | 40 (26–93) | 38 (27–66) |
| Pro time (s) | 12.8 ± 0.3 | 11.9 ± 0.1 |

[a] Median time from variceal bleed to hospital admission (non-sclerotherapy group) or to sclerotherapy.
[b] Major bleeding episode is characterized by one of the following: 1) greater than 1000 ml blood transfusion requirement, 2) decrease in hematocrit to 30% or 3) > 10% fall in hematocrit while under observation or treatment. A minor bleeding episode was bleeding which did not meet the above criteria.
[c] Median (innerquartile range).
Reprinted with permission, from Ref. 12.

## Results

### Patient classification

The percentages of patients with non-alcohol- and alcohol-related causes of esophageal varices, the specific diseases of the non-alcohol causes for esophageal varices (Table 2), and the distribution of Child's classes within the non-sclerotherapy and sclerotherapy groups were remarkably similar. Further, some factors which have been previously identified as adversely affecting survival [21] were similar among patients of the non-sclerotherapy and sclerotherapy groups (Table 3; degree of ascites and encephalopathy). Although several measurements related to bleeding appeared to be slightly decreased in the non-sclerotherapy group (number of previous bleeds and percent of major index bleeds), within the non-sclerotherapy and sclerotherapy groups no association for survival or rebleeding with the number of previous bleeds or severity of index bleed was detected (Table 3). Several indicators of liver function (hyperbilirubinemia and prolonged prothrombin time) appeared worse in the non-sclerotherapy group and are associated with survival and rebleeding as they are part of Child's classification.

### Survival

#### Association with severity of liver disease
Survival was significantly associated with severity of underlying liver disease (Child's grade) in both non-sclerotherapy and sclerotherapy patients ($P < 0.0005$;

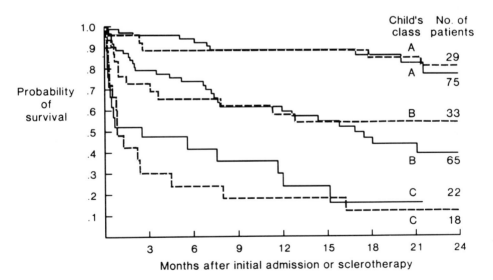

FIG. 1 Survival probabilities for non-sclerotherapy (– – –) and sclerotherapy (———) patients related to hepatic function (Child's class). Differences among Child's class within non-sclerotherapy and sclerotherapy groups was highly significant ($P < 0.0005$, A vs B vs C, log rank test). Reprinted with permission, from Ref. 12.

TABLE 4 One- and 2-year survival and bleeding free interval probabilities for severity of hepatic function (Child's Class), etiology (alcohol and non-alcohol related) and combined Child's Class and etiology. The 2-year probabilities for the Child's Class C patients are based on very small numbers of patients. For that reason probability ranges are given for this group.

| | Non-sclerotherapy | | | | Sclerotherapy | | | |
| | Survival | | Bleeding free interval | | Survival | | Bleeding free interval | |
| | 1-year | 2-year | 1-year | 2-year | 1-year | 2-year | 1-year | 2-year |
|---|---|---|---|---|---|---|---|---|
| **Child's Class** | | | | | | | | |
| A | 0.89 | 0.82 | 0.92 | 0.75 | 0.89 | 0.77 | 0.56 | 0.56 |
| B | 0.58 | 0.55 | 0.68 | 0.63 | 0.62 | 0.40 | 0.39 | 0.30 |
| C | 0.18 | 0.12 | 0.35 | 0.35 | 0.30 | 0.00–0.16 | 0.21 | 0.00–0.21 |
| **Etiology** | | | | | | | | |
| Alcoholic | 0.68 | 0.64 | 0.76 | 0.60 | 0.71 | 0.49 | 0.42 | 0.36 |
| Non-alcoholic | 0.57 | 0.50 | 0.72 | 0.65 | 0.69 | 0.56 | 0.49 | 0.47 |
| **Etiology and Child's Class** | | | | | | | | |
| Alcoholic A + B | 0.74 | –[a] | 0.77 | – | 0.73 | – | 0.44 | – |
| Alcoholic C | 0.50 | – | 0.75 | – | 0.64 | – | 0.32 | – |
| Non-alcoholic A + B | 0.73 | – | 0.84 | – | 0.81 | – | 0.52 | – |
| Non-alcoholic C | 0 | – | 0 | – | 0 | – | 0 | – |

[a] Number of patients under observation too small for reliable estimate.
Reprinted with permission, from Ref. 12.

Fig. 1 and Table 4). The one year survival probabilities decreased with increasing disease severity in both the sclerotherapy and non-sclerotherapy patients (Table 4). In sclerotherapy and non-sclerotherapy groups, survival probabilities remained relatively stable after one year (Fig. 1). At 2 years, the approximate survival probability for Child's A patients was 77%, 40% for Child's B patients and 16 – 20% for Child's C patients. Survival of patients in the non-sclerotherapy group who were treated with a surgical shunt ($N = 18$; 17 of 18 were A or B patients) was not significantly different from the other A and B patients of the non-sclerotherapy group.

*Association with etiology of bleeding esophageal varices*
Overall, the etiologies (alcohol versus non-alcohol) of esophageal varices was not associated with survival in either sclerotherapy or non-sclerotherapy patients. A and B patients of either non-alcoholic or alcoholic etiology have better survival than C patients (Fig. 2, Table 4). C patients who had non-alcohol-related etiology of esophageal varices had an extremely poor survival – in both non-sclerotherapy ($n = 11$) and sclerotherapy ($n = 10$) groups, all patients were dead within one year (Fig. 2). By contrast, alcoholic C patients in both groups of patients have remarkably high one year survival probabilities (50 and 64%; Table 4). Survival was not associated with the number of previous bleeds and severity of bleeds in either the non-sclerotherapy or sclerotherapy groups of patients.

*Probability of remaining free of bleeding: association with severity of liver disease and underlying etiology of esophageal varices*

The estimated probabilities for rebleeding indicated an association with severity and

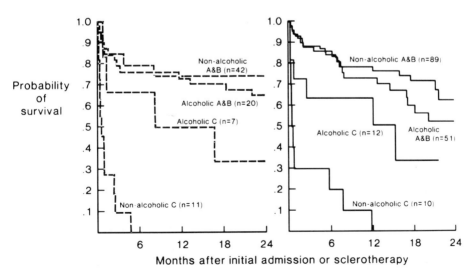

FIG. 2 Survival probabilities for non-sclerotherapy (– – –) and sclerotherapy (———) related to etiology and severity of liver disease. Reprinted with permission, from Ref. 12.

30

etiology ($P < .01$; Table 4, Fig. 3) similar to that indicated by the survival analysis. Patients with less severe liver disease (A and B patients) in both sclerosed and non-sclerosed groups, were free from bleeding for longer time intervals than C patients. The underlying etiology of esophageal varices did not appear to be associated with the duration of time free from rebleeding. A and B patients who had alcoholic and non-alcoholic etiology of varices had longer bleeding free intervals than C patients. However, alcoholic C patients had a greater probability of remaining free of bleeding than nonalcoholic C patients.

*Obliteration of esophageal varices by sclerotherapy and the association of the duration of sclerotherapy, survival and bleeding free interval probabilities*

Forty-five patients (27%; 42 Child's grade A or B, three Child's grade C) had their varices obliterated. The median time to obliteration of varices for all patients who attained this goal was 187 days (inner quartile range was 17 to 342 days). When the survival curves for the 42 A + B patients who achieved obliteration of varices (top line, Fig. 4) and the 98 A + B patients who did not achieve variceal obliteration in response to sclerotherapy (bottom line, Fig. 4) were compared, a difference in survival was suggested. However, when survival of those A + B patients whose varices were not totally obliterated by sclerotherapy but who survived at least 187 days, (the median time to obliteration, middle line, Fig. 4), was examined there was no apparent difference in their survival from the A + B patients achieving obliteration. Furthermore, after the median time of obliteration (the portion of Fig. 4 represented by 7 to 24 months on the time scale), the slopes of the three curves are

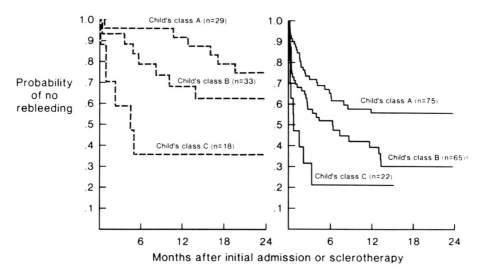

FIG. 3  Probability of no rebleeding in non-sclerotherapy (– – –) and sclerotherapy (——) patients related to hepatic function (Child's class). Reprinted with permission, from Ref. 12.

similar suggesting that there was no difference in survival regardless of the status of the varices (obliterated or non-obliterated) if the patient lived at least 187 days.

Non-sclerosed patients bled infrequently during the first 187 days (an estimated 91% chance of not rebleeding). Obliterated and non-obliterated patients had similar probabilities of not rebleeding (0.64, 0.56) by the median time (187 days) to obliteration of varices (Table 5). Bleeding free interval probabilities one year following

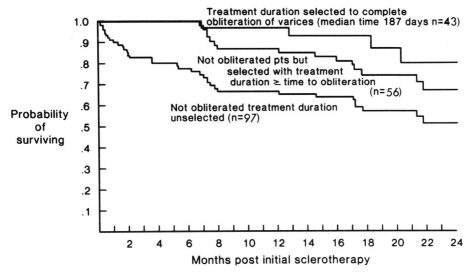

FIG. 4   Survival probabilities in sclerotherapy patients of A + B Child's class. – – –, upper line = patients with obliterated varices (median time to obliteration = 187 days). – – –, middle line = subgroups of sclerotherapy patients who lived at least 187 days but whose varices were not obliterated by sclerotherapy. ——— = all A + B sclerotherapy patients whose varices were not obliterated (57 patients of the middle curve and the 41 A + B patients who did not live 187 days). Reprinted with permission, from Ref. 12.

TABLE 5   Bleeding free interval probabilities and the number and percent of Child's class in sclerotherapy and non-sclerotherapy patients who lived at least 187 days.

| | Probability | | Child's Class | | | |
|---|---|---|---|---|---|---|
| | 187 days[a] | 552 days[b] | A(%) | B(%) | C(%) | Total |
| Sclerotherapy | | | | | | |
| Obliterated varices | 0.64 | 0.79 | 25(56) | 17(37) | 3(7) | 46 |
| Non-obliterated varices | 0.56 | 0.79 | 30(48) | 26(43) | 6(9) | 62 |
| Non-sclerotherapy | 0.91 | 0.75 | 24(52) | 18(39) | 4(9) | 46 |

[a] Bleeding free interval probabilities at 187 days (the median time to obliteration) for all groups.
[b] Bleeding free interval probabilities for one year after obliteration of varices (obliterated varices patients) or for one year following the initial 187 days, the median time to obliteration of varices (patients with non-obliterated varices and non-sclerotherapy patients). Reprinted with permission, from Ref. 12.

obliteration of varices or one year after 187 days (non-obliterated and non-sclerotherapy patients) were 0.75, 0.79 and 0.79 for non-sclerotherapy, non-obliterated and obliterated sclerotherapy patients, respectively (Table 5).

## Discussion

As a result of these data we concluded [12] "that the hepatic reserve (Child's criteria), determines survival, and predicts the length of bleeding free interval. In our population of patients who had bleeding esophageal varices, the estimated probabilities for survival and bleeding free intervals when related to Child's classes were similar regardless of whether they received sclerotherapy. We also confirmed that decreased survival is most pronounced during the first several months and then stabilizes [20, 21]. This same general pattern was present for bleeding free interval probabilities, but the decline of the bleeding free interval probability curves were steeper than survival curves and only leveled off after one year.

We also found that patients with relatively good hepatic reserve had similar survival and bleeding free time intervals regardless of the underlying etiology of the liver disease. However, patients with poor hepatic reserve (Child's class C) due to alcoholic liver disease had better survival and less bleeding than patients with non-alcoholic causes of liver disease. The probability of surviving of our alcoholic C patients was 0.50 to 0.64 over 2 years which is greater than that reported previously [20 – 22]. Virtually all of our patients with alcoholic liver disease ceased drinking alcohol which likely accounts for their remarkably high survival. By contrast, none of the non-alcoholic C patients survived a year. Most of the non-alcoholic C patients had liver diseases which were irreversible and have no known effective treatment (primary biliary cirrhosis, sclerosing cholangitis)".

Although there is increasing enthusiasm [1, 2] for sclerotherapy as the treatment of choice in patients with bleeding esophageal varices and published controlled trials have shown that sclerotherapy improves survival and reduces rebleeding [9, 10, 23], our data and two control trials [8, 11] fail to support this position. To reconcile these differences is difficult. It is impossible to make comparisons among studies since no other studies have related survival and rebleeding data to hepatic reserve and etiology of liver disease. Because there are marked differences in survival and rebleeding among Child's classes and subgroups of patients with different etiologies (C patients who have alcohol- and non-alcohol-related liver disease), overall survival and rebleeding rates are difficult to interpret in the published control trials because different mixtures of Child's classes and etiologies comprise the sclerotherapy and non-sclerotherapy treatment groups. For example, in one trial, practically all patients had alcoholic liver disease [8], whereas in another there were 20% more patients with non-alcoholic liver disease in the control group [9, 10] which may account for the relatively poor survival of the control patients.

The importance of hepatic reserve in determining bleeding free interval probabilities can be inferred from one published control trial [11]. In this trial there was no significant difference in survival or bleeding free interval probabilities in patients only sclerosed during acute bleeding episodes (control) and patients who were sclerosed at 2 week intervals (sclerotherapy treatment group). The control group had significantly more C patients (Child's score 8.95) and the sclerotherapy group had more B patients (score 7.75). The percent of patients free from recurrent bleeding at one year (estimated from fig. in Ref. 11) for the control group was 0.22 and for the sclerotherapy group was 0.36 which corresponds quite closely to bleeding free interval probabilities of 0.26 and 0.39 for our B and C patients, respectively.

A difference among some studies is the choice of sclerosants and the timing of sclerotherapy. We sclerosed our patients with ethanolamine at 4 to 6 week intervals, whereas many sclerotherapists now use sodium morrhuate and sclerose at weekly intervals or less until varices are obliterated. However, mean interval between the first and second sclerotherapy was 28 days and the sclerosant (ethanolamine) and the interval between sclerotherapies in our study was similar to both of the controlled trials [9 – 11]. Moreover, our data and one trial [11] suggest that neither the interval to nor the presence of obliterated varices influences overall survival (Fig. 4) or rebleeding (Table 5). Nevertheless, all these variables need to be considered when studies are compared.

Although our study was not a controlled trial and has possible selection biases, the sclerotherapy and non-sclerotherapy groups were similar according to liver function (Child's class), the etiology of esophageal varices, and factors which have been associated with decreased survival [7] such as the severity of hemorrhage, ascites, encephalopathy, bilirubin > 2.5 mg%, SGOT > 100 and prothrombin time > 14 s (Table 3). After beginning sclerotherapy, we examined more patients with bleeding varices. However, the similarities among the non-sclerotherapy and sclerotherapy groups indicate that the overall type of patient was unchanged. A potential bias may be that more non-sclerotherapy patients (22%) underwent a surgical shunt procedure than sclerotherapy patients (3%). However, there was no significant difference in the survival and bleeding free interval probabilities of the shunted non-sclerotherapy patients (17 of 18 were A or B patients) when compared to the other A and B non-sclerotherapy patients.

At the present time I believe that repeated esophageal variceal sclerosis to increase survival and reduce further bleeding is an unproven procedure. Since hepatic reserve and etiology of the underlying liver disease are significantly associated with mortality and rebleeding, these factors must be considered in future treatment trials on patients with bleeding esophageal varices.

Thus, what is the role of sclerotherapy in clinical practice today? In my opinion, sclerotherapy should be used to treat actively bleeding varices. I do not favor *elective* repetitive sclerotherapy to obliterate varices as a treatment to reduce rebleeding or in an attempt to prolong survival. If regular repetitive sclerotherapy affects the natural history of esophageal varices that have bled, as suggested by several control trials, the effects as pointed out above are small. Furthermore, patients treated with repeated sclerotherapy only if and when they rebleed appear to have as frequent rebleeding and the same survival as patients who are resclerosed at regularly scheduled intervals [11].

This approach would be particularly applicable to Child's class A and B patients with alcoholic or non-alcoholic liver disease who have relatively low rebleeding rates and relatively good survival. However, in these patients who do not have ascites, which is difficult to control, some authorities are again recommending a splenorenal shunt [24]. History repeats itself! In class C patients perhaps repeated regularly scheduled sclerotherapy is warranted because of very frequent rebleeding and poor operative risk for shunt surgery [24]. The ultimate treatment, however, for patients with bleeding esophageal varices secondary to liver disease is a new liver (e.g., transplantation).

Finally, prophylactic sclerosis should not be performed unless this treatment is part of a controlled randomized trial. This treatment is particularly hazardous in male patients who have alcoholic cirrhosis. A recent prospective Veterans Administration Hospital cooperative study, thus far published in abstract form [25], reported excess mortality (42 of 143 vs. 23 of 7139; $P = 0.009$) and bleeding (32 vs. 22; $P = 0.02$) in sclerotherapy vs. medically treated patients. As a result the study was closed.

## References

1   Editorial. Bleeding oesophageal varices. Lancet 1984; i: 141.
2   Reynolds TB. Editorial. What to do about esophageal varices. N Engl J Med 1984; 309: 1575 – 1577.
3   Resick RH, Iber FL, Ishihara Am, et al. A controlled study of therapeutic portacaval shunt. Gastroenterology 1974; 67: 843 – 857.
4   Jackson FL, Perrin EB, Felix WR, et al. A clinical investigation of the portacaval shunt. V. Surgical analysis of the therapeutic operation. Ann Surg 1971; 174: 672 – 701.
5   Reynolds TB, Donovan AJ, Mikkelsen WP, et al. Results of a 12-year randomized trial of portal caval shunting in patients with alcoholic liver disease and bleeding varices. Gastroenterology 1981; 80: 1005 – 1011.
6   Reuff R, Prand D, Degos F, et al. A controlled study of the therapeutic portacaval shunt in alcoholic cirrhosis. Lancet 1976; i: 655 – 659.
7   Terblanche J, Bornman P, Yakoob H, et al. Prospective randomized controlled trial of sclerotherapy after esophageal variceal bleeding (Abstr). Gastroenterology 1980; 79: 1128.
8   Korula J, Balart LA, Radvan G, et al. A prospective randomized controlled trial of chronic esophageal variceal sclerotherapy. Hepatology 1985; 5: 554 – 589.
9   MacDougall BRD, Theodoss A, Westaby D, Dawson JL, Williams R. Increased long-term survival in variceal hemorrhage using injection sclerotherapy. Lancet 1982; i: 124 – 127.
10  Westaby D, MacDougall BRD, Williams R. Improved survival following injection sclerotherapy for esophageal varices: final analysis of a controlled trial. Hepatology 1985; 5: 827 – 830.
11  Terblanche J, Bornman PC, Kahn D, Jonker MAT, Campbell JAH, Wright J, Kirsch R. Failure of repeated injection sclerotherapy to improve long-term survival after oesophageal variceal bleeding. Lancet 1983; ii: 1328 – 1332.
12  DiMagno EP, Zinsmeister AR, Larson DE, Viggiano TR, Clain JE, Laughlin B, Hughes RW. Influence of hepatic reserve and etiology of esophageal varices on survival and rebleeding before and after introduction of sclerotherapy: a retrospective analysis. Mayo Clin Proc 1985; 60: 149 – 157.
13  Terblanche J, Northover JMA, Bornman P, et al. A prospective controlled trial of sclerotherapy in the long term management of patients after esophageal variceal bleeding. Surg Gynecol Obstet 1979; 148: 323 – 333.

14   Child GG III, Turcotte SG. Surgery and portal hypertension. In: Major problems in clinical surgery: the liver and portal hypertension, Vol. 1. Philadelphia, PA: WB Saunders, 1964; 1 – 85.

15   Soloway RD, Summerskill WHJ, Baggenstoss AH, Geall MG, Gitnick GL, Elveback LR, Schoenfield LJ. Chemical, biochemical and histologic remission of chronic active liver disease: a controlled study of treatments and early prognosis. Gastroenterology 1972; 63: 820 – 833.

16   Dickson ER, Fleming CR, Ludwig J. Primary biliary cirrhosis. In: Popper H, Schaffner F, eds. Progress in Liver Diseases, Vol. 6. New York: Grune and Stratton, 1979; 487 – 502.

17   Wiesner RH, LaRusso NF. Clinicopathologic features of the syndrome of primary sclerosing cholangitis. Gastroenterology 1980; 79: 200 – 206.

18   Kalbfleisch JD, Prentice DL. The Statistical Analysis of Failure Time Data. New York: J. Wiley, 1980.

19   Hughes RW, Viggiano TR, van Heerden JA, Larson DE, Adson MA, Reeves CB. Endoscopic variceal sclerosis: a one year experience. Gastrointest Endoscopy 1982; 28: 62 – 66.

20   Nachlas MM, O'Neil JE, Campbell AJA. The life history of patients with cirrhosis of the liver and bleeding esophageal varices. Ann Surg 1955; 141: 10 – 23.

21   Graham DY, Smith JL. The course of patients after variceal hemorrhage. Gastroenterology 1981; 90: 800 – 809.

22   Ratnoff OD, Patek AJ Jr. The natural history of Laennec's cirrhosis of the liver. An analysis of 386 cases. Medicine 1942; 21: 207 – 268.

23   The Copenhagen Esophageal Varices Sclerotherapy Project. Sclerotherapy after first variceal hemorrhage in cirrhosis. A randomized multicenter trial. N Engl J Med 1984; 311: 1594 – 1600.

24   Cello JP, Crass RA, Grendell JH, Trunkey DD. Management of the patient with hemorrhaging esophageal varices. J Am Med Assoc 1986; 256 (11): 1480.

25   Gregory P, Hartigan P, Amodeo D, Baum R, Camara D, Colcher H, Fye C, Gebhard R, Goff J, Kruss D, McPhee M, Meier P, Rankin R, Reichelderfer M, Sanowski R, Shields D, Silvis S, Weesner R, Winship D, Young H. Prophylactic sclerotherapy for esophageal varices in alcoholic liver disease: results of a VA cooperative randomized trial. Gastroenterology 1987; 92: 1414.

—

© 1988 Elsevier Science Publishers B.V. (Biomedical Division)
Treatment of esophageal varices
Y. Idezuki, editor

Chapter 3

# Indication and results of injection sclerotherapy

Eizo Okamoto, Akiyoshi Shu and Yoshiyuki Nakai

Department of Surgery, Hyogo College of Medicine, 1-1 Mukogawa-cho, Nishinomiya, Hyogo 663, Japan

## Introduction

During the past six years since the introduction of sclerotherapy into our department of surgery in 1981, a revolutionary change has occurred in the modality of treatment for esophageal varices. Esophageal transection, a modified Sugiura procedure, was our main procedure adopted for esophageal varices. Excellent results were obtained in patients with good liver function; however, results were very poor in patients with acute variceal bleeding and/or severe hepatic dysfunction. Since 1981, acute variceal bleeding has been controlled by sclerotherapy in 90% of patients, resulting in a remarkable reduction in the number of patients who need emergency operation. Since 1983, elective and prophylactic sclerotherapies have been tried. With the advancement of techniques and improvements of instruments and sclerosing drugs, this method seems capable of replacing the major part of surgery in the treatment of esophageal varices. In this paper, our experiences of sclerotherapy and its long-term results in the past six years will be reviewed and discussed.

## Materials and methods

From October 1980, to December 1987, a total of 463 patients with esophageal varices were treated by endoscopic sclerotherapy in our department. Two hundred of these were emergency cases, 149 were elective and 114 were prophylactic. For the first few years the indication for sclerotherapy was limited to emergency cases and those in whom esophageal transection was not indicated due to severe hepatic dysfunction; therefore the incidence of emergency sclerotherapy was relatively high in our series.

An Olympus EF B3 or GIF Q10 fixed with fiberscopic balloon was used in this series. 1 − 2 ml of 50% glucose, 3 − 5 ml of 1% aethoxysclerol and 500 − 1000 units of thrombin were consecutively injected intra-variceally. Intra-variceal injection was performed at an apex of the varices at the level 1 − 3 cm above the esophago-gastric junction using a Teflon-coated 23-gauge needle. The sclerotherapy was repeated every week until the red color signs disappeared. Routine endoscopic follow-up observation was carried out one week, one month and three months after the red color signs had disappeared.

## Results and discusssion

### Sclerotherapy for emergency cases

A total of 200 cases with acute esophageal variceal bleeding underwent the emergency sclerotherapy. One hundred and sixty-eight patients, excluding 32 who died within two weeks due to hepatic failure, were used for evaluation. Variceal bleeding was successfully stopped by the sclerotherapy in 153 of 168 patients (91%) for more than two weeks. Eighteen of these effective cases underwent elective surgery within a few months after sclerotherapy. No operative death was encountered. The remaining 135 patients were observed without undergoing the surgery; rebleeding occurred in 24 of these patients, a rate of 17.8%. In 15 of 168 patients (9%), variceal bleeding could not be stopped by the sclerotherapy. Two of these non-effective patients underwent an emergency operation. One died within one month after the operation.

Fig. 1 shows the proportion of emergency, elective and prophylactic cases in all the operative cases before and after the introduction of injection sclerotherapy in our department (1981). Before 1980, nearly 1/4 of operative cases were emergency, while this proportion abruptly reduced to only 1.0% after 1981. Instead of the reduction of emergency operation cases, the rate of elective operation has markedly

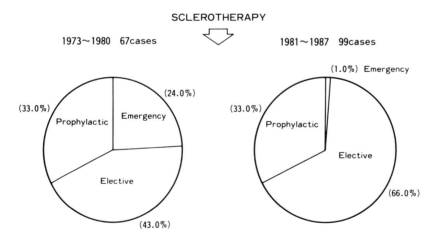

FIG. 1   Change of operations before and after introduction of sclerotherapy.

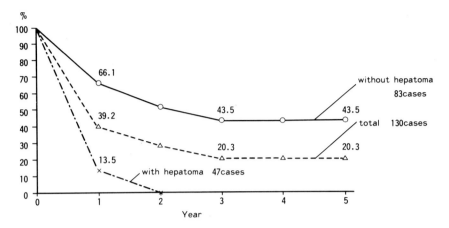

FIG. 2   Long-term survival of emergency cases (sclerotherapy).

increased since 1981. This fact will indicate the definite contribution of sclerotherapy in avoiding emergency operation, the results of which were extremely poor.

The long-term survival curves of the patients with acute esophageal variceal bleeding treated by sclerotherapy are shown in Fig. 2. The overall survival rates at one, three and five years were 39.2, 20.3 and 20.3%, respectively. The survival rates of the patients who were not suffering from hepatocellular carcinoma were 66.1% at one year, 43.5% at three years and 43.5% at five years. None of the patients associated with hepatocellular carcinoma survived more than two years.

*Sclerotherapy for non-emergency cases*

Repeated endoscopic follow-up observation is essential for evaluation of the efficacy of prophylactic as well as of elective sclerotherapy. In one week after the sclerotherapy, ulcer formation at the point of needle puncture for injection was frequently seen. Either flattening or vanishing of the varices with intravariceal thrombus was also observed and the red color signs disappeared. One month after the sclerotherapy, varices almost disappeared and the ulcer, erosion and other inflammatory reactions also subsided. These observations suggest that evaluation of the efficacy of sclerotherapy should be done one month after the sclerotherapy.

Serial endoscopic observation was performed on 112 patients for more than six months after prophylactic and elective sclerotherapies (Table 1). According to the endoscopic findings one month after the sclerotherapy, the patients were classified into three groups. In 40 of 112 patients (35.7%), the endoscopic features of the varices improved to F0-1 with negative red color signs one month after the sclerotherapy. In only 4 of these 40 patients, red color signs reappeared after 6 months; two of these patients rebled later. In 41 patients (35.6%), F2 varices still remained but no red color sign was observed at one month. In 14 of these 41 patients (14.0%) the forms of the varices were aggravated to F2-3 with positive red color

TABLE 1    Endoscopic findings after sclerotherapy

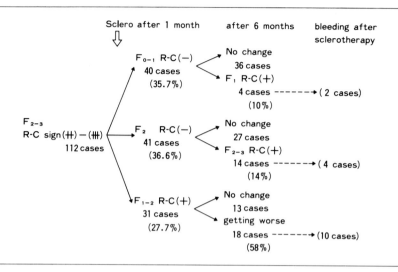

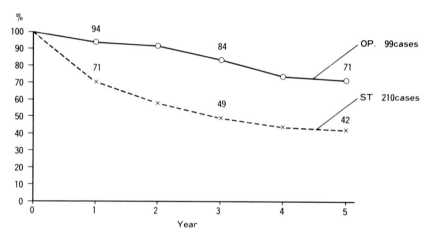

FIG. 3    Long-term survival (operation cases and sclerotherapy cases).

signs at 6 months after the sclerotherapy and 4 of them rebled later. In the remaining 31 patients (27.7%), F1-2 varices with positive red color signs still remained. In 18 of these patients (58.0%), the F scores and positive red color signs worsened at 6 months after the sclerotherapy, and 10 of them rebled later. These observations suggest that repeated sclerotherapy is mandatory whenever the follow-up endoscopy indicates positive red color signs.

Long-term survival curves of the patients who underwent esophageal transection were compared with those who underwent the sclerotherapy (Fig. 3). Since the sclerotherapy, either prophylactic or elective, was adopted mainly for the patients

who would not tolerate the major surgery due to severe impairment of liver function, it seems to be acceptable that the long-term survival curve of the patients
treated with sclerotherapy is much worse than those with esophageal transection.

The long-term survival curves of the patients who underwent sclerotherapy were
compared among the emergency, elective and prophylactic cases (Fig. 4). The survival rate was lower in the emergency cases after 3 years; however, no significant
difference was seen among the three groups 4 and 5 years after the sclerotherapy.

The long-term survival curves of the patients who underwent sclerotherapy were
then compared according to Child's grades (Fig. 5). The survival rates per year
declined in the order of Child's grade A, B and C. This suggests that the long-term

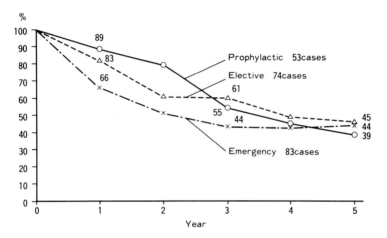

FIG. 4   Long-term survival I (sclerotherapy).

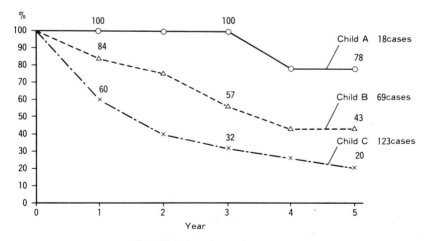

FIG. 5   Long-term survival II (sclerotherapy).

survival rates of the patients who underwent sclerotherapy, whether emergency, elective or prophylactic, were largely influenced by the degree of hepatic impairment of the patients. It is also worthy of note that the survival curves of the patients with sclerotherapy categorized as Child's A and B are not inferior to those with esophageal transection in this series.

*Prospective randomized trial – transection (OP) vs. sclerotherapy (ST)*

Since 1983 a prospective randomized study comparing the efficacy of the sclerotherapy with that of the esophageal transection has been carried out, using patients with the backgrounds given in Table 2. The timing of treatment, grading of Child's category, sex, age, liver function test estimated by ICG tests and period of follow-up observation did not differ between the groups. The results are shown in Fig. 6. No bleeding was encountered in the surgery group and the only bleeder in

TABLE 2   Prospective randomized trial: nonshunting op. vs. sclerotherapy (ST)

|  | OP. (10cases) | ST (10cases) |
|---|---|---|
| Prophylactic | 5 | 5 |
| Elective | 5 | 5 |
| Child A | 5 | 5 |
| Child B | 5 | 5 |

|  | M : F | Age | $ICGR_{15}$ (mean±SEM) | $K_{ICG}$ (mean±SEM) | follow up period (month) |
|---|---|---|---|---|---|
| OP. | 8 : 2 | 48.0 (35~60) | 21.8 ±1.47 | 0.105 ±0.006 | 26 (13~36) |
| ST | 8 : 2 | 50.2 (40~61) | 23.8 ±1.40 | 0.106 ±0.004 | 25 (14~39) |

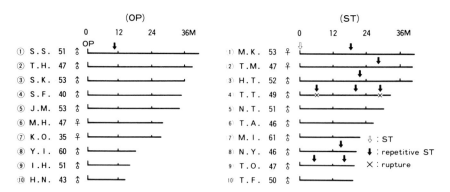

FIG. 6   Prognosis: nonshunting op. vs. sclerotherapy (ST).

the sclerotherapy group was controlled by additional sclerotherapy. Worsening of the endoscopic features of varices was seen in one of the surgical group and six, including one bleeder, of the sclerotherapy group. All of them were controlled by additional or repeated sclerotherapy and no death was seen in either group so far at up to 39 months after the treatment.

## Summary

1. Acute variceal bleeding was successfully controlled by sclerotherapy in 91% of patients.
2. Introduction of sclerotherapy has reduced the incidence of emergency surgery cases from 24% to only 1%.
3. Additional and repeated sclerotherapies are mandatory to prevent rebleeding, whenever the follow-up endoscopy indicates positive red color signs.
4. Long-term survival rates were not influenced by the mode of sclerotherapy, emergency, elective or prophylactic, but by the degree of hepatic impairment.
5. In the prospective randomized study aimed at comparing the efficacy of sclerotherapy with that of esophageal transection, the surgical treatment provided a lower frequency of rebleeding but no better survival rates than the sclerotherapy.
6. In conclusion, sclerotherapy can be the treatment of first choice, replacing surgical treatment for cirrhotic patients with acute variceal bleeding or potentially at risk of bleeding.

## References

1    Sugiura M, Futagawa S. A new technique for treating esophageal varices. J Thorac Cardiovasc Surg 1973; 66: 677 – 685.
2    Sugiura M, Futagawa S. Further evaluation of the Sugiura procedure in the treatment of esophageal varices. Arch Surg 1977: 112: 1317 – 1321.
3    Kuwata K, Okamoto E, Toyosaka A, et al. Indication and limitation of esophageal transection for esophageal varices. J Jpn Soc Clin Surg 1982; 43: 612 – 615 (in Japanese).
4    Crafoord C, Freckner P. New surgical treatment of varicose veins of the esophagus. Acta Otolaryngol 1939; 27: 422 – 429.
5    Shu A, Okamoto E, Kashitani M, et al. Clinical evaluation of endoscopic embolization for the patients with esophageal varices. Gastroenterol Endosc 1984; 26: 381 – 390 (in Japanese with English abstract).

© 1988 Elsevier Science Publishers B.V. (Biomedical Division)
*Treatment of esophageal varices*
*Y. Idezuki, editor*

Chapter 4

# Endoscopic sclerotherapy for esophageal varices by combined injection technique with 1% Polidocanol

Y. Watanabe[1], M. Kohyama[1], R. Ohmasa[1], K. Masuda[1], H. Suzuki[2] and O. Miho[2]

*Departments of [1] Endoscopy and [2] Surgery, Aoto Hospital, Jikei University School of Medicine, Tokyo, Japan*

Endoscopic sclerotherapy is gaining increasing acceptance in the control of variceal bleeding. In this paper the technique we use and results of our sclerotherapy are described in patients with esophageal varices observed over an 8-year period (1979 – 1987).

## Materials and methods

Since March 1979, we have practised endoscopic sclerotherapy not only to control acute variceal bleeding but also to prevent possible rebleeding by eradication of varices. We have performed 878 therapies in total on 276 patients. There were 94 emergency, 92 elective and 90 prophylactic cases.

The constitution of cases according to Child's classification was 166 cases in Child A or B, and 110 in Child C, with the majority of them not being candidates for surgery (Table 1).

Emergency sclerotherapy consisted of volume resuscitation according to the gradation of bleeding (Nagao's) followed by endoscopy. The nature and source of bleeding were defined with emergency endoscopy and treated by sclerotherapy at one time in most cases.

Fig. 1 illustrates our ordinary injection technique and typical course of eradication of varices after therapy. We use 1% Polidocanol as the safest sclerosant. It has very low toxicity and in addition its viscosity is low. The injections are first made into a submucosal site between the varices and then into each variceal channel, 3 ml in each portion. This combined injection technique was first reported by us in 1980 [1]. Total dose of sclerosant is limited to 30 ml at one session of therapy. We perform the sclerotherapy by freehand technique without any sheath or balloon, using a flexible 23 or 25 gauge fine needle under intravenous sedation and topical anesthesia.

46

TABLE 1   Constitution of cases according to the timing of therapy and the Child's classification

| Timing of therapy | No. of cases | Child's classification | No. of cases |
|---|---|---|---|
| Emergent | 94 | A | 37 |
| Elective | 92 | B | 129 |
| Prophylactic | 90 | C | 110 |
| Total | 276 | | 276 |

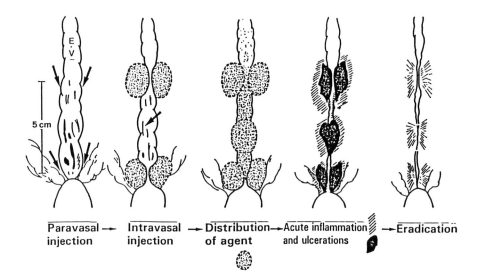

FIG. 1   Injection techniques and typical course of eradication of varices after therapy.

All patients receive standard anti-ulcer therapy with both $H_2$ blockers and antacids after the therapy. Per oral feeding is permitted from the next day, gradually changing from liquid meal to soft meal.

Typically one or two weeks later after the therapy, ulcerations occur on and around the varices and finally varices are remarkably diminished or have even disappeared.

As a rule, 3 sclerotherapies are performed every week in a series of therapy, and a follow-up study is done every 3 months for either additional therapy or observation.

## Results

### Hemostatic effects in emergency variceal bleeding

Hemostatic effects of our sclerotherapy were studied in 94 emergency cases in relation to endoscopic findings. There were 57 cases with active bleeding at the emergency endoscopy. Bleeding could be stopped for more than 72 hours in 52 cases, so the hemostatic rate was as high as 91%. There were 33 cases with blood spurting in these cases. Even in such serious cases, a high hemostatic rate of 88% was obtained.

Other than these, there were 37 cases of red or fibrin emboli without active bleeding at the time of endoscopy, and bleeding could be controlled in all of them (Table 2). Only in 5 cases could bleeding not be stopped.

TABLE 2   Hemostatic effects in emergency variceal bleeding

| At emergency endoscopy (n = 94) | Endoscopic findings (No. of cases) | Hemostatic effects (No. of cases (%)) | |
|---|---|---|---|
| Active bleeding (n = 57) | Blood spurting (33) | 29 (88) | 52 (91) |
| | Blood oozing (24) | 23 | |
| Non-active bleeding (n = 37) | Red emboli | | |
| | Fibrin emboli | | |

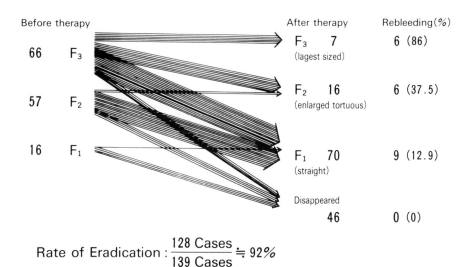

Before therapy

66  F₃

57  F₂

16  F₁

After therapy

F₃   7
(lagest sized)

F₂   16
(enlarged tortuous)

F₁   70
(straight)

Disappeared
46

Rebleeding(%)

6  (86)

6  (37.5)

9  (12.9)

0  (0)

$$\text{Rate of Eradication}: \frac{128\ \text{Cases}}{139\ \text{Cases}} \fallingdotseq 92\%$$

FIG. 2   Eradicating effects on varices and prevention of rebleeding.

*Eradicating effects on varices*
Next, we studied the eradicating effects on varices of sclerotherapy. We consider that the merits of sclerotherapy are not only its hemostatic effect but also its eradicating effect on varices which is connected to prophylaxis of possible bleeding.

One hundred and thirty-nine cases followed up for more than 3 months after therapy were studied.

The forms, namely F number of varices classified by the Japanese Society of Portal Hypertension, are shown in Fig. 2, before treatment on the left and those after treatment on the right. Lines declining to the right show an improvement in grade of varices, i.e., an eradicating effect. On the whole, the eradicating effect could be obtained in 128 cases of a total of 139 cases, with an efficacy rate of 92%. The column on the right shows the rate of rebleeding in terms of postoperative F number. It is worth noting that in successfully treated cases of $F_1$ or less, there is extremely little danger of rebleeding.

*Long-term survival*
The long-term survival curve studied by the Kaplan-Meier method from the view point of timing of therapy in all cases is shown in Fig. 3.

Survival for more than 5 years was obtained in 77% of elective or prophylactic cases. As compared with them, just 33% of emergency cases survived.

Then the results of long-term management particularly in the emergency cases were studied from the view point of Child's classification (Fig. 4). Child A group could survive in all cases and Child B group had 68% survival rate for more than 5 years even in emergency cases. On the other hand, Child C group in emergency cases survived in barely 18% of them.

In other words, the prognosis of the patients treated by sclerotherapy is decided by both the timing of therapy and the gradation of liver damage.

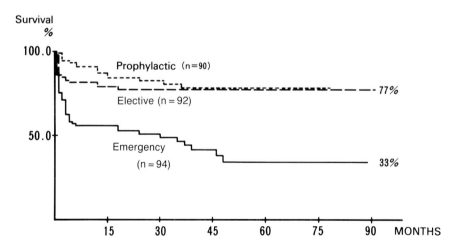

FIG. 3   Long-term survival curve.

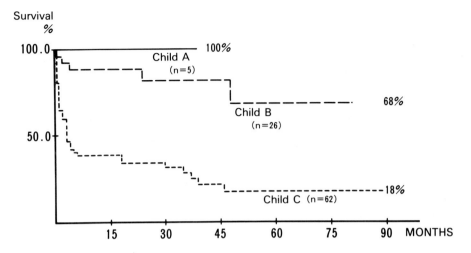

FIG. 4   Long-term survival in emergency cases.

## Discussion

In recent years, endoscopic injection sclerotherapy has become widely accepted in the control of acute variceal bleeding.

Endoscopic injection sclerotherapy is a palliative treatment for esophageal varices because it cannot improve the background disease of the liver. However, by eliminating the recurrent bleeding, the chances of survival can be increased. Furthermore, the purpose of the sclerotherapy for esophageal varices, we consider, is not only to control the acute bleeding but also to prevent possible bleeding by eradication of varices.

Many controversies exist concerning sclerotherapy on such points as the timing of therapy or the technique. Westaby [2] reported his timing to be within 12 hours of the initial control of bleeding by balloon tamponade.

Terblanche [3] notes his timing to be in the bleeding-free interval under general anesthesia at a convenient time in daylight hours and he also selects balloon tamponade for the initial control of active variceal bleeding.

Fig. 5 shows our contingent plan to control acute bleeding from esophageal varices. Commonly in day time, we select the sclerotherapy as the first-choice procedure to control the bleeding, but at the weekend or at night balloon tamponade should be selected because of its simplicity and certainty for operation. We perform sclerotherapy as a continuation of the emergency endoscopy under intravenous sedation without general anesthesia.

In our study, 57 active bleeders (33 blood spurting and 24 blood oozing) were detected by emergency endoscopy in 94 cases. Even in such serious cases bleeding could be stopped in 91%. If the bleeding point can be detected at the emergency endoscopy, we consider the efficacy of subsequent sclerotherapy on liberation from the distress accompanied by balloon tamponade.

50

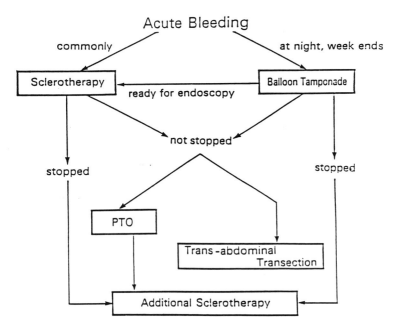

FIG. 5   Contingent plan to control acute bleeding from esophageal varices.

With regard to the injection technique, the King's College group employs the esophageal sheath (Williams tube) as injection apparatus and 5% ethanolamine oleate as the sclerosant. Takase [4] also selects 5% ethanolamine oleate with contrast medium to embolize the varices using the balloon attached to the end of the fiberscope.

Our injection technique with 1% Polidocanol, a so-called combined injection technique (para- and intra-variceal injection), is more simple, using neither balloon nor esophageal sheath [4].

## Conclusions

Sclerotherapy is an important new treatment both for acute variceal bleeding and for the prevention of recurrent or possible bleeding. According to recent trends, this procedure will be more actively and widely used. We consider, in conclusion, that the simplification of technique is one of the important points for popularizing this therapy, and the additional sclerotherapy to eradicate the varices is the other important point for prophylaxis of rebleeding.

## References

1.   Suzuki H, Kohyama M, Nagata T, Watanabe Y. and Nagao F. Endoscopic sclerotherapy for the control of bleeding from esophageal varices. Endoscopic Surgery (Okabe H, Honda T, Ohshiba S. eds), Amsterdam: Excerpta Medica, 1984; 23 – 30.

2.  Westaby D. and Williams R. Injection sclerotherapy for the long-term management of variceal bleeding. World J. Surg. 1984; 8: 667 – 672.

3.  Terblanche J, Bornman P.C, Kahn D. and Kirsh R.E. (1986) Sclerotherapy in acute variceal bleeding: technique and results. Endoscopy 18, 23 – 27.

4.  Takase Y, Ozaki A, Orii K. et al. (1982) Injection sclerotherapy of esophageal varices for patients undergoing emergency and selective surgery. Surgery, 92, 474 – 476.

© 1988 Elsevier Science Publishers B.V. (Biomedical Division)
Treatment of esophageal varices
Y. Idezuki, editor

Chapter 5

# Endoscopic injection sclerotherapy: application, results and prediction of recurrence after the treatment

YASUYUKI YAZAKI, HIROYUKI MAGUCHI, SHIGEYUKI OKANO, YOSHIHARU TOMINAGA, TAKAHISA SUZUKI, MASAMI MIZUNO, CHIHIRO SEKIYA, AKIRA UEHARA AND MASAYOSHI NAMIKI

*Third Department of Internal Medicine, Asahikawa Medical College, Nishikagura 4-5, Asahikawa 078, Japan*

## Introduction

Esophageal varices develop as a complication of portal hypertension mainly related to liver cirrhosis. Clinically, acute variceal bleeding is one of the major life-threatening complications observed in liver cirrhosis, and the management of esophageal varices is of great importance.

From 1983 to 1987, we performed endoscopic injection sclerotherapy (EIS) on 171 patients with esophageal varices. In addition, we used $^{201}$Tl enema as a possible means for the prediction of recurrence of esophageal varices following EIS. We report here the detailed results of our experience.

## Materials and Methods

The subjects were 171 Japanese cirrhotics with esophageal varices who received EIS at Asahikawa Medical College Hospital between 1983 and 1987. In all 171 patients liver cirrhosis was histologically confirmed. Etiologically, 45 cases were alcoholic liver cirrhosis while 120 were viral cirrhosis (35 with B type and 85 with non-A non-B type) and six were others. Hepatitis B (HB) virus-related markers were determined by radioimmunoassay. The diagnosis of alcoholic liver cirrhosis was based upon the histological finding of micronodular change together with the alcoholic intake history of more than 80 g alcohol per day over a period of 10 years or longer. Non-A

All correspondence should be mailed to: Yasuyuki Yazaki, M.D., Ph.D., Third Department of Internal Medicine, Asahikawa Medical College, Nishikagura 4-5, Asahikawa 078, Japan.

non-B type viral liver cirrhosis was diagnosed by excluding involvement of HB virus, alcohol, drugs, parasites, autoimmune hepatitis and idiopathic portal hypertension. The severity of liver disease was graded A, B and C, according to a modified Child's classification [1].

EIS was performed according to the method of Takase et al. [2, 3] with modification. We have used contrast medium + 5% ethanolamine oleate as the sclerosant and a flexible fiberoptic endoscope (Olympus QW, K-10 or GF-V10) as the esophagoscope. As shown in Fig. 1, a balloon attached to the distal end of the endoscope is inflated to stop blood flow in a varix, and the sclerosant is gradually injected into the varix and its feeding vein(s) under X-ray monitoring. When an abnormal shunt is observed, we immediately discontinue the injection and then re-inject the sclerosant from a different site of the varix. If the sclerosant leaks outside the varix, we limit the injection volume to 2 ml and re-inject in the same way, as described previously [4]. Bleeding from the injected site is easily controlled by tamponading

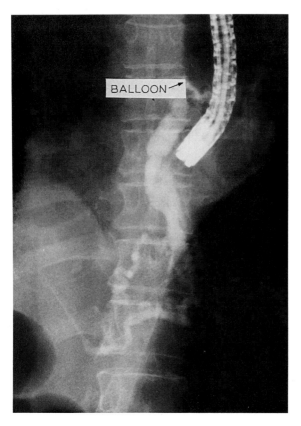

FIG. 1   The injection of the sclerosant, contrast medium + 5% ethanolamine oleate, under X-ray monitoring. An inflated balloon attached to the distal end of a flexible fiberoptic endoscope stops blood flow in a varix, and the sclerosant is injected into the varix and its feeding veins in a sufficient amount.

the injection area with the inflated balloon. The total amount of the sclerosant used in each treatment is usually less than 20 ml. We repeat EIS at one-week intervals until all the varices completely disappear. Complete thromboses of main variceal channels and small venous channels required three to five sessions of EIS, therefore taking approximately a month.

The heart/liver count ratio (H/L ratio) in [201]Tl-chloride per-rectal scintigraphy was calculated according to the method of Tonami et al. [5]. Briefly 1 mCi of [201]Tl-chloride was injected into the area of suprarectal vein in the rectal space through a plastic tube after the rectum was emptied by glycerine enema 60 min before injection. After administration, radioactivity was measured every 5 min up to 25 min by a scintillation camera with a large detection field (Toshiba GCA-401) which had been placed over the upper abdominal area of a patient examined. Data were recorded by a data processing apparatus (Toshiba DAP 5000N). The sequential count of the liver, heart, spleen and lungs was then determined. The H/L ratio at 20 min after [201]Tl injection was used as an index of porto-systemic shunts. The changes in the H/L ratio before and after EIS were examined in 11 patients in terms of the recurrence of esophageal varices. Recurrence of varices after EIS was defined as the reappearance of enlarged tortuous varices ($F_2$), or of straight varices ($F_1$) with positive red color sign.

## Results

Table 1 summarizes the results of all 171 patients who received EIS. Forty-five patients underwent initial injections of the sclerosant in acute conditions (emergency group) and 19 in elective conditions (elective group); 107 were given prophylactic injections (prophylactic group). In 42 out of the 45 emergency cases (93%), bleeding was successfully controlled. The definition of successful control of hemorrhage was that rebleeding did not occur for more than 2 weeks after the treatment. Re-bleeding

TABLE 1    Patients treated with EIS between 1983 and 1987

|  | n | Bleeding stopped | Re-bleeding | Recurrence of varices | Death during 1983–1987 | Death due to variceal bleeding |
|---|---|---|---|---|---|---|
| Emergency cases | 45 (26%) | 42 (93%) | 8 (18%) | 13 (29%) | 25 (56%) | 7 (16%) |
| Elective cases | 19 (11%) |  | 1 (5%) | 2 (11%) | 5 (26%) | 0 (0%) |
| Prophylactic cases | 107 (63%) |  |  | 39 (36%) | 18 (17%) | 3 (3%) |
| Total | 171 (100%) |  |  | 54 (32%) | 48 (28%) | 10 (6%) |

happened in seven cases in the emergency group and one case in the elective group. During a follow-up period of 5 years, recurrence of esophageal varices was observed in 32% of all the patients, most of whom have received additional EIS once or twice. Although 48 cases (28%) died during this follow-up period, only 10 (6%) of them were due to variceal bleeding.

As shown in Table 2, serious complications related to EIS were observed in seven

TABLE 2   Complications of EIS

| Complication | N | Outcome |
|---|---|---|
| Perforation | 1 | Dead |
| Stricture | 2 | Cured by endoscopic dilation |
| Bleeding from ulcer | 2 | Treated with blood transfusion |
| Pleural effusion | 2 | Disappeared without special treatment |
| Total | 7/171 (4%) | |

TABLE 3   Etiology of liver disease and results of the emergency group

| Diseases | Child's Class. at first EIS | n | Bleeding stopped | Re-bleeding | Hepatoma | Death during 1983 – 1987 | Death due to variceal bleeding |
|---|---|---|---|---|---|---|---|
| NB-LC | A | 10 | 10 | 2 | 5 | 4 | 0 |
| 26 (58%) | B | 4 | 4 | 1 | 1 | 1 | 0 |
| | C | 12 | 11 | 2 | 2 | 10 | 2 |
| B-LC | A | 1 | 1 | 0 | 0 | 0 | 0 |
| 7 (16%) | B | 0 | 0 | 0 | 0 | 0 | 0 |
| | C | 6 | 4 | 0 | 3 | 5 | 1 |
| AL-LC | A | 1 | 1 | 0 | 0 | 0 | 0 |
| 10 (22%) | B | 5 | 5 | 1 | 0 | 1 | 1 |
| | C | 4 | 4 | 1 | 0 | 2 | 2 |
| Others | A | 0 | 0 | 0 | 0 | 0 | 0 |
| 2 (4%) | B | 0 | 0 | 0 | 0 | 0 | 0 |
| | C | 2 | 2 | 1 | 1 | 2 | 1 |
| Total | | 45 (100%) | 42 (93%) | 8 (18%) | 12 (27%) | 25 (56%) | 7 (16%) |

NB-LC, non-A non-B type viral liver cirrhosis; B-LC, B type viral liver cirrhosis; AL-LC, alcoholic liver cirrhosis.

cases out of all the cases (4%): esophageal perforation, esophageal stricture which required endoscopic dilatation, massive bleeding from esophageal ulcer which needed blood transfusion and pleural effusion. Although the perforation case died, other complications were conservatively controlled.

The emergency group consisted of 45 patients who received EIS within 48 h following the rupture of esophageal varices after conventional therapy such as Sengstaken-Blakemore (S-B) tube failed to control the variceal bleeding. As to the etiology of accompanied liver disease, 58% of this group had non-A non-B type viral liver cirrhosis (Table 3). There was the tendency that the severity of liver cirrhosis was positively correlated to the frequency of variceal bleeding. However, it was characteristic that a number of non-A non-B type liver cirrhosis experienced variceal rupture even in the Child's Class A group.

TABLE 4   Child's classification and results of the emergency group

| Child's class. at first EIS | (n) | Bleeding stopped | Re-bleed-ing | Treatment and out-come of re-bleeding | | Death during 1983 – 1987 | Death due to variceal bleeding |
|---|---|---|---|---|---|---|---|
| A | 12 | 12 (100%) | 2 (17%) | PTO[a] Re-EIS | (1) (1) | 4 (33%) | 0 (0%) |
| B | 9 | 9 (100%) | 2 (22%) | Operation Death due to bleeding | (1) (1) | 2 (22%) | 1 (11%) |
| C | 24 | 21 (88%) | 4 (17%) | Re-EIS Death due to bleeding | (1) (3) | 19 (79%) | 6 (25%) |
| Total | 45 | 42 (93%) | 8 (18%) | | | 25 (56%) | 7 (16%) |

[a] PTO, percutaneous transhepatic obliteration.

TABLE 5   Mortality and cause of death in the emergency group

| Alive | 20 (44%) | | |
|---|---|---|---|
| | | *Cause of death* | |
| Dead | 25 (56%) | hepatic failure | 9 (20%) |
| | | hepatoma | 8 (18%) |
| | | hemorrhagic gastritis | 1 (2%) |
| | | death due to variceal bleeding | 7 (16%) |
| Total | 45 (100%) | | 25 (56%) |

58

Table 4 shows the results of the emergency group, according to the Child's classification. Variceal bleeding was successfully controlled in all Child's A and B cases, while acute variceal hemorrhage of three cases (12%) in Child's Class C was not. With respect to the frequency of re-bleeding after first EIS, there was no significant difference among these three classes. Although the majority of re-bleeding cases led to death, three cases who survived received additional EIS, percutaneous transhepatic obliteration or surgical treatment.

During the follow-up period of 5 years, the survival rate of the emergency group was 44%, as shown in Table 5. Among 25 cases who died, seven occurred because of variceal bleeding (three from the initial bleeding and four from re-bleeding or further re-bleeding).

Table 6 illustrates the long-term results of the emergency group, according to the Child's classification. The patients in Child's Class A and B demonstrated relatively long survival periods once they survived the first bleeding episodes, while most cases in Child's Class C died within 6 months. There were nine patients who survived for more than 3 years.

The elective group consisted of 19 cases receiving EIS in elective conditions after acute variceal bleeding had been controlled by conventional treatment such as the S-B tube. Etiologically, eight patients had non-A non-B type viral cirrhosis, four had B type viral liver cirrhosis and seven alcoholic liver cirrhosis. Table 7 shows the rate of re-bleeding, recurrence and death in the elective group, according to the Child's classification. There was no significant difference in these parameters be-

TABLE 6   Child's classification and long-term results of the emergency group during a follow-up period of each case

| Child's class. at first EIS | 0 M | 6 M | 12 M | 18 M | 24 M | 30 M | 36 M | 42 M | 48 M | 54 M |
|---|---|---|---|---|---|---|---|---|---|---|
| A 12 cases | ○ | ○ ★★ | | | | ○ | ○○ | ○○ ★ | ○ ★ | |
| B 9 cases | ○ ▼ | ◇○ | ○ | | ○○ | ○ | ○ | | | |
| C 24 cases | ○○ ●● ●●●● ★★★ ★★★★ ▲▲▼▼ ▲ | ▼ | ○ | | ● | | ○ | | | |

○, alive; ●, death due to hepatic failure; ★, death due to hepatoma; ▲, death due to first variceal bleeding; ▼, death due to re-bleeding from varices; ◇, dropped out.

tween each Child's class. Although re-bleeding occurred in one case and recurrence was observed in another case, neither died of variceal bleeding. The long-term results of the elective group are demonstrated in Table 8.

Prophylactic EIS was performed on 107 patients with esophageal varices which were at high risk of rupture, as indicated by moderate or huge size ($F_2$ or $F_3$) and positive red-color sign under endoscopic observation. In this prophylactic group, non-A and non-B type liver cirrhotics comprised half of the 107 cases (Table 9). As anticipated, the percentage of Child's Class A was higher in this group, compared with the emergency group and elective group.

TABLE 7  Child's classification and results of the elective group

| Child's class. at first EIS | n | Re-bleeding | Recurrence | Death during 1983 – 1987 | | |
|---|---|---|---|---|---|---|
| A | 9 | 0 | 0 | 2 | hemorrhagic gastritis | (1) |
| | | | | | acute pancreatitis | (1) |
| B | 4 | 1 | 0 | 0 | | |
| C | 6 | 0 | 1 | 3 | hepatic failure | (2) |
| | | | | | uterus carcinoma | (1) |
| Total | 19 | 1 (5%) | 1 (5%) | 5 (26%) | | |

TABLE 8  Child's classification and long-term results of the elective group during a follow-up period of each case

| Child's class. at first EIS | 0 M | 6 M | 12 M | 18 M | 24 M | 30 M | 36 M | 42 M | 48 M | 54 M |
|---|---|---|---|---|---|---|---|---|---|---|
| A 9 cases | ○ ■■ | | | ○ | ○ | ○○ | | ○○ | | |
| B 4 cases | ○ | | | ○ | | | ○ | ○ | | |
| C 6 cases | ○○○ | ● | ○ | | | | ○ | | | |

○, alive; ●, death due to hepatic failure, ■, death due to other causes.

TABLE 9  Etiology of liver disease and results of the prophylactic group

| Diseases | Child's class. at first EIS | | Bleeding | Recurrence | Hepatoma | Death during 1983 – 1987 | Death due to variceal bleeding |
|---|---|---|---|---|---|---|---|
| NB-LC 51 (48%) | A | 25 | 3 | 5 | 4 | 2 | 1 |
| | B | 15 | 1 | 8 | 3 | 3 | 0 |
| | C | 11 | 1 | 4 | 2 | 1 | 0 |
| B-LC 24 (22%) | A | 15 | 1 | 6 | 5 | 5 | 0 |
| | B | 4 | 0 | 2 | 1 | 0 | 0 |
| | C | 5 | 0 | 1 | 1 | 3 | 0 |
| AL-LC 28 (26%) | A | 15 | 1 | 1 | 3 | 2 | 1 |
| | B | 7 | 1 | 1 | 0 | 0 | 0 |
| | C | 6 | 3 | 0 | 0 | 3 | 1 |
| Others 4 (4%) | A | 2 | 0 | 0 | 0 | 0 | 0 |
| | B | 0 | 0 | 0 | 0 | 0 | 0 |
| | C | 2 | 0 | 0 | 0 | 2 | 0 |
| Total | | 107 (100%) | 11 (10%) | 28 (26%) | 19 (17.5%) | 21 (20%) | 3 (3%) |

NB-LC, non-A non-B type viral liver cirrhosis; B-LC, B type viral liver cirrhosis; AL-LC, alcoholic liver cirrhosis.

Table 10 shows the rate of recurrence, bleeding and death observed in the prophylactic group, according to the Child's classification. Recurrence and bleeding were seen in 28 cases (26%) and 11 cases (10%) out of the 107 cases, respectively. Only three patients died of variceal bleeding. In this group the death rate was highest in Child's Class C, but only one Child's C case died from variceal bleeding. The long-term results of the prophylactic group are illustrated in Table 11.

Table 12 demonstrates the long-term results of all 171 patients given EIS. It was indicated that death due to variceal bleeding rarely occurred once esophageal varices were successfully managed for the first 12 months after initial EIS. Thirty-one out of 66 patients who were followed up for more than 2 years received additional EIS once or twice (1.3-times on average).

TABLE 10   Child's classification and results of the prophylactic group

| Child's class. at first EIS | $n$ (%) | Recurrence | Bleeding | Death during 1983 – 1987 | Death due to variceal bleeding |
|---|---|---|---|---|---|
| A | 56 (52) | 12 (21%) | 5 (9%) | 9 (16%) | 2 (4%) |
| B | 27 (25) | 11 (41%) | 2 (7%) | 3 (11%) | 0 (0%) |
| C | 24 (23) | 5 (21%) | 4 (17%) | 9 (38%) | 1 (4%) |
| Total | 107 (100) | 28 (26%) | 11 (10%) | 21 (20%) | 3 (3%) |

TABLE 11   Child's classification and long-term results of the prophylactic group during a follow-up period of each case

○, alive; ●, death due to hepatic failure; ★, death due to hepatoma; ▲, death due to variceal bleeding; ■, death due to other causes.

62

TABLE 12  Child's classification and long-term results of all the patients receiving EIS during a follow-up period of each case

Child's class.
at first EIS

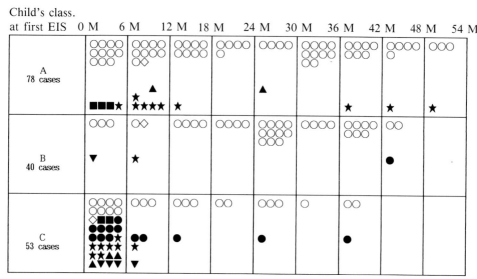

○, alive; ●, death due to hepatic failure; ★, death due to hepatoma; ▲, death due to first variceal bleeding; ▼, death due to re-bleeding from varices; ■, death due to other causes; ◇, dropped out.

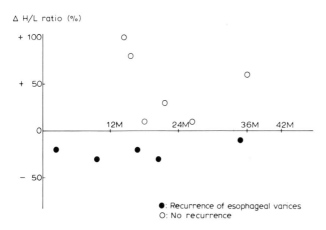

FIG. 2  The changes in the H/L ratio of $^{201}$Tl enema before and after EIS. The vertical axis and horizontal axis indicate the change in the H/L ratio (Δ H/L ratio, %) and the follow-up period of each case, respectively. Open circles mean no recurrence of esophageal varices and closed ones mean recurrence.

The changes in the H/L ratio of $^{201}$Tl enema before and after EIS were examined in 11 patients in Child's Class A and B whose varices were completely obliterated by first EIS. The follow-up period of these cases was 12 to 37 months. As shown in Fig. 2, no recurrence was observed in six cases which demonstrated an increase or no significant change in the H/L ratio. An increase in the H/L ratio indicated increased porto-systemic shunts. On the other hand, recurrence was found in five cases which showed a decrease in the H/L ratio, indicating that a decrease in the porto-systemic shunts followed and that the treated varices had been the main shunt channel(s).

## Discussion

It has been reported that EIS is effective for controlling variceal bleeding and that the success rate for stopping hemorrhage ranges between 84 and 94% [3, 6 – 10]. Our result was 93%, comparable to that of other investigators. Paquet and Fuessner showed, in their controlled randomized trial study [11], that EIS was more effective than the S-B tube in terms of the management of variceal bleeding and the long-term survival rate.

As to the frequency of variceal bleeding, there was the tendency that the severity of liver cirrhosis was positively correlated to the frequency of variceal rupture. It should be noted, however, that a number of non-A non-B type liver cirrhosis suffered variceal bleeding even in Child's Class A group (Table 3).

Nineteen patients received elective EIS. The long-term results of those patients were satisfactory, with no death due to variceal bleeding observed during the follow-up period of 5 years (Tables 7 and 8).

We have actively performed prophylactic EIS on patients with esophageal varices who were at high risk of rupture. Our criteria for prophylactic EIS are the presence of esophageal varices with moderate or huge size ($F_2$ or $F_3$) and positive red-color sign. Principally, these are in accord with those of other researchers [12, 13].

It is still under debate, however, whether or not prophylactic EIS should be actively performed. Paquet et al. [12, 13] reported that prophylactic EIS could largely prevent variceal hemorrhage and was able to prolong the life of chronically ill patients with esophageal varices to an appreciable extent. Our results also suggested that prophylactic EIS was effective for the prevention of variceal bleeding and death due to it (Tables 10 and 11). Since variceal bleeding can cause the rapid deterioration of liver function especially in liver cirrhosis in Child's Class C, it is critically important to prevent the rupture of esophageal varices. However, since the procedures of EIS on their own could be dangerous, we usually exclude patients with hepatoma in the terminal stage, serum total bilirubin levels of over 10 mg/dl or hepatic coma even though they meet our criteria for prophylactic EIS.

Several controlled randomized trials of EIS on the long-term survival have been published [14 – 17] and all agreed with a decrease in the frequency of re-bleeding following EIS. The Copenhagen Group [15] and Westaby et al. [16] further reported the significant improvement of cumulative survival rate in EIS-treated groups. Although our present study was not a controlled randomized trial, it seemed that the long-term results of our study were generally comparable to those of other investigators.

Esophageal varices develop as a complication of portal hypertension mainly related to liver cirrhosis. Therefore, the long-term survival of patients with esophageal varices is influenced not only by the rupture of esophageal varices, but also by the progression of hepatic failure and the development of hepatoma. This should be taken into consideration especially in our country, where the major cause of liver cirrhosis is persistent viral infection.

At least two papers have been published as to the method of prevention of rebleeding or recurrence of esophageal varices after EIS. Obara et al. [18] emphasized the importance of complete obliteration of esophageal varices, while Kitano et al. [19] reported the effectiveness of circumferential eradication of lower esophageal mucosa. Fleig et al. [20] showed that the administration of propranolol was significantly effective after EIS.

It is still difficult to precisely predict recurrence of esophageal varices since complete disappearance of varices does not necessarily guarantee the absence of later recurrence. We have used the change in the H/L ratio of [201]Tl-enema before and after EIS as a possible means of predicting recurrence. There was no recurrence of esophageal varices in cases which showed an increase or no change in the H/L ratio following EIS. An increase in this ratio indicated escalation or further generation of porto-systemic shunts, and no change in this index suggested that the treated varices were not the main shunt channel(s). This speculation was directly confirmed by percutaneous transhepatic portography in a few cases. On the other hand, recurrence of esophageal varices was briefly observed in cases which showed a decrease in the H/L ratio, indicating that the obliterated varices had been the main shunt channel(s). These results suggested that the measurement of the change in the H/L ratio of [201]Tl enema before and after EIS would provide useful information on the prediction of recurrence. In addition, surgical treatment may be considered for further management of recurrent esophageal varices in the case of a decrease in the H/L ratio following EIS.

**Summary**

From 1983 to 1987, we performed endoscopic injection sclerotherapy (EIS) on 171 liver cirrhotics with esophageal varices; 45 patients received EIS under acute conditions, 19 under elective conditions and 107 were given prophylactic EIS. In 42 of the 45 emergency cases (93%), acute variceal hemorrhage was successfully controlled by EIS. There was the tendency that the severity of liver disease was positively correlated to the frequency of variceal bleeding. It was, however, characteristic that patients with non-A non-B type viral liver cirrhosis in the emergency group suffered variceal hemorrhage even in the Child's Class A group. During a follow-up period of 5 years, recurrence of esophageal varices was observed in 54 out of all 171 patients (32%), most of whom underwent additional EIS once or twice. Although 48 patients (28%) died during this follow-up period, only 10 (6%) were due to variceal bleeding. Once esophageal varices were managed for more than 12 months after first EIS, death due to variceal hemorrhage rarely occurred.

The changes in the heart/liver (H/L) ratio of $^{201}$Tl-chloride per-rectal scintigraphy before and after EIS were examined in 11 cases. During a follow-up period of 12 – 37 months, no recurrence was observed in cases which showed an increase or no significant change in the H/L ratio. On the other hand, recurrence was briefly observed in cases which demonstrated a decrease in this ratio. It is suggested that the measurement of the change in the H/L ratio might provide useful information on the prediction of recurrence of esophageal varices following EIS.

## References

1   Pugh RNH, Murray-Lyon IM, Dawson JL, Pietroni MC, Williams R. Transection of the oesophagus for bleeding esophageal varices. Br J Surg 1973; 60: 646 – 649.
2   Takase Y, Ozaki A, Orii K, Nagoshi K, Okamura T, Iwasaki Y. Injection sclerotherapy of esophageal varices for patients undergoing emergency and elective surgery. Surgery 1982; 92: 474 – 479.
3   Takase Y, Kobayashi Y, Chikamori F, Iwasaki Y. Endoscopic sclerotherapy for esophageal varices. Its practice and prognosis. Stomach and Intestine 1985; 20: 481 – 487 (in Japanese).
4   Yazaki Y, Okuno K, Ishikawa Y, et al. Studies on various esophageal lesions due to paravariceal injections of 5% ethanolamine oleate during endoscopic injection sclerotherapy of esophageal varices. Gastroenterol Endoscopy 1986; 28: 2257 – 2267 (in Japanese).
5   Tonami N, Nakazima K, Mitigishi T, et al. Evaluation of portal circulation by $^{201}$Tl-chloride per-rectal scintigraphy. Kaku Igaku (Jpn J Nucl Med) 1981; 18: 205 – 209 (in Japanese).
6   Terblanche J, Bornman PC, Kahn D, Kirsh RE. Sclerotherapy in acute variceal bleeding: techniques and results. Endoscopy 1986; 18 (Suppl 2): 23 – 27.
7   Paquet K-J, Oberhammer E. Sclerotherapy of bleeding esophageal varices by means of endoscopy. Endoscopy 1978; 10: 7 – 12.
8   Makuuchi H, Tanaka Y, Sugihara T, et al. Endoscopic sclerothrombotherapy (ETP) for esophageal varices: technique and long-term follow-up of ETP. Stomach and Intestine 1985; 20: 497 – 505 (in Japanese).
9   Suzuki H, Inagaki Y, Kohyama M, et al. Endoscopic sclerotherapy for esophageal varices: its practice and prognosis. Stomach and Intestine 1985; 20: 489 – 495 (in Japanese).
10  Soehendra N, de Heer K, Kempeneers I, Runge M. Sclerotherapy of esophageal varices: acute arrest of gastrointestinal hemorrhage or long term therapy? Endoscopy 1983; 15: 136 – 140.
11  Paquet K-J, Fuessner H. Endoscopic sclerosis and esophageal balloon tamponade in acute hemorrhage from esophagogastric varices: a prospective controlled randomized trial. Hepatology 1985; 5: 580 – 583.
12  Paquet K-J. Prophylactic endoscopic sclerosing treatment of the esophageal wall in varices: a prospective controlled randomized trial. Endoscopy 1982; 4: 4 – 5.
13  Paquet K-J, Koussouris P. Is there an indication for prophylactic paravariceal injection sclerotherapy in patients with liver cirrhosis and portal hypertension? Endoscopy 1986; 18 (Suppl 2): 32 – 35.
14  Terblanche J, Bornman PG, Kahn D, et al. The failure of long term injection sclerotherapy after variceal bleeding to improve survival. Lancet 1983; ii: 1328 – 1331.

15  The Copenhagen Esophageal Varices Sclerotherapy Project. Sclerotherapy after first variceal hemorrhage in cirrhosis. A randomized multi-center trial. N Engl J Med 1984; 311: 1594 – 1600.

16  Westaby D, Macdougall BRD, Williams R. Improved survival following injection sclerotherapy for esophageal varices: final analysis of a controlled trial. Hepatology 1985; 5: 827 – 830.

17  Westaby D, Williams R. Elective sclerotherapy. Techniques and results. Endoscopy 1986; 18 (Suppl 2): 28 – 31.

18  Obara K, Masaki M, Sakamoto H, et al. Studies on prognosis of patients with esophageal and gastric varices treated with injection sclerotherapy using EO or EO-AS combination method. Gatroenterol Endoscopy 1987; 29: 2232 – 2236 (in Japanese).

19  Kitano S, Koyanagi N, Iso Y, Higashi H, Sugimachi K. Prevention of recurrence of esophageal varices after endoscopic injection sclerotherapy with ethanolamine oleate. Hepatology 1987; 7: 810 – 815.

20  Fleig WE, Stange EF, Huncke R, et al. Prevention of recurrent bleeding in cirrhotics with recent variceal hemorrhage: prospective randomized comparison of propranolol and sclerotherapy. Hepatology 1987; 7: 355 – 361.

© 1988 Elsevier Science Publishers B.V. (Biomedical Division)
*Treatment of esophageal varices*
*Y. Idezuki, editor*

Chapter 6

# Clinical evaluation of endoscopic injection sclerotherapy for esophageal varices

KYUICHI TANIKAWA AND ATSUSHI TOYONAGA

*Second Department of Medicine, Kurume University School of Medicine, Kurume 830, Japan*

## Introduction

Repeated endoscopic injection sclerotherapy (EIS) for treatment of variceal bleeding and elective-prophylactic purposes is now adopted worldwide with good results as reported many times in the literature [1 – 5].

The purpose of the present study is to assess the hemostatic efficacy of EIS in emergency cases, and the efficacy, safety and complications in patients given elective-prophylactic EIS, and an attempt was also made to predict the cases which would be resistant to EIS by endoscopic and portographic studies.

## Materials and methods

From March 1981 to May 1986, 371 consecutive patients with esophageal varices were seen and included for study, consisting of 231 cases with acute variceal bleeding and 140 cases receiving elective-prophylactic treatment (Table 1). All had nonalcoholic liver cirrhosis (LC) (mainly posthepatitic).

*Injection technique* In the early stage in the course of repeated EIS, the complete eradication of esophageal varices was the aim with delicate and precise intravariceal injection of an adequate volume of 5% ethanolamine oleate (EO) into the variceal channels.

In the later stage, careful injection of a small amount of EO into the submucosa was done in an area with atypical red color sign [5, 6] such as small intramucosal venous dilatation and/or telangiectasia on the smooth surface of the lower esophageal wall. Small ulcers in this stage were intentionally formed because ulcer healing with fibrosis greatly contributes to strict eradication of small venous channels.

The repeated EIS would end when eradication of atypical red color signs was completed by injections into the surrounding submucosa of the thrombosclerosed varices, which eliminated residual venous channels in the mucosal and submucosal layers [7].

Indications for EIS included emergency variceal bleeding and elective situation following cessation of hemorrhage.

Patients with blue varices of moderate ($F_2$) or huge ($F_3$) size and showing one of the following, red wale marking ($+ +, + + +$), cherry red spot ($+ +, + + +$) and hematocystic spot ($+$), or who had rapid exacerbation of the variceal condition in a short time, were given prophylactic injections according to our criteria [5, 6].

Fifty-four out of 140 elective prophylactic cases were subjected to endoscopic and portographic studies before and after the EIS.

Forty-two of 140 were also planned for portographic study of the cases resistant to EIS.

TABLE 1   Endoscopic injection sclerotherapy for esophageal varices (EIS)

Subjects: 371 nonalcoholic liver cirrhosis (1981 – 1986);
 sex m:f = 263:108; age 54.3 (18 – 76) years

EIS: Intravariceal injection of 5% ethanolamine oleate (EO) by free-hand method

Occasion for EIS:
 Emergency (acute bleeding) 231
  Child A: 28, Child B: 91, Child C: 112
 Elective (22) and Prophylactic (118)
  Child A: 12, Child B: 97, Child C: 13

Studies carried out
 Emergency: hemostatic effect and late efficacy
 Elective-prophylactic: portographic study and efficacy

TABLE 2   Hemostatic effect (emergency cases, $n = 231$; intravariceal injection of 5% ethanolamine oleate by free-hand method)

Combination with
 Sengstaken-Blakemore tube                    :   58 (32.0%)
 Percutaneous transhepatic obliteration       :   15 (8.3%)
 S-B tube and PTO                             :    9 (5.0%)

| Complete (no re-bleeding for 1 week) | Effective (repeated EIS in 1 week) | Failed or died[a] | Hemostatic ratio |
|---|---|---|---|
| 205 (88.7%) | 11 (4.7%) | 15 (6.4%) | 216 (93.3%) |

[a] Cases of failure or death were all Child's Class C ($n = 15$), including 5 with DIC and 7 with shock on arrival. 6 of these 15 had hepatocellular carcinoma (HCC).

## Results

*(1) Emergency cases: control of acute bleeding (Table 2)*
Successful hemostasis was achieved in 216 patients (93.3%) by EIS, in whom 58 had combination treatment with Sengstaken-Blakemore tube (S-B tube), 15 with percutanous transhepatic obliteration (PTO) and 9 with both S-B tube and PTO. Fifteen out of 231 failed in hemostasis or died within 2–3 days. All the 15 had Child's class C liver function. Six of these 15 cirrhotics and hepatocellular carcinoma (HCC) and 7 were in shock on arrival at our emergency service.

*(2) Elective-prohylactic cases*
Details of EIS include an average of 48.3 (23–188) ml of total amount of EO used, 6.1 (2–14) sessions and 2.7 (1.5–6) month period (cf. Table 4).

*(3) Portographic studies before and after EIS in 54 out of 140 (Table 3)*
Portal pressure decreased in 27, remained unchanged in 2 and rose in 25 after EIS. Variceal recurrence was seen less in the cases with decreased portal pressure after EIS, although this was not statistically significant. However, in the cases with new and/or enlarged collaterals after EIS, there was significantly less recurrence of varices.

TABLE 3   Portal pressure change and recurrence after EIS ($n = 54$)

| Portal venous pressure | Recurrence of varices | |
|---|---|---|
| | + ($n = 16$) | – ($n = 38$) |
| Drop         ($n = 27$) | 7 | 20[a] |
| Unchanged  ($n = 2$) | 0 | 2 |
| Elevated     ($n = 25$) | 9 | 16 |

[a] Not significant (Chi-square test).

Collateral change and recurrence after EIS ($n = 54$)

| | Recurrence of varices | |
|---|---|---|
| Collateral change | + ($n = 16$) | – ($n = 38$) |
| New and /or enlarged | | |
| + ($n = 32$) | 6 | 26[b] |
| – ($n = 22$) | 10 | 12 |

[b] $P < 0.05$ (Chi-square test).

*(4) Cases resistant to EIS in portographic study (Table 4)*
When esophageal varices were the only collateral fed by the large left gastric vein, more sessions, more total EO used and a longer period were needed in the treatment with EIS.

*(5) Typical portogram (Fig. 1) and endoscopic view (Fig. 2) of the same patient with esophageal varices (pipeline varix) resistant to EIS*
Fig. 1 shows that the esophageal varix was fed by the large left gastric vein and a single, large varix ran directly upward to the esophagus resembling a pipeline without the bamboo-blind appearance (parallel pattern) usually seen in the ordinary varices [5, 10, 11].

Fig. 2 shows endoscopic views of the pipeline varix of the same patient. As shown by the portogram, a varix came into existence at the gastric cardia running directly upward to a high location in the esophagus.

TABLE 4   Portographic study of 5 cases which were resistant to EIS ($n = 42$)

| Collaterals | | EIS session $\geq 7$ | Total EO $\geq 50$ ml | EIS period $\geq 4$ months |
|---|---|---|---|---|
| A: Esophageal varices (EV) only | ($n = 9$) | 5 (55.6%) | 5 (55.6%) | 5 (55.6%) |
| B: EV + Paraumbilical vein (PUV) | ($n = 6$) | 2 (33.3%) | 3 (50.0%) | 1 (16.7%) |
| C: EV + Paraesophageal vein (PEV) | ($n = 10$) | 1 (10.0%) | 2 (20.0%) | 0 ( 0.0%) |
| D: EV + PUV + PEV | ($n = 10$) | 2 (20.0%) | 1 (10.0%) | 0 ( 0.0%) |
| E: EV + Spleno-renal shunt + others | ($n = 7$) | 3 (42.8%) | 0 ( 0.0%) | 1 (14.3%) |

(Ordinary average of EIS: 6.1(2 – 14) session; total EO used 48.3(23 – 188) ml; period 2.7(1.5 – 6) months)

Portal pressure and size of left gastric vein ($n = 42$)

| | Portal pressure (mmH$_2$O) (splenic pulp pressure) | Size of left gastric vein (mm) |
|---|---|---|
| Cases resistant to EIS ($n = 5$) | 483.3 ± 11.6 | 13.0 ± 1.7[a] |
| Ordinary cases ($n = 37$) | 457.9 ± 78.6 | 8.5 ± 3.4[a] |

[a] $P < 0.025$ (mean ± SD).

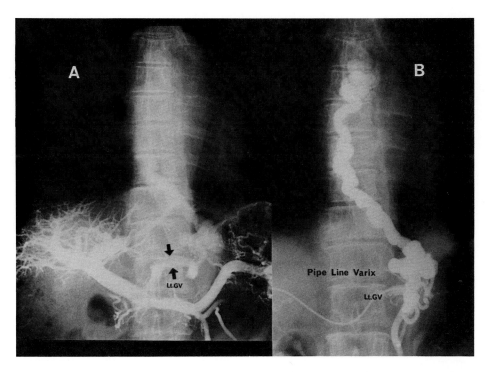

FIG. 1   Percutaneous transhepatic portogram of a patient with pipeline varix. A, total portography; B, selective left gastric venogram.

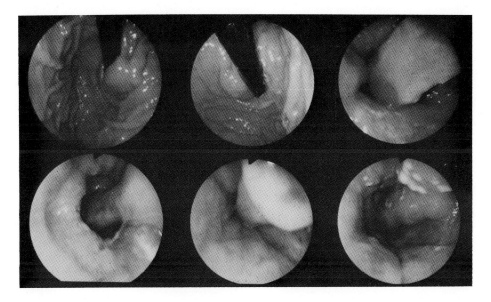

FIG. 2   Endoscopic views of pipeline varix.

72

*(6) Complications in 140 elective prophylactic cases*
Bleeding from the esophageal ulcer of puncture sites was encountered in 3 cases and
2 of these died of massive bleeding associated with liver failure. Gastric bleeding was
seen in 2 patients and one died of uncontrolled hemorrhagic gastritis in whom
hepatocellular carcinoma (HCC) and tumor thrombus of the portal trunk were
found at autopsy. We had one case with esophageal stricture which was successfully
treated by bougienage without sequelae.

*(7) Cumulative survival rate in 122 compliant patients in the elective-
prophylactic group of EIS (Fig. 3)*
The 3 — 4 year cumulative survival rate was 63.4% in the 122 cases (LC 99, LC +
HCC 23), which was almost equal to 62.3% in the surgery group. The group of 99
with LC showed a rate of 80.7%, while it was 8.8% in HCC group.

**Discussion**

EIS is effective for controlling variceal bleeding. Paquet [8] and others [9, 10] showed the superiority of prophylactic EIS in the management of patients with
esophageal varices.
    Prophylactic EIS is justified in high-risk patients with endoscopic criteria for im-
pending bleeding [5, 8 – 10]. Complete eradication of varices by repeated EIS is important for preventing variceal recurrence and recurrent bleeding.
    As for the injection procedure, after 3 – 5 main submucosal varices are throm-
bosclerosed later in the course of repeated EIS, intentional submucosal injections
with a small volume of EO at the area with atypical red color sign [10] are required
to eliminate residual small venous channels in the distal esophagus, ensuing fibrotic
change in the mucosa and the submucosa with epithelialization.
    In the present study portographic and endoscopic evaluation revealed that 5 cases
with esophageal varices resistant to EIS were present and most of the endoscopists

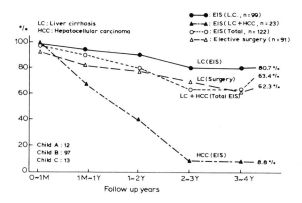

FIG. 3   Cumulative survival rate (elective and prophylactic cases, *n* = 122).

had an empirical impression of the presence of such cases, although they were few in number [10]. These cases had a dominant single varix and high grade in form and location which was supposed to have a high speed and large volume of intravariceal blood flow. Consequently the sclerosant did not work enough to damage the endothelial cells of blood vessels because of the dilution effect, not causing thrombus formation.

In the histopathological studies of autopsied specimens, the angioarchitecture of ordinary esophageal varices [10, 11] was apparently different from that of esophageal varices (pipeline varix) resistant to EIS. However, they could be treated with a combination of PTO or a device of sclerosant. The cumulative survival rate was satisfactory compared with that following elective-prophylactic surgery in our institute.

EIS could be the first choice of treatment in management of patients with esophageal varices in any condition.

## Conclusions

1. Emergency EIS is the first choice of treatment in acute bleeding.
2. Prophylactic EIS is justified in high-risk patients with endoscopic criteria.
3. The efficacy of EIS depends not only upon the technique but somewhat upon the directional flow pattern of portal collaterals.
4. A few cases which would be resistant to EIS could be predicted by endoscopic and portographic examinations.
5. EIS could be the first choice of treatment in the management of patients with esophageal varices in any condition.

## References

1　Macdougall BRD, Westaby D, Theodossi A, et al. Increased long-term survival in variceal haemorrhage using injection sclerotherapy. Results of a controlled trial. Lancet 1982; i: 124 – 127.

2　Terblanche J, Bornman PHC, Kahn D, et al. Failure of repeated injection sclerotherapy to improve long-term survival after esophageal variceal bleeding. A five-year prospective controlled clinical trial. Lancet 1983; ii: 1328 – 1332.

3　The Copenhagen Esophageal Varices Sclerotherapy Project. Sclerotherapy after first variceal hemorrhage in cirrhosis. N Eng J Med 1984; 311: 1594 – 1600.

4　Korula J, Balart LA, Radvan G, et al. A prospective, randomized controlled trial of chronic esophageal variceal sclerotherapy. Hepatology 1985; 5: 584 – 589.

5　Toyonaga A, Tanikawa K. Endoscopic injection sclerotherapy for esophageal varices. Intern Med 1986; 58: 420 – 428 (Tokyo, Japan).

6　Japanese Research Society for Portal Hypertension: The general rules for recording endoscopic findings on esophageal varices. Japanese Surg 1980; 10: 84 – 87 (correspondence).

7　Arakawa M, Toyonaga A, Kage M, et al. Esophageal varices treated with endoscopic injection sclerotherapy – a pathological study. Kurume Med J 1985; 32: 131 – 139.

74

8   Paquet KJ. Prophylactic endoscopic sclerosing treatment of esophageal wall in varices − a prospective randomized trial. Endoscopy 1982; 14: 4 − 5.

9   Toyonaga A. The treatment of esophageal varices. Shin-Naikagaku Taikei 1986; '86 − A: 143 − 170.

10  Fukuda K, Toyonaga A, Yasumoto M, et al. Endoscopic observation of esophageal varices and its clinical significance. Gastroenterol Endosc. 1981; 23: 212 − 223.

11  Noda T. Angioarchitectural study of esophageal varices: with special reference to variceal rupture. Virchows Arch (Pathol Anat) 1984; 404: 381 − 389.

© 1988 Elsevier Science Publishers B.V. (Biomedical Division)
*Treatment of esophageal varices*
*Y. Idezuki, editor*

Chapter 7

# A combination method for endoscopic injection sclerotherapy with ethanolamine oleate and polidocanol on esophageal varices

REIJI KASUKAWA, MORIO MASAKI, KATSUTOSHI OBARA AND HIKOYA MITSUHASHI

*Second Department of Internal Medicine, Fukushima Medical College Fukushima, Japan*

## Introduction

Several injection methods, using different sclerosants, are reported for the endoscopic injection sclerotherapy against esophageal varices.

We have recently been using a combined injection method of intravariceal ethanolamine oleate (EO) and paravariceal polidocanol (Aethoxysklerol, AS) for the sclerotherapy. The results obtained in 150 variceal patients treated with the sclerotherapy are presented here. In addition, experiments carried out in animal models are reported.

## Materials and Methods

*Patients*
The 150 patients treated included 140 (93%) with liver cirrhosis, of which 16 (11%) were alcoholic and 124 (89%) were post-hepatitic, nine of the others had idiopathic portal hypertention and one had extrahepatic portal obstruction as seen in Table 1. Using Child's classification, 95 (63%) were A, 36 (24%) were B and 19 (13%) were C. The clinical state of the patients at the moment of the sclerotherapy was emergency in 24 (16%), elective in 43 (29%) and prophylactic in 83 (55%).

---

Correspondence to: R. Kasukawa, 2nd Dept. of Int. Med., Fukushima Medical College, 1, Hikarigaoka, Fukushima 960-12, Japan.

*Sclerosants*
Ethanolamine oleate (EO) (5%), prepared in the Department of Pharmacy of our Hospital was injected intravariceally in one or two channels at up to 20 ml (0.4 ml/kg) maximum and 1% polidocanol (Aethoxysklerol, AS) was injected paravariceally at up to 20 ml maximum.

*Damage of canine veins injected with EO or AS*
The subcutaneous veins in the legs of dogs were tied at two points at a distance of 5 cm apart and the blood within this region was replaced by EO or AS at various concentrations diluted in human blood (ranging from 90 to 50%; 5% EO and 1% AS were each considered to be 100%). The sclerosants were allowed to remain for 30 s and were then washed out by saline and normal blood circulation resumed. These injections of sclerosants were done at various times before excision of veins: 1 min, 1 h, 2 h and 12 h on one group of dogs; and then 24 h, 1, 2 and 4 weeks, on a second group of dogs. Of the excised veins some were cut cross-sectionally and some longitudinally and were examined macroscopically and microscopically for endothelial destruction and thrombus formation.

*Ulcer formation in rabbit ear by intracutaneous injection of EO or AS*
Five per cent EO or 1% AS was injected intracutaneously into rabbit ears. Four days after the injection, rabbit ears were cut off and histological examination was performed.

TABLE 1   150 patients treated by EIS (1981 – 1987; 6 years)

| | | *n* |
|---|---|---|
| Diagnosis | | |
| Liver cirrhosis | | 140 (93%) |
| alcoholic (including one case with HCC) | | 16 (11%) |
| post hepatitic (including 15 cases with HCC) | B type | 14 (89%) |
| | non-B type | 110 |
| Idiopathic portal hypertension | | 9 |
| Extrahepatic portal obstruction | | 1 |
| | | |
| Child's classification | | |
| A | | 95 (63%) |
| B | | 36 (24%) |
| C | | 19 (13%) |
| | | |
| Treatment | | |
| emergency | | 24 (16%) |
| elective | | 43 (29%) |
| prophylactic | | 83 (55%) |

## Results and Discussion

During the past 6 years, from 1981 to 1987, 150 patients with esophageal varices were treated by endoscopic injection sclerotherapy (EIS).

Out of these patients, 54 were treated by the intravariceal injection of 5% ethanolamine oleate (EO) alone, 12 were treated by the paravariceal injection of 1% polidocanol (Aethoxysklerol AS) alone and 68 patients were treated by the combination of intravariceal injection of EO and paravariceal injection of AS. The method of EO alone was used in the early period of our experience with sclerotherapy and recently the combination method of EO and AS has been used.

The effectiveness of these three methods was 88.9% (48/54) in EO alone, 75.0% (9/12) in AS alone and 98.6% (67/68) in combination of EO and AS as seen in Table 2. The treatment was evaluated as effective when the varices produced a negative red-color sign, or the varices were reduced from $F_2$ or $F_3$ to $F_1$ and no rebleeding occurred within 2 weeks after EIS.

From our clinical experience combined with results obtained from the animal experiments, we considered the indications for EO and AS to be as follows (Table 3): EO can be used intravariceally against varices which have enough inside space to be injected as are moderated to large-sized varices. Gastric varices can occasionally be treated by EO and initial esophageal varices should be treated exclusively by EO. On the other hand, AS can be used paravariceally against small varices and

TABLE 2   Efficacy of the sclerotherapy

|  | 5% ethanolamine oleate (EO) intravariceal | 1% polidocanol (AS) paravariceal | Combination of EO and AS |
|---|---|---|---|
| No. of patients treated | 54 | 12 | 68 |
| No. of patients with effective results (%) | 48 (88.9) | 9 (75.0) | 67 (98.6) |

TABLE 3   Indication of EO and AS for EIS

| EO | AS |
|---|---|
| Intravariceal | Paravariceal |
| Varices which have enough intravariceal space to be injected | Varices which have not enough intravariceal space to be injected |
| Moderate to large-sized varices | Small-sized varices, telangiectasia |
| Gastric varices | Remnant varices after EO-EIS |
| Initial varices | Recurrent varices |

telangiectasia. The varices which remain after EO treatment and those which are recurrent should be treated by AS.

Prognosis of esophageal varices treated with EIS was considered to depend on the completeness of disappearance of all channels of the varices. As seen in Table 4, in 51 patients who received a complete eradication of their varices, lower frequencies of recurrence (17.6%) and rebleeding (5.9%) were observed, whereas in 19 patients who stopped their treatment at a stage of incomplete eradication, higher frequencies of recurrence (100%) and rebleeding (31.6%) were observed. Obviously more frequent repetition (4.5-times) of EIS and a longer period (50.0 days) are needed for complete eradication than those (2.5-times and 32.9 days) for incomplete eradication.

There was no great difference in the rates of both recurrence and rebleeding between the complete and incomplete eradication groups. Comparing the methods for treatment of EIS, complete eradication was achieved in 24 by EO alone and also in 24 by the combination of EO and AS, whereas there was incomplete eradication in 14 of the EO group and in only two of the combination group. In the complete eradication group rebleeding was seen in three cases: one case of cardiac rebleeding, one of fornical and one of bulbar. In those with incomplete eradication there were five cases of esophageal rebleeding and one case of cardiac rebleeding (see Table 4).

Twenty-two deaths were observed in 140 cirrhotic patients who were treated with

TABLE 4    Prognosis of varices treated by EIS

|  | Complete eradication (51) | | | Incomplete eradication (19) | | | Total (70) |
|---|---|---|---|---|---|---|---|
|  | EO (24) | AS (3) | EO + AS (24) | EO (14) | AS (3) | EO + AS (2) |  |
| Mean no. of treatments | 4.5 | | | 2.5 | | | |
| Mean period (days) | 50.0 | | | 32.9 | | | |
| Recurrence no. of patients | 9 (17.6%) | | | 19 (100%) | | | 28 (40%) |
| mean interval (months) | 14.2 | | | 13.2 | | | |
| Rebleeding no. of patients | 3 (5.9%) | | | 6 (31.6%) | | | 9 (12.9%) |
| mean interval (months) | 19.3 | | | 15.7 | | | |
| Sites of rebleeding | cardiac 1 fornical 1 fulbar 1 | | | esophageal 5 cardiac 1 | | | |

TABLE 5   Causes of 22 deaths in 140 cirrhotic patients treated with EIS

| | 14 of 124 patients without HCC (11.3%) | | | 8 of 16 patients with HCC (50%) | | |
|---|---|---|---|---|---|---|
| | Hemorrhage from varices | Hepatic failure | Total | Hemorrhage from varices | Hepatic failure | Total |
| No. of patients died (%) | 2 (17%) | 10 (83%) | 12 | 6 (75%) | 2 (25%) | 8 |
| Child's classification | | | | | | |
| A | 1 | 2 | 3 | 0 | 0 | 0 |
| B | 1 | 4 | 5 | 1 | 1 | 2 |
| C | 0 | 4 | 4 | 5 | 1 | 6 |
| Mean survival period after EIS (months) | 26.5 | 13.5 | 20.0 | 1.7 | 0.77 | 1.5 |
| Grade of eradication | | | | | | |
| complete | 1 | 7 | 8 | 0 | 0 | 0 |
| incomplete | 1 | 3 | 4 | 6 | 2 | 8 |

TABLE 6   The mechanisms for intractability of varices

| Extremely large esophageal varices (one case) | Isolated fornical varices (two cases) | Varices with portal obstruction with HCC (four cases) | |
|---|---|---|---|
| ↓ | ↓ | ↓ | |
| large amount of blood | high blood flow | increased blood flow | |
| ↓ | ↓ | ↙ ↘ | |
| diluteness of sclerosant | no stagnation of sclerosant | high blood flow | bleeding from untreated varices or ulceration caused by EIS |
| ↓ | ↓ | ↓ | |
| no destruction of endothelium | no destruction of endothelium | no thrombi | |

EIS and followed up for one or more years. The causes of their death, conditions of their hepatic lesion and grade of eradication are shown in Table 5. The mortality rate was as low as 11.3% (14 of 124) in patients without hepatocellular carcinoma (HCC), whereas it was as high as 50% (eight of 16) in patients with HCC. Patients without HCC died mostly of hepatic failure (83%, ten of 14), whereas patients with HCC died mostly of hemorrhage from varices (75%, six of 8). The mean survival time was longer in patients without HCC (26.5 months) than in patients with HCC (1.7 months). The ratio of complete and incomplete eradication of the varices was 8 : 4 in patients without HCC, whereas it was 0 : 8 in patients with HCC.

In seven of our patients the varices showed no improvement in form or rebled within 2 weeks even after extensive sclerotherapy. There was one case with extremely large esophageal varices, two cases with isolated fornical varices and four with varices acompanied by portal obstruction with HCC. Insufficient concentration of sclerosants in the large varices and increased blood flow in the fornical varices and the varices with portal obstruction were considered to be the reasons for intractability of the varices (Table 6).

In a total of 426 treatments with EIS in 150 patients, no fatal complications were observed except in one patient with cirrhosis and HCC who suffered from necrosis of intestine after the injection of EO and died 7 days after the injection (Table 7).

TABLE 7   Complications of EIS in two methods

| Complication | EO | AS |
|---|---|---|
| | 319 times of treatment with EO | 107 times of treatment with AS |
| | $n$ % | $n$ % |
| Esophageal ulcer | 124 (38.9) | 76 (71.0) |
| Bleeding from esophageal varices | 2 (0.6) | 0 |
| Bleeding from esophageal ulcer | 7 (2.2) | 0 |
| Perforation (penetration) | (1) (0.3) | 0 |
| Esophageal stenosis | 2 (0.6) | 0 |
| Pleural effusion & mediastinitis | 7 (2.2) | 0 |
| Pulmonary emboly | 3 (0.9) | 0 |
| Hemorrhagic gastritis | 3 (0.9) | 0 |
| Portal thrombosis | 3 (0.9) | 0 |
| Hepatic coma | 2 (0.6) | 0 |
| Renal damage | 2 (0.6) | 0 |
| Shock | 4 (1.3) | 0 |
| Necrosis of intestine (died) | 1 (0.3) | 0 |
| Chest pain | 98 (30.7) | 12 (11.2) |
| Fever | 130 (40.8) | 18 (16.8) |

TABLE 8   Intensity of endothelial damage and thrombus formation of canine leg veins treated with EO or AS

| | Concentration of sclerosant (%) | | | | | | | |
| | Original sclerosant 100 | diluted with human blood | | | | | | |
| | | 90 | 80 | 70 | 60 | 50 | 40 | 30 |
|---|---|---|---|---|---|---|---|---|
| 5% Ethanolamine oleate (EO) | | | | | | | | |
| Endothelial destruction | + + + | + + + | + + + | + + | + | − | − | − |
| Thrombus formation | + + + | + + + | + + | + | ± | − | − | − |
| 1% Aethoxysklerol (AS) | | | | | | | | |
| Endothelial destruction | + + | + | − | − | − | − | − | − |
| Thrombus formation | + + | + | − | − | − | − | − | − |

+ + +, always happens; + +, on many occasions happens; +, sometimes happens; ± seldom happens; −, never happens.

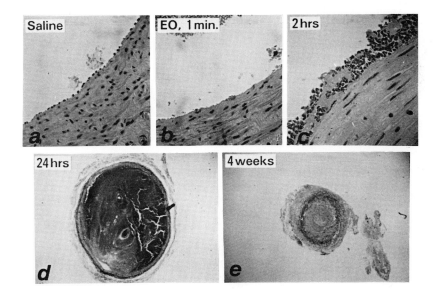

FIG. 1   Microscopic findings of canine leg vein treated with saline (a), treated with 70% EO for 30 s and taken out 1 min later (b) and 2 h later (c) (× 400). Microscopic findings of canine vein treated with 70% EO for 30 s and taken out 24 h later (d) and 4 weeks later (e) (× 20).

In order to understand the pharmacological effects of the sclerosants, several experiments were done in animal models.

In the experiments on canine veins, endothelial destruction was severely caused by the 60% or more concentrations of 5% EO, whereas it was caused to a lesser extent by the 90% concentration of 1% AS. The intensity of the thrombus formation was in parallel to the intensity of the endothelial damage as shown in Table 8.

Complete disappearance of one layer of endothelial cells of the canine vein occurred as early as 1 min after a 30 s blood replacement with an 80% concentration of 5% EO as seen in Fig. 1b. Then, 2 h later, mural thrombus was observed (Fig. 1C). The vein was completely obstructed by a red thrombus within 24 h, and 4 weeks later the vein with white thrombus shrunk to approximately half its previous diameter (Fig. 1d, e) [2].

Two sclerosants, EO and AS, were injected intracutaneously into rabbit ears at concentrations of 5 and 1%, respectively. Severe ulceration reaching to the cartilage of the ear was observed 4 days after injection with 5% EO as seen in Fig. 2a, whereas moderate ulceration which left arteries intact but caused necrosis in veins was observed with 1% AS (Fig. 2b) [1].

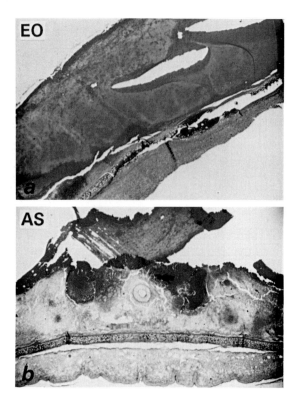

FIG. 2   Microscopic findings of rabbit ear 4 days after subcutaneous injection with EO (a) and AS (b) (× 20).

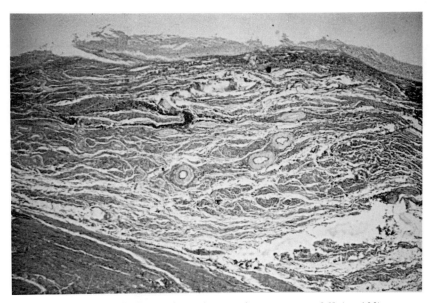

FIG. 3   Microscopic findings of esophagus of autopsy case MI (× 100).

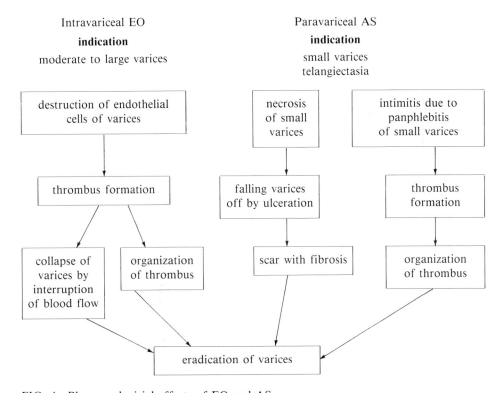

FIG. 4   Pharmacologicial effects of EO and AS.

84

In one autopsy case (37-year-old male patient, MI) who had received a complete eradication of his esophageal varices with the combination sclerotherapy with EO and AS and died one year later because of hemorrhage from gastric fornical varices, the submucosal vein of his esophagus was completely organized as seen on the left side of Fig. 3 which might be caused by intravariceally injected EO. The submucosal tissue which can be seen on the right side of Fig. 3 was thoroughly replaced by fibrous tissues which observed all the small veins leaving only the arteries, and which were considered to be caused by the paravariceally injected AS.

From the observations obtained in both animal experiments and autopsy, the pharmacological effects of EO and AS were tentatively presented in Fig. 4. Intravariceally injected EO causes destruction of endothelial cells of varices and forms a thrombus which brings about collapse of the varices and then organization. On the other hand, paravariceally injected AS causes (a) necrosis of tissues including small varices and ulceration causing scar formation and fibrosis and (b) intimitis of small veins from the outside and organization of thrombus. Using these procedures, it is possible to carry out complete eradication of varices as shown in Fig. 4.

**Summary**

Combined injection sclerotherapy, intravariceal EO against large to moderate-sized varices and paravariceal AS against small varices or telangiectasia, seems to be the most effective method against the esophageal varices. In addition, repeated injection until complete eradication of the varices is achieved is considered to be most important to prevent the recurrence and rebleeding of the varices.

**References**

1   Obara K, Masaki M, Sakamoto H, et al. Studies on prognosis of patients with esophageal and gastric varices treated with injection sclerotherapy using EO or EO-AS combination method. Gastroenterological Endoscopy 1987; 29: 2232 – 2236 (Japanese).
2   Masaki M, Obara K. Mechanisms of action and process of effect of sclerosants (ethanolamine oleate and Aethoxysklerol®) against esophageal varices. In: Takase Y, ed. Injection Sclerotherapy. Tokyo: Chugai Igaku Co. 1986; 23 – 44 (Japanese).

© 1988 Elsevier Science Publishers B.V. (Biomedical Division)
*Treatment of esophageal varices*
*Y. Idezuki, editor*

Chapter 8

# Indication and technique of endoscopic injection sclerotherapy

Keizo Sugimachi, Seigo Kitano, Makoto Hashizume and Hirohiko Yamaga

*Department of Surgery II, Kyushu University Faculty of Medicine, Japan*

## Introduction

The most effective treatment for variceal bleeding in patients with portal hypertension remains controversial; nevertheless new techniques, including various operative and endoscopic procedures, have been introduced. Patients are referred for control of acute variceal bleeding and/or prevention of further bleeding.

A portacaval shunt does not appear to prolong survival and may be followed by encephalopathy even in patients with good liver function [1]. Since this procedure was abandoned in Japan, direct interruption procedures and selective shunts, both related to the concept of portal nondecompression surgery, have been widely used to prevent variceal bleeding, without causing Eck's syndrome. Techniques used for direct interruption include esophageal transection [2], cardial resection [3], Hassab's operation [4] and so on. Selective shunts include left gastric venacaval shunt [5] and distal splenorenal shunt [6].

In recent years, endoscopic injection sclerotherapy [7, 8] has come to be widely accepted as an alternative to surgery for management of patients with esophageal varices. However, there are also variants of techniques of sclerotherapy with regard to the type of endoscope used, sclerosants and the volume injected, injection sites and intervals, and the endpoint.

## Indications for sclerotherapy

Our current policy for treating esophageal varices is shown in Table 1. Endoscopic injection sclerotherapy is the treatment of choice for patients with acute variceal bleeding, because of the high control rate which ensues. Patients with poor liver function, recurrence of varices after surgery and concomitant hepatoma who could not tolerate surgery are given sclerotherapy. Eighty to ninety per cent of such patients have undergone sclerotherapy, as an absolute indication in our institution. In the remaining 10–20%, sclerotherapy has been used as a relative indication, because this treatment is an alternative to surgery in patients with good liver function. In some patients, sclerotherapy was performed to halt bleeding from gastric varices, and to prevent recurrent bleeding.

## Techniques, sclerosants and endopoint

### New over-tubes

Our technique of endoscopic injection sclerotherapy is summarized in Table 2. The initial and second sessions of sclerotherapy are performed using a newly designed transparent over-tube [9]. This tube provides a clear field of vision and facilitates

TABLE 1  Our current policy for treating esophageal varices

| | |
|---|---|
| Absolute indication | |
|   Acute bleeders | |
|   Poor liver function (Child C) | 80–90% |
|   Recurrence after surgery | |
|   Hepatoma | |
| Relative indication | |
|   Good liver function (Child A, B) | 10–20% |
|   Gastric varices | |

TABLE 2  Technique of endoscopic injection sclerotherapy

| | | | | | |
|---|---|---|---|---|---|
| Premedication | : | Diazepam | 5 | mg | iv |
| | | Pentazocine | 30 | mg | iv |
| | | Buscopan | 20 | mg | iv |
| | | 4% Xylocaine | | | topical |
| Fiberscope | : | Olympus GIF Q or K series | | | |
| Over-tube | : | Double-lumened transparent over-tube (K-S tube) used in the 1st and/or 2nd session | | | |
| Sclerosant | : | 5% Ethanolamine oleate | | | |
|   each injection | | ;  1 to 3 ml | | | |
|   maximum volume | | ;  30 ml (1st) | | | |
| | | 20 ml (2nd) | | | |
| | | 10 ml (3rd ~ ) | | | |
| Repeated EIS | : | One week intervals | | | |
| End-point | : | Removal of mucosa for prevention of recurrence of esophageal varices | | | |

precise injection of the sclerosant into varices, even in patients with massive bleeding.

At the late stage of repeated sclerotherapy, further injections are given into the thrombosed varices and surrounding submucosa. The objective is the production of a superficial, circumferential ulcer in the lower esophagus, which will prevent a recurrence of the varices [10].

The new transparent over-tube (Fig. 1) has a slit measuring 7 × 30 mm in the lower end. The external diameter is 20 mm and the internal one 16 mm. The second lumen for the flexible injection needle runs adjacent to the inside of the main lumen from the proximal end to the rim of the slit. The lumen for the injection needle facilitates accurate and rapid injection of the sclerosant, because the injection needle is lined up with the varix protruding into the main lumen through the slit.

Recently, a new double-ballooned tube was fabricated. This tube facilitates precise injection into small size varices, by making use of a distal balloon.

The over-tube is placed over the fiberoptic scope at the proximal end, before insertion of the scope. After topical anesthesia with 4% xylocaine, the Olympus GIF Q10 fiberoptic scope is inserted through the oral cavity into the stomach. The tube is then gently slid over the fiberscope. There will be some resistance in the first stricture portion of the esophagus; however, thereafter the tube can be easily inserted, as shown here.

Once the tube is inserted, the control of bleeding is achieved by compression of the bleeding point and this is confirmed endoscopically through the transparent wall. After rotation of the tube, the active bleeding point emerges and is fixed within the slot. Injection of the sclerosant can be readily performed via the injection needle through the second channel, under a clear field of vision. Thus, the active bleeding is readily controlled. This procedure can be performed much more readily in elective cases.

Results of our prospective randomized trial [11] comparing the two injection techniques showed that the over-tube technique takes less time to accomplish; at the initial session of treatment, time and bleeding during these techniques were an

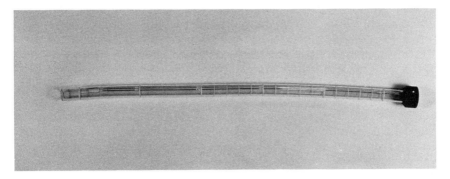

FIG. 1   K-S tube: a transparent over-tube with the slit (7 × 30 mm) at the distal end with the second channel for the injection needle. The external diameter is 20 mm and the internal one 16 mm.

88

average of 11.5 min and 7.3 ml in the over-tube technique, and 20.4 min and 45.1 ml in the free-hand technique. Complications directly related to these procedures are less frequent when the over-tube technique is used. We found that use of the over-tube is a rapid and easier method for sclerosing esophageal varices.

*Removal of esophageal mucosa to prevent variceal recurrence*
Fig. 2A – E are illustrations of the technique we use to treat repeated injection sclerotherapy to prevent recurrent bleeding and recurrence of the esophageal varices. At the initial and second sessions of sclerotherapy, A and B, a precise injection of 5% ethanolamine oleate into varices is required. At the third session, C, injection of the sclerosant into the submucosal tissue of the esophagus plus an injection into the thrombosed varices are given. At the fourth and/or fifth sessions, the sclerosant is injected into the surrounding submucosa, visible after removal of the necrotizing, thrombosed varices. After a sufficient number of sessions, the superficial ulcer in the lower esophagus indicates disappearance of the mucosa. One week after a sufficient number of sessions, re-epithelialization occurs over the area, hence there are no areas where varices can recur.

Endoscopic views taken before and 3 years after sclerotherapy are shown in Fig. 3A and B. Esophageal varices never recurred during the follow-up time, but this particular patient died of a concomitant hepatoma.

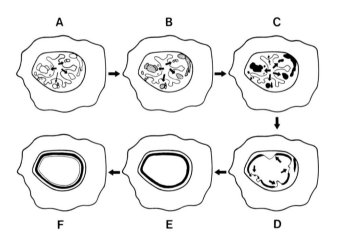

FIG. 2 Illustrations of our modified technique of repeated injection sclerotherapy to prevent recurrent bleeding and recurrence of esophageal varices. (A, B) the initial and second session of sclerotherapy: a precise injection of the sclerosant (5% ethanolamine oleate) into varices using a K-S tube. (C) The third session of sclerotherapy: injection of the sclerosant into the submucosal tissue of the esophagus plus injection into the thrombosed varices. (D) The fourth and/or fifth session of sclerotherapy: injection into the surrounding submucosa, visible after removal of the necrotizing, thrombosed varices. (E) After a sufficient amount of sclerotherapy: the superficial ulcer in the lower esophagus indicates disappearance of the mucosa. (F) A few weeks after a sufficient number of sclerotherapy sessions: epithelialization occurs over area, hence no varices can form. (Reproduced from Hepatology 1987; 5: 810 – 815.)

Fig. 3C shows a section of the esophageal wall from this same patient. There is a marked fibrosis mainly in the mucosa and the submucosal layers, and the lamina muscularis mucosae has disappeared. All possible areas where varices could form in the submucosal layer of the esophagus have been eliminated [10].

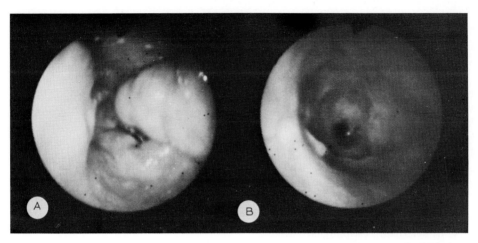

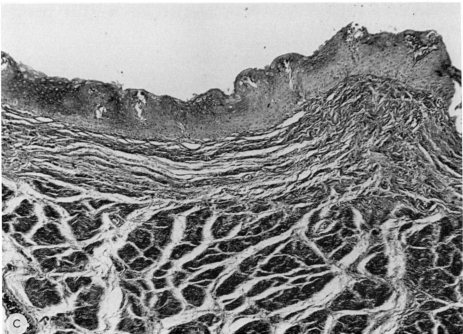

FIG. 3   Endoscopic views taken before (A) and 3 years after (B) sclerotherapy, and a section of the esophageal wall taken from this same patient (C). Note the marked fibrosis in the mucosal and submucosal layers. All areas where varices could form in the submucosal layers were eliminated.

*Sclerosants*

Comparative data on the three sclerosants in clinical use, 5% ethanolamine oleate, 1% aethoxysklerol [12] and 2% sodium tetradecyl sulfate, are shown in Table 3. Eradication of esophageal varices was achieved with repeated injections using any of these sclerosants, and esophageal varices were all eradicated with 4 or 5 sessions of sclerotherapy in a little over one month. However, use of aethoxysklerol or sodium tetradecyl sulfate led to early esophageal bleeding and ulceration. We found that 5% ethanolamine oleate is superior to aethoxysklerol and sodium tetradecyl sulfate, when administered intravariceally.

In our randomized trial on the volume of sclerosant injected, the volumes of 5% ethanolamine oleate used for the first, second and third sessions of sclerotherapy were 15 ml, 10 ml and 5 ml, in the small volume group, and up to 30, 20 and 10 ml in the large volume group. The large volume group showed a significantly high rate of disappearance of red color signs on varices, one week after the initial session of sclerotherapy (14/15 vs. 8/15). The period and number of sessions for eradication of esophageal varices were significantly less in the larger volume group (3.7 sessions in 4.1 weeks vs. 5.5 sessions in 6.3 weeks on average). There was no statistically significant difference in frequency of occurrence of complications between the two groups. We found that the larger volume injection method is superior for the purpose of sclerosing esophageal varices.

TABLE 3   Comparison of three sclerosants: 5% ethanolamine oleate (EO), 1% aethoxysklerol (AS) and 2% sodium tetradecyl sulfate (STD)

|  | EO | AS | STD |
|---|---|---|---|
| No. of patients | 18 | 16 | 17 |
| Sex (male:female) | 13:5 | 13:3 | 14:3 |
| Mean age (years) | 54.7 | 57.7 | 54.8 |
| Child's grading |  |  |  |
| A | 3 | 5 | 3 |
| B | 11 | 8 | 10 |
| C | 4 | 3 | 4 |
| Occasion |  |  |  |
| Acute | 6 | 5 | 4 |
| Elective | 4 | 3 | 5 |
| Prophylactic | 8 | 8 | 8 |
| No. of sessions | 4.0 | 4.8 | 4.4 |
| No. of weeks | 4.7 | 5.4 | 4.9 |
| Complications |  |  |  |
| Early bleeding | 0/18 | 6/16 | 4/17 |
| Early ulcer | 0/18 | 7/16 | 7/17 |
| Stricture | 2/18 | 2/18 | 1/17 |

*Our overall results*

Between January 1982 and July 1987, we treated 500 Japanese patients with injection sclerotherapy. There were 90 with Child's A, 265 with Child's B, and 145 with Child's C liver function. There were 117 patients in acute condition and 143 in elective condition. Prophylactic injection was given to 240 patients who had huge varices with marked red color signs.

Control of variceal bleeding was attained in 98.3% of 117 acute bleeders. In the group of 335 patients who underwent sclerotherapy with our current method, two patients had variceal bleeding after the initiation of sclerotherapy, one in the early stage of repeated sclerotherapy and another noncompliant patient 9 months later.

Fig. 4 shows the cumulative survival rate of the patients who underwent sclerotherapy. One and 3 year survival rates in patients with concomitant hepatoma were 51.8% and 10.2%, respectively, while in those without hepatoma the rates were 91.6% and 76.8%, respectively.

The difference in cumulative survival rates for patients without concomitant hepatoma after sclerotherapy between Child's A and B patients was not statistically significant, while the survival rate of Child's C patients was significantly lower than those of Child's A or B. Three year survival rates were 95.7%, 89.8% and 51.1% in Child's A, B and C patients, respectively.

*Comparative data on surgical treatment and sclerotherapy (Table 4)*

We use two types of surgical procedure to treat esophageal varices, both of which have been performed in our ongoing prospective randomized clinical trials done to compare the effects of three different modalities; distal splenorenal shunt, esophageal transection and endoscopic injection sclerotherapy for patients with good liver function. Total pancreatic disconnection is a requisite in making a distal splenorenal shunt to prevent the occurrence of postoperative malcirculation in the

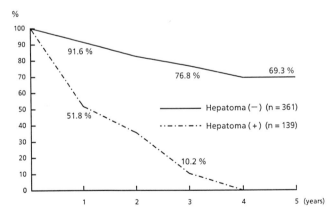

FIG. 4 Cumulative survival rates of 500 patients who underwent sclerotherapy. One and 3 year survival rates in the patients with concomitant hepatoma were 51.8% and 10.8%, respectively. Five year survival rate in patients without hepatoma was 69.3%.

TABLE 4   Comparative data of three different treatment modalities: distal splenorenal shunt (DSRS), esophageal transection (ET) and endoscopic injection sclerotherapy (EIS) (April 1985 – )

|                      | DSRS  | ET    | EIS   |
|----------------------|-------|-------|-------|
| No. of patients      | 16    | 15    | 16    |
| Sex (male:female)    | 12:4  | 10:5  | 11:5  |
| Child's grading      |       |       |       |
| A                    | 9     | 10    | 11    |
| B                    | 7     | 5     | 5     |
| Occasion             |       |       |       |
| Elective             | 7     | 7     | 6     |
| Prophylactic         | 9     | 8     | 10    |
| Late survival        | 15/16 | 14/15 | 15/16 |
| Variceal bleeding    | 1/16  | 0/15  | 0/16  |

portal system. Esophageal transection is performed using an EEA stapler, after esophago-gastric devascularization and splenectomy.

Two groups comparable with regard to age, sex, severity of liver disease and clinical condition were studied. One patient in each group died. One died of liver failure following thrombosis of the portal vein in the distal splenorenal shunt group. One patient in the ET group had gastric bleeding, and one died of an unknown cause in the EIS group. Variceal bleeding occurred in one of the DSRS group after the shunt occluded one month postoperatively.

At this point in time, we find no statistically significant differences among the three groups with regard to survival and bleeding rates.

## Discussion

Esophageal varices are treated to control acute bleeding and to prevent recurrent bleeding. Although bleeding can almost always be halted using a Sengstaken tube, 60% of these patients have a recurrence of bleeding in the near future [13]. Emergency portacaval shunts and emergency non-shunting procedures carry a high mortality, 40% [14] and 25% [15], respectively. Simple and effective injection sclerotherapy is recommended for patients who otherwise would have undergone emergency surgery and also for patients who are poor candidates for surgery.

In elective cases, repeated injection sclerotherapy can completely eradicate esophageal varices and with no varices there is no recurrent bleeding. The prognosis of patients with esophageal varices is much improved in those given repeated injection sclerotherapy.

Bleeding from esophageal varices is a major life-threatening sequal of portal hypertension and the mortality rate for the initial episode of variceal bleeding is generally high. Therefore, it is most important to prevent variceal bleeding in the long-term management of patients with esophageal varices. Not all patients with esophageal varices bleed and surgery may well bring on death in patients with advanced liver cirrhosis. The risk of variceal bleeding can be determined using endoscopy. We follow the criteria of the Japanese Research Society for Portal Hypertension [16].

Prophylactic injection sclerotherapy for patients who have not yet bled from varices is expected to be approved following further testing in properly designed prospective, controlled trials.

'New' varices recurred after the initial obliteration of varices in 60% of 45 patients with repeated injection sclerotherapy, and rebleeding occurred in half the number of patients [17]. We found no recurrence of varices in the area of the esophageal ulcer produced by injecting the sclerosant into submucosal tissue of the esophagus at the later stage of repeated injection sclerotherapy [10]. Ulcer formation – removal of the mucosa is an endpoint of sclerotherapy at the later stage to prevent the recurrence of esophageal varices and rebleeding.

We propose that endoscopic injection sclerotherapy be the first choice of treatment to halt acute variceal bleeding and to prevent recurrent bleeding, particularly in patients with poor liver function. In patients with good liver function, distal splenorenal shunt, esophageal transection and endoscopic injection sclerotherapy seem to be equally efficacious.

# References

1   Conn HO. Therapeutic portacaval anastomosis. To shunt or not to shunt. Gastroenterology 1974; 67: 1065 – 1973.
2   Sugiura M, Futagawa S. Further evaluation of the Sugiura procedure in the treatment of esophageal varices. Arch Surg 1977; 112: 1317 – 1321.
3   Yamamoto S, Hidemura R, Sawada M, Takeshige K, Iwatsuki S. The late result of terminal esophago-proximal gastrectomy (TEPG) with extensive devascularization and splenectomy for bleeding esophageal varices in cirrhotics. Surgery 1976; 80: 106 – 114.
4   Hassab MA. Gastrooesophageal decongestion and splenectomy in the treatment of oesophageal varices in bilharzial cirrhotics: further studies with a report on 355 operations. Surgery 1967; 61: 169 – 176.
5   Inokuchi K, Kobayashi M, Kusaba A, Ogawa Y, Saku M, Shiizaki T. New selective decompression of esophageal varices by a left gastric venous-caval shunt. Arch Surg 1970; 100: 157 – 162.
6   Warren WD, Zeppa R, Fomon JJ. Selective transsplenic decompression of gastro-esophageal varices by a distal splenorenal shunt. Ann Surg 1967; 166: 437 – 455.
7   Crafoord C, Frenckner P. New surgical treatment of varicose veins of the esophagus. Acta Otolaryngol 1939; 27: 422 – 429.
8   Terblanche J, Northover JMA, Bornman P, et al. A prospective evaluation of injection sclerotherapy in the treatment of acute bleeding from esophageal varices. Surgery 1979; 85: 239 – 245.
9   Kitano S, Sugimachi K. A rapid and relatively safer method of sclerosing esophageal varices utilizing a new transparent tube. Am J Surg 1987; 153: 317 – 320.
10  Kitano S, Koyanagi H, Iso Y, Higashi H, Sugimachi K. Prevention of recurrence of

esophageal varices after endoscopic injection sclerotherapy with ethanolamine oleate. Hepatology 1987; 7: 810 – 815.

11  Kitano S, Koyanagi N, Iso Y, et al. Prospective randomized trial comparing two injection techniques for sclerosing esophageal varices: over-tube and free-hand. Br J Surg 1987; 67: 603 – 606.

12  Kitano S, Iso Y, Koyanagi N, et al. Ethanolamine oleate is superior to polidocanol (aethoxysklerol) for endoscopic injection sclerotherapy of esophageal varices: a prospective randomized trial. Hepato-gastroenterol 1987; 34: 19 – 23.

13  Novis BH, Duys P, Barbezat GO, et al. Fibreoptic endoscopy and the use of the Sengstaken tube in acute gastrointestinal haemorrhage in patients with portal hypertension and varices. Gut 1976; 17: 258 – 262.

14  Orloff MJ, Bell RHjr, Hyde PV, et al. Long-term results of emergency portacaval shunt for bleeding esophageal varices in unselected patients with alcoholic cirrhosis. Ann Surg 1980; 192: 325 – 340.

15  Inokuchi K. Present status of surgical treatment of esophageal varices in Japan: a nationwide survey of 3,588 patients. World J Surg 1985; 9: 171 – 180.

16  Japanese Research Society for Portal Hypertension. The general rules for recording endoscopic findings on esophageal varices. Jap J Surg 1980; 10: 84 – 87.

17  Westaby D, Macdougall BRD, Williams R. Improved survival following injection sclerotherapy for esophageal varices: final analysis of a controlled trial. Hepatology 1985; 5: 827 – 830.

© 1988 Elsevier Science Publishers B.V. (Biomedical Division)
*Treatment of esophageal varices*
*Y. Idezuki, editor*

Chapter 9

# Elective treatment of esophageal varices by injection sclerotherapy

Yasuhiro Takase, Yukio Kobayashi and Susumu Shibuya

*Department of Surgery, Institute of Clinical Medicine, University of Tsukuba, Tsukuba City, Ibaraki Pref., 305 Japan*

## Introduction

Sclerotherapy on esophageal varices is a therapeutic method widely used presumably owing to the fact that, once one has attained proficiency in the technique, its application is easy. Relatively recently there has been a revival of interest in sclerotherapy, but data available about the long-term effects of treatment by the technique are scarce. We report here on results of elective sclerotherapy for cases with a history of bleeding.

## Method and patients

### Method

Our method is intended to embolize esophageal varices, the route of hematic supply being by injection of sclerosant (Figs. 1 and 2) [1 – 3]. As premedication, adult cases were given 15 – 30 mg of pentazocine and 25 – 50 mg of hydroxyzine hydrochloride intramuscularly 30 min before the main procedure, 1A of scopolamine butyl-bromide and 1A of 0.5% atropine sulfate 15 min before and anesthetized pharyngeally immediately prior to the operation, with xylocaine as jelly or spray. Infant cases were anesthetized generally by endotracheal intubation. The following endoscopes were used successfully: Olympus EF-B3, GIF-XQ10 and GIF-P10 fiberscopes. A contrast medium, iopamidol or meglumine amidotrizoate, was added (Table 1) [4] to 5% ethanolamine oleate (EO) or 5% EOMA [5] and injected into the varices.

During injection of 5% EOI or 5% EOMA, the balloon (oral side balloon) fitted to the tip of the scope is inflated so that the sclerosant cannot flow out from the varices (Figs. 1 and 3). The dose of 5% EOI or 5% EOMA to be injected into an esophageal varix is 4 – 36 ml, decided under fluoroscopic observation. Injection is discontinued if the sclerosant begins to escape into the portal vein or other unrelated areas (Fig. 3). Accordingly, the dose of the sclerosant to be injected was not constant in our method. When the injection needle penetrates a varix, 0.5 – 3 ml is injected directly into the variceal area. The injection needle size was 20 G, 21 G, 22 G or 23 G depending on the size of the forceps-opening on the endoscope. Before insertion of the fiberscope, the anal side balloon, a kind of pressure tube, is inserted into the stomach. This acts to restrict hemorrhage from the injection site for 0.5 – 3 hours after removal of the scope. This procedure usually allows injection of 1 – 3 varices but, depending on total numbers, the procedure usually must be repeated. The endoscopic procedure is thus conducted a number of times, at intervals of 1 day to 2 weeks (mean interval 1 week). Oxygen inhalation was done intranasally (3

TABLE 1    Patient data (148 cases of esophageal varices in patients with liver cirrhosis; October 1977 – December 1987)

| Age (mean) | 4 – 80 (50.2) |
|---|---|
| Sex | |
|    male | 119 |
|    female | 29 |
| Child's classification | |
|    Grade A | 49 |
|    Grade B | 60 |
|    Grade C | 39 |

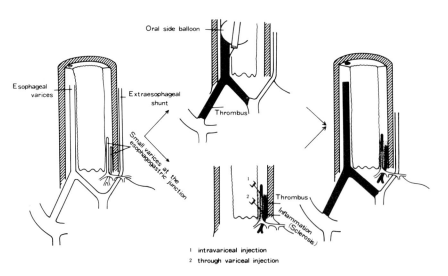

FIG. 1    Technique for treatment of esophageal varices.

litres/min) for 24 hours after the treatment, and an antibiotic was administered intravenously for 3 days. After removal of the anal side balloon, a mucosal protective agent and anti-ulcer agent were administered orally. The patients were not allowed food on the day of treatment, and feeding following treatment was conducted as follows: liquids for 1 – 2 days, 30% gruel for days 3 – 4, and 50% gruel for days 5 – 6. Observation of the course after treatment was made half-yearly to yearly.

*Patients*

The patients assessed in the present study were 148 cases of esophageal varices with liver cirrhosis (Child A, 49 cases; B, 60 cases; and C, 39 cases) treated by this

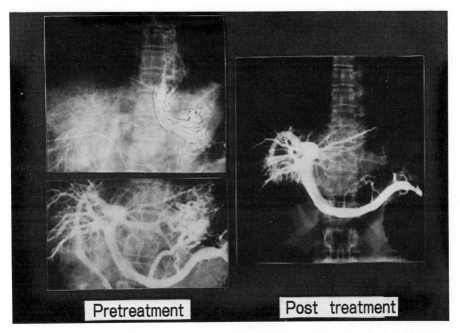

FIG. 2   Percutaneous transhepatic portography before (left) and after (right) endoscopic embolization. The varices were embolized together with the blood supply route.

TABLE 2   Premedication injection: Ethanolamine oleate (contrast medium iopamidol)

| | |
|---|---|
| Monoethanolamine | 0.91 g |
| Oleic acid | 4.23 g |
| Benzyl alcohol | 2.0 ml |
| Iopamidol | 50.0 ml |
| Water for injection | q.s. |
| | 100 ml |

method at the University of Tsukuba Hospital and its affiliated hospitals, during the approximately ten years from October, 1977, to December, 1987 (Table 2). The ages of these 148 cases were distributed between 4 and 80 years (mean 50.2). Long-term therapeutic results were assessed, and charted according to cumulative 5-year survival rate, incidence of major complications, ultimate cause of death, and recurrence/rebleeding rates.

**Results**

The following results were obtained from the 148 cases assessed.
  *Cumulative 5-year survival rate:*  the rates were 80% in 49 cases in Child A, 58%

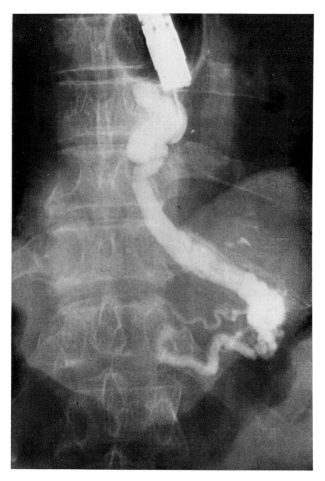

FIG. 3  Sclerosing agent (5% EOI) is injected into varices. EOI is flowing from the varices into LGV, which is its blood supply route.

in 60 cases in B and 29% in 39 cases in C (Fig. 4), thus suggesting that this survival rate is influenced mainly by degree of hepatic function.

*Incidence of major complications:* 5 cases out of 148, i.e. 3.4% (Table 3). The complications in these 5 cases were: 2 cases of esophageal erosion and/or ulcerous bleeding, occurring due to penetration of small varices, where sclerosant (4 ml) was injected into underlying tissue; stenosis of the esophagus resulting from injection into the muscular layer of the esophageal wall in approximate cross-sectional placement (resulting in narrowing); renal dysfunction due to injection of sclerosant which travelled from varices to unrelated areas; and hypotension for approx. 10 min occurring because the sclerosant (in an amount estimated as 5 ml) flowed into the main portal vein. However, these cases with major complication were subsequently cured through conservative (non-surgical) treatment. We provided follow-up, and there was no case which developed complication of any kind after a lapse of more than 1 month after the treatment. Therefore, it is presumed that this treatment method is safe.

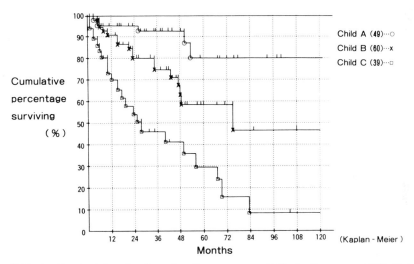

FIG. 4   Survival data for the sclerotherapy group (148 elective cases, 1977, October − 1987, 12 December).

TABLE 3   Major complications (five cases)

| No. | Sex | Age (yr) | Complication |
| --- | --- | --- | --- |
| 1 | M | 38 | Bleeding at esophageal erosions and/or ulcers |
| 2 | M | 51 | Bleeding at esophageal erosion and/or ulcer |
| 3 | F | 60 | Esophageal stenosis |
| 4 | M | 48 | Renal dysfunction |
| 5 | F | 65 | Transitional hypotension |

TABLE 4   Cause of death (42 cases)

| Cause of death | No. of patients (Child A, B, C) |
| --- | --- |
| Hepatic failure | 22 (1, 6, 15) |
| Gastric and/or intestinal bleeding | 4 (0, 3, 1) |
| Hepatocellular carcinoma | 3 (0, 3, 0) |
| Cardiac failure | 2 (0, 1, 1) |
| Renal failure | 2 (0, 1, 1) |
| Esophageal variceal bleeding | 2 (0, 2, 0) |
| Myocardiac infarction | 1 (0, 0, 1) |
| Pneumonia | 1 (1, 0, 0) |
| Cerebral bleeding | 1 (1, 0, 0) |
| Sheehan's disease | 1 (0, 0, 1) |
| Esophageal carcinoma | 1 (1, 0, 0) |
| Operation death | 1 (0, 1, 0) |
| Accident | 1 (0, 0, 1) |
| | 42 (4, 17, 21) |

*Ultimate cause of death:*   during the period of assessment, 42 cases out of 148 died (Table 4). The causes were: hepatic failure in 22 cases (52.4%); gastric and intestinal bleeding in 4 cases (9.5%); hepatoma developed during the course in 3 cases (7.1%); variceal bleeding in 2 cases (4.8%); cardiac failure in 2 cases (4.8%); renal dysfunction in 2 cases (4.8%); myocardial infarction, etc. in 7 cases (16.7%); and unknown cause in 1 case. From these data it appears that the cumulative 5-year survival rate is strongly influenced by degree of hepatic function, and also that this treatment is preventing a large number of possible deaths due to variceal bleeding.

*Recurrence and rebleeding rates:*   recurrences were observed in 27 cases out of 148 (18.2%), and treatment was done using the same technique as in the initial treatment. Rebleeding was observed in 6 cases out of the 27 and two patients died because of this bleeding.

To summarize the above results, we can conclude that this treatment (1) is a relatively safe therapeutic measure and (2) can prevent a large number of possible deaths due to variceal rebleeding.

## Discussion

The history of injection sclerotherapy started with the report by Crafoord et al. and Frenckner [6] in 1939 on the cases treated by the intravariceal injection method, but the technique almost disappeared from the general clinical field in the 1950s when surgical procedures such as shunt operations were developed. However, with the report by Johnston and Rodgers in 1973 [7] as impetus, an opportunity for reconsidering the technique arose, and injection sclerotherapy (including the paravariceal injection method [8, 9] devised by this time) has thus found its place in the clinical field. Injection sclerotherapy is now performed not only as an emergency hemostatic operation in cases with esophageal varices but also electively and prophylactically. It has been reported that injection sclerotherapy reduces the bleeding rate to levels lower than those with the standard medical treatments [10, 11] and improves the survival rate significantly [12]. However, Sarles et al. [13] report that survival in Child A and B patients may be improved with sclerotherapy but Child C patients are unaffected. Also, the long-term effects of sclerotherapy have not yet been fully assessed, because the method has been applied only to inoperable cases. Accordingly, we have assessed long-term therapeutic effects in the elective cases to which we applied our technique.

We began to perform sclerotherapy on esophageal varices, centering on the cases in which surgery was not possible, in October, 1977. There was no unified name for sclerotherapy at this time, and the general name for the 'treatment by injection to esophageal varices endoscopically' was subsequently defined as 'injection sclerotherapy', while our technique has been defined as 'endoscopic embolization', a further clarification of the therapy itself [1, 3].

We reported in 1981 that the effect of sclerotherapy continues for 1 year [14]. In assessing the results of long-term sclerotherapy this time, we selected cases of esophageal varices mostly from patients with liver cirrhosis as their primary disease, omitting cases of esophageal varices resulting from diseases scarce in number or with severely complicated primary diseases, such as hepatocellular carcinoma. As a result, cumulative 5-year survival rates were measured as 80%, 58% and 29% for Child A, B and C, respectively, and the fact that the cause of death in 52.4% of cases was hepatic failure suggested that the factor which influences the prognosis after treatment is mainly the degree of hepatic function. Death due to variceal rebleeding was 4.8% (2/42), or, conversely, the ultimate cause of death in 95.2% (40/42) was not from variceal bleeding. The variceal rebleeding rate of 4.1% (6/148) is quite low, and points to the relative attractiveness of this treatment, where the incidence of complications leading to death is low. Overall, sclerotherapy is presumed to be a useful therapeutic measure for achieving the purpose of prevention of rebleeding. However, in the light of the fact that the recurrence rate was 18.2% (27/148), we do not find sclerotherapy alone to be a fully satisfactory treatment, when the influence of re-treatment (requiring approx. 1 month) is taken into account. Future assessment regarding long-term effects and cause(s) of recurrence should be conducted.

## Conclusions

We have performed sclerotherapy on esophageal varices electively over a ten-year period. Long-term effects were assessed in 148 cases of esophageal varices in patients with liver cirrhosis as primary disease (child A, 49 cases; B, 60 cases; and C, 39 cases, Oct. 1977 – Dec. 1987). As a result, the following conclusions were obtained:

1. Cumulative 5-year survivial rates of 148 cases assessed were 80% in Child A, 58% in B and 29% in C.

2. Long-term follow-up of patients found 42 deaths, of which 22 cases (52.4%) were death due to hepatic failure, and the proportion of total deaths due to lethal variceal bleeding was 4.8%.

3. Incidence of major complications in 148 cases assessed was 3.4% (5/148), consisting of: esophageal erosions and/or ulcerous bleeding, 2 cases; esophageal stenosis, 1 case; renal dysfunction, 1 case; and transient hypotension, 1 case; all of which were, however, cured.

4. The following rates were also observed: recurrence, 18.2% (27/148); rebleeding, 4.1% (6/148); and lethal rebleeding, 1.4% (2/148).

5. From the above, it is presumed that this method is relatively safe and can effectively prevent many cases of variceal rebleeding. Future research into the causes of recurrent cases might be beneficial.

## References

1   Takase Y, Nakahara A. Treatment of bleeding esophageal varices by endoscopic embolization. Progr Digest Endoscopy 1978; 13: 34 – 37 (in Japanese).

2   Takase Y, Ozaki A, Orii K, Nagoshi K, Okamura T, Iwasaki Y. Injection sclerotherapy of esophageal varices for patients undergoing emergency and elective surgery. Surgery 1982; 92: 474 – 479.

3   Takase Y, Ozaki A. Injection sclerotherapy for esophageal varices (clinical experience of 6 years). In: Okabe H, Honda T, eds. Endoscopic surgery. Amsterdam, New York, Oxford: Elsevier Science Publishers B.V., 1984; 11 – 20.

4   Takeda M, Arai K, Ieta J, Yoshino K, Machishima H, Takase Y, Iwasaki Y. Injection sclerotherapy (Endoscopic Embolization) for esophageal varix. 2. Stability of sclerosing agent mixed with contrast medium. Byoin Yakugaku 1984; 10: 446 – 449 (in Japanese).

5   Takeda M, Suga H, Ieta J, Yoshino K, Machishima H, Takase Y, Iwasaki Y. Stability of agent for injection sclerotherapy (endoscopic emobolization) for esophageal varix. Byoin Yakugaku 1984; 10: 35 – 38 (in Japanese).

6   Crafoord C, Frenckner P. New surgical treatment of varicose veins of the esophagus. Acta Otolaryngol 1939; 27: 422 – 429.

7   Johnston GW, Rodgers HW. A review of 15 years' experience in the use of sclerotherapy in the control of acute haemorrhage from oesophageal varices. Br J Surg 1973; 60: 797 – 800.

8   Wodak E. Oesophagusvarizen-Blutung bei portaler Hypertension; ihre Therapie und Prophylaxe. Wien Med Wschr 1960; 110: 581 – 583.

9   Paquet KT, Oberhammer E. Sclerotherapy of bleeding oesophageal varices by means of endoscopy. Endoscopy 1978; 10: 7 – 12.

10  Clark AW, Macdougall BRD, Westaby D, Mitchell KJ, Silk DBA, Straunin L, Dawson JL, Williams R. Prospective controlled trial of injection sclerotherapy in patients with cirrhosis and recent variceal heamorrhage. Lancet 1980; ii: 552 – 554.

11  Macdougall BRD, Westaby D, Theodossi A, Dawson JL, Williams R. Increased long term survival in variceal haemorrhage using injection sclerotherapy. Lancet 1982; i: 124 – 127.

12  Williams R, Westaby D. Endoscopic sclerotherapy for esophageal varices. Digest Dis Sci 1986; 31: 108S – 121S.

13   Sarles HE, Sanowski RA, Talbert G. Course and complications of endoscopic variceal sclerotherapy: a prospective study of 50 patients. Am J Gastroenterol 1985; 80: 595 – 599.

14   Takase Y, Orii K, Todoroki T, Takeshima T, Ozaki A, Iwasaki Y. A clinical report of injection sclerotherapy for esophageal varices. Jpn J Gastroenterol Surg 1981; 14: 455 – 450 (in Japanese).

© 1988 Elsevier Science Publishers B.V. (Biomedical Division)
Treatment of esophageal varices
Y. Idezuki, editor

Chapter 10

# Indications of injection sclerotherapy for varices of the cardia

Yoshiya Kumagai[1] and Hiroyasu Makuuchi[2]

[1] Mitsukoshi Health and Welfare Foundation Clinic and [2] Surgical Department Medical School, Tokai University, Japan

## Summary

Since the 1979 report by the authors various methods described in the literature have been attempted for the treatment of esophageal varices. Recently the authors treated a series of over 400 cases by consecutive intravascular injections of anhydrous ethanol, 1% polidocanol (EPT) and human thrombin by means of a 23 gauge needle passed via a flexible fiberscope.

## Method of EPT injection sclerotherapy

The inflatable balloon on the fiberscope is usually fully inflated during the injection sclerotherapy (IS) procedure. Injections are performed on the summit of the most noticeable varices (Fig. 1).

First, 3 ml of 1% polidocanol is injected and, in cases in which no swelling of the varices is recognized, negative pressure is applied to the syringe; if blood is seen to flow back into the lumen of the catheter, puncture of the blood vessels is thereby verified, and 3 – 5 ml of anhydrous ethanol can be injected. Injections are made rapidly with application of negative pressure at 1 ml intervals to confirm the continued maintenance of the needle in the vascular lumen by recognition of backflow of blood.

Further injection of ethanol should be stopped when the backflow has significantly diminished or halted; 3 ml 1% polidocanol is then injected, followed by a final additional injection of human thrombin (200 units).

In most cases in which treatment is carried out over a 3-week period, the varices almost completely disappear, subsequently becoming undetectable at 8 weeks. However, some cases may require more treatment in the outpatient clinic.

106

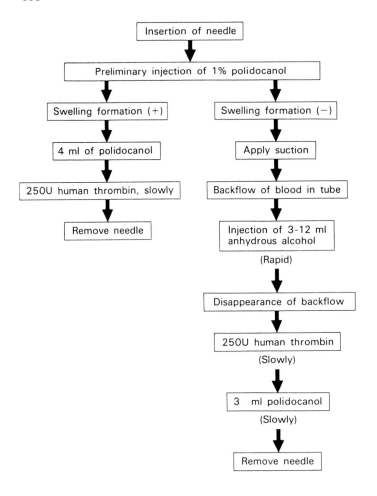

FIG. 1    Injection method procedure.

TABLE 1    Injection sclerotherapy for esophago-cardiac varices

| | |
|---|---|
| Total cases of ETP method | 416 |
| With complete endoscopic data of gastric lesion | 276 |
| Co-existing gastric varices | 191 (71.3%) |
|     Cardiac varices (CV) | 163 |
|     Fundic varices (FD) | 28 |
|     Unclassified | 8 |

(1982,3, Keio Cancer Detection Center, Tokai University Hospital)

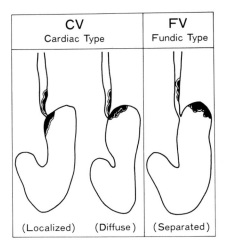

FIG. 2   Gastric varices were classified by the authors into two groups: cardiac varices (CV) and fundic varices (FV). In the former (CV) gastric varices surround the cardia and in the latter (FV) varices are located separately from the former in the greater curvature, and no continuity between the two was found endoscopically.

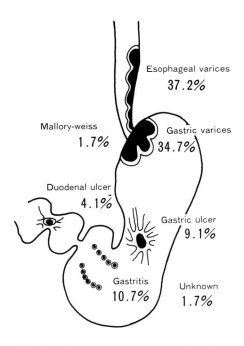

FIG. 3   The endoscopic records of 138 bleeding cases with esophageal varices were studied. This figure shows the site of bleeding: in almost one-third of cases, bleeding originated from gastric varices. These data suggest that more attention should be paid to gastric varices.

**Treatment of gastric varices by IS**

Of these 416 cases, 276 cases in which the endoscopic findings of the gastric lesion were completely evaluable were studied in this paper. In 191 (71.3%) of 276 cases, gastric varices were observed to some extent (Table 1).

These gastric varices were classified into two groups, i.e. cardiac varices (CV) and fundic varices (FV) (Fig. 2). The former (CV), in which the varices were located around the cardia, were found in 163 cases, whereas in 28 cases varices were found at the greater curvature at separate sites from cardiac ring (Fig. 3).

For the former IS was performed from the esophageal varices (Table 3). Injections were made intravasally, to make some amount of sclerosant flow down into the cardiac varices (Fig. 4). This indirect injection method was not effective for FV, because of the discontinuity of the varices.

**Results**

The esophageal varices disappeared completely in 85% of cases following three IS treatments, while in the remainder, in which small varices remained, periodical addi-

TABLE 2   Treatment of gastric varices (CV, FV)

| Method | Indication | Cases |
|---|---|---|
| Indirect IS (sclerosant flows downward from esophageal varices) | CV elective or prophylactic | 144 |
| Direct IS | CV, FV, bleeding or emergency | 13 |
| Operation (Hassab) | FV prophylactic | 7 |
| No treatment | FV only | 17 |

(1982,3, Keio Cancer Detection Center, Tokai University Hospital)

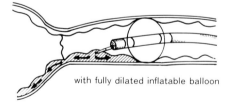

with fully dilated inflatable balloon

FIG. 4   For cardiac varices the indirect method of injection was performed in 144 cases. The figure shows the technique of injection from the lowermost esophageal varices to make the sclerosant flow downward into the lumen of the cardiac varices. The inflatable balloon should be fully dilated with 20 ml of air.

TABLE 3   Results of endoscopic sclerotherapy for cardiac varices

|  |  | Good | Effective | No effect | Residual FV |
|---|---|---|---|---|---|
| Indirect IS from esophageal varices | Emergency | 32 | 4 | 2 | 1 |
|  | Elective or prophylactic | 95 | 7 | 1 | 2 |
| Direct IS | Emergency | 8 | 1 | 1 | 0 |
|  | Elective or prophylactic | 1 | 0 | 2 | 0 |

(1982,3, Keio Cancer Detection Center, Tokai University Hospital)

tional sclerotherapy injecting small amounts of 1% polidocanol at our outpatient clinic was necessary. The results were satisfactory for esophageal varices but for gastric varices results were not as successful. IS is effective in cases of cardiac varices (CV), for which injection should be done in the lower portion of the esophageal varices. As a result of the sclerosant flowing downward into the cardia varices, cardia varices become more flat, diminish in size or disappear (Table 3).

For 6 cases of FV, the indirect injection method was not effective or fundic varices remained to some degree.

For 10 FV cases and 3 bleeding CV the direct injection method was employed. In 10 cases it was effective but in 3 cases it was not effective.

## Discussion

Table 3 shows the results of treatment of IS for cardiac varices and fundic varices. Indirect IS was effective in 96% of cardiac varices but was not effective in 6 cases. Direct IS was effective for 10 cases of fundic varices, but in 3 cases it was not effective and these cases subsequently succumbed.

While direct injection sclerotherapy is not always effective, in certain emergency FV cases it can be a life-saving procedure.

Our results have also shown that our indirect IS method is a safe and effective procedure in the treatment of cardiac varices.

© 1988 Elsevier Science Publishers B.V. (Biomedical Division)
*Treatment of esophageal varices*
*Y. Idezuki, editor*

Chapter 11

# Pathological findings after endoscopical injection sclerotherapy for esophageal varices

MASAHIRO ARAKAWA AND MASAYOSHI KAGE

*The First Department of Pathology, Kurume University School of Medicine, Kurume, Japan*

## Introduction

There is a comparatively large number of reports [1 – 3] concerning pathological findings in early deaths after endoscopical injection sclerotherapy (EIS). These reports mainly discuss changes in the esophageal wall caused by sclerosant, formation of intravarix red thrombi and their organization, and complications of EIS, etc. Our department autopsied more than 70 cases of EIS and reported histological changes taking place over periods of time in the gastric/esophageal wall [4], and the extent of intravarix thrombi formation [5] in emergency cases.

However, since more EIS is expected to be carried out in the future to prevent bleeding from varices and to eradicate varices, pathological studies must be done on such problems as pathological changes in cases of long-term survival after EIS, and in recurrence of varices. This paper reports on the results of our studies on cases which resulted in death for various reasons after survival for longer than three months after EIS, on pathological changes in the esophageal and gastric walls, particularly on the changes and distribution of intravarix thrombi, and on discussions concerning the distribution and causes of death and recurrence of varices.

## Material and methods

A total of 15 cases of EIS were studied; in eight of these EIS was applied for emergency bleeding, and in seven as prophylactic treatment. These cases had survived for more than three months after initial EIS was applied.

A summary is given in Table 1 indicating an age group between 43 and 73; nine cases of males and six of females; underlying diseases including nine cases of liver cirrhosis with hepatocellular carcinoma, and six cases of liver cirrhosis. In the six cases of liver cirrhosis a case of esophageal carcinoma and a case of multiple myeloma are combined.

For EIS, 5% ethanolamine oleate was used as a sclerosant, and intravarix injection by the free-hand method was employed. For elective and prophylactic treatment cases, from three to eight injections were carried out to completely eradicate varices endoscopically.

The period from the first application of EIS to death varied from 4 to 46 months. In cases towards the top end of this scale, additional EIS was carried out from one to three times because of endoscopical appearance of atypical red-color sign, intensified telangiectasia, recurrence of varices and bleeding due to rupture of varices. Causes of death included 10 cases of combined malignant tumor; eight cases of hepatocellular carcinoma, a case of esophageal carcinoma, a case of multiple myeloma, five cases of upper gastro-intestinal bleeding (three cases of varix rupture and two cases of hemorrhagic gastritis).

In the above 15 cases, a specimen was taken from eight places on the gastric and esophageal walls as shown in Fig. 1, and hematoxylin eosin (HE) stain and elastica Van Gieson (EVG) stain were applied. The extent of esophageal intravarix thrombi formation was studied microscopically while bearing in mind the angioarchitecture of esophageal varices (Fig. 2).

TABLE 1   Summary of 15 autopsy cases

| Case | Age | Sex | Underlying disease | Period (M.)[a] | Additional EIS | Cause of death |
|------|-----|-----|--------------------|----------------|----------------|----------------|
| 1 | 52 | M | LC + HCC | 4 | 0 | HCC |
| 2 | 73 | F | LC | 5 | 0 | Varix rupture |
| 3 | 57 | M | LC | 5 | 0 | Esophageal carcinoma |
| 4 | 73 | F | LC | 6 | 0 | Multiple myeloma |
| 5 | 53 | F | LC | 8 | 0 | Hemorrhagic gastritis |
| 6 | 60 | M | LC + HCC | 10 | 0 | HCC |
| 7 | 68 | F | LC + HCC | 12 | 0 | HCC |
| 8 | 62 | F | LC + HCC | 13 | 1 | Varix rupture |
| 9 | 59 | M | LC + HCC | 16 | 0 | HCC |
| 10 | 51 | M | LC + HCC | 16 | 0 | HCC |
| 11 | 46 | M | LC | 16 | 2 | Varix rupture |
| 12 | 43 | M | LC | 22 | 2 | Hemorrhagic gastritis |
| 13 | 66 | M | LC + HCC | 23 | 2 | HCC |
| 14 | 59 | F | LC + HCC | 31 | 2 | HCC |
| 15 | 49 | M | LC + HCC | 46 | 3 | HCC |

[a] Period: from initial EIS to death.

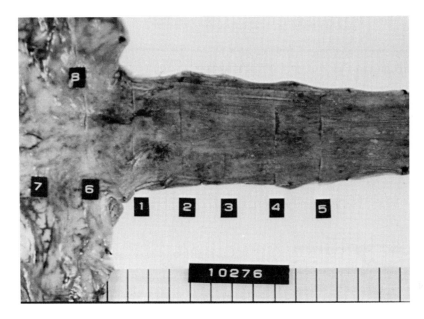

FIG. 1   The position and identity number of the sections taken from the esophagus and proximal stomach.

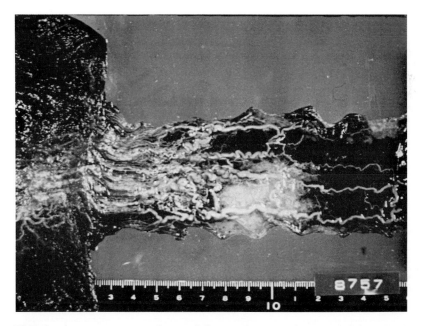

FIG. 2   A transparent specimen of the esophagus and stomach injected with gelatin plus barium in a representative case with varices.

114

## Results

*(1) Macroscopic and histological findings on the gastric/esophageal wall*
Macroscopically, many cases of sclerotic changes were observed on the esophagus, particularly in the lower esophagus. Mucosa were slightly dipped, forming bridging formations in some cases. The four cases showed intensified telangiectasia although there was no projection of varices. There was some petechia noted in the cardiac region of the stomach. This was particularly notable in Cases 5 and 12, where hemorrhagic gastritis was considered the cause of death.

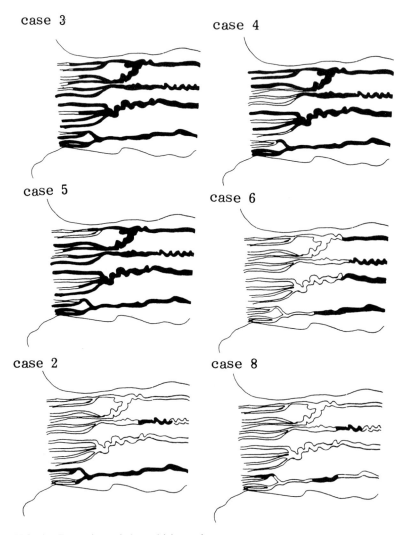

case 3   case 4

case 5   case 6

case 2   case 8

FIG. 3   Extension of thrombi in varices.

Histologically, excluding two cases discussed later (Cases 8 and 11), no acute changes due to EIS were observed. Varices clearly identified by EVG stain were fully obliterated by organized thrombus with recanalization of various degrees. HE stain failed to demonstrate the existence of varices, because of severe fibrosis around varices.

While most veins in the submucosa were obliterated by organized thrombi, there were four cases where no thrombi were found on veins of the lamina propria mucosae and where dilatation of the veins was even noted, for example near the esophago-cardiac (EC) junction in the lower esophagus. Fibrosis was observed mostly on submucosa, but in some cases it extended to the muscularis propria. However, even in the extreme cases, it was found within a quarter range around the esophageal wall. There were many cases of disappearance of lamina muscularis mucosa; this area corresponded to the injection site of EIS, presenting a repair to ulcer.

Three cases of death due to the rupture of varix (Cases 2, 8 and 11) showed different findings from the above cases; in two cases (Cases 8 and 11) EIS carried out immediately before death showed macroscopical varix and red thrombi inside one variceal vein.

Histologically, two cases also showed acute changes in the condition of the patient after EIS, such as the formation of intravarix red thrombi, hemorrhage around the

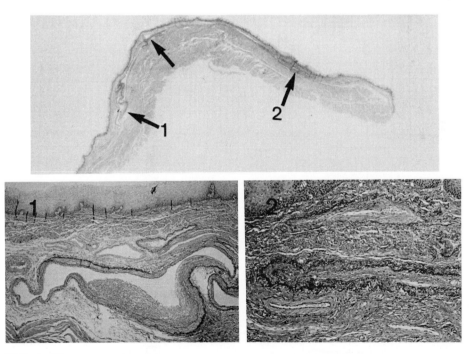

FIG. 4   The cross-section of the lower esophagus in Case 2 and a close-up view. The arrows indicate variceal veins. 1, dilated vein and its thickened wall; 2, obliterated vein due to organized thrombi.

116

varix, edema, inflammatory cellular infiltration, and necrosis of the muscularis propria. Other varices were organized thrombi and remained obliterated.

### (2) Distribution of intravarix thrombus formation

Thrombi were found in most cases at about $10-12$ cm from the EC junction on the side of the esophagus. On the stomach side, they were found in areas not going beyond the EC junction, and where gastric coronary veins pass through the gastric wall.

Fig. 3 shows schematically the range of intravarix thrombus formation in six cases, and a similar search revealed organized thrombus on all four variceal veins in 13 cases out of 15. In Cases 2 and 8, the range of thrombus formation was insufficient and findings clearly indicated the dilatation of veins which were not obliterated, and varices such as thickened walls.

### Two representative cases

(1) Case 2: (one case of two where intravarix thrombus formation was insufficient) the patient was hospitalized because of hematemesis. Endoscopic findings before EIS indicated F3 Cb Ls, CRS +, RWM + + according to the general rules for recording endoscopic findings on esophageal varices [6]. After applying EIS three times and administering a total of 14 ml of 5% ethanolamine oleate, improvement of varix form and disappearance of red-color sign were endoscopically noted in ad-

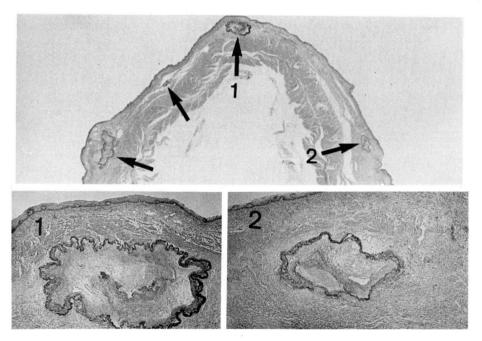

FIG. 5  The cross-section of the lower esophagus in Case 10 and a close-up view. Four variceal veins (arrows) were obliterated by organized thrombi (1 and 2).

dition to hemostasis, but the patient died of hematemesis five months after initial injection. As shown in Fig. 4, in two esophageal variceal veins out of three, no thrombi were found, and dilatation of veins and thickening of the walls were observed. Obliteration due to organized thrombi was noted in one.

(2) Case 10: (one case out of 13 showing sufficient distribution of intravarix thrombus formation) in prophylactic treatment cases, endoscopic findings before EIS were F2, Cb, Ls, CRS + +, RWM +.

EIS was applied over two months, eight times, and a total of 60 ml of 5% ethanolamine oleate was injected, resulting in the complete eradication of endoscopical varices. The patient died 16 months later of a complication from an intra-abdominal rupture of the hepatocellular carcinoma. As shown in Fig. 5, all four variceal veins were obliterated by organized thrombi.

### (3) Case of revarication
Case 11: (a case where one varix recurred while organized thrombi formed on four variceal veins) the patient was hospitalized with hematemesis, and endoscopic findings before EIS were F3 Cb Ls CRS +, RWM + +. EIS was carried out six times over approximately two months and a total of 90 ml of 5% ethanolamine oleate was injected, resulting in complete endoscopic eradication of esophageal varices.

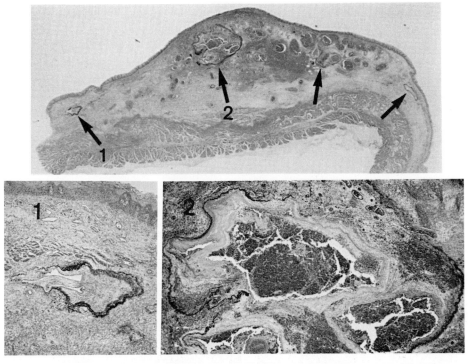

FIG. 6   The cross-section of the lower esophagus in Case 11 and a close-up view. One of the variceal veins (arrow No. 2) consisted of significantly dilated fine vessels in organized thrombi.

118

Against the doctor's advice, however, the patient continued drinking and working. About a year later when he visited the hospital complaining of general malaise, a recurrence of varix was suspected and additional EIS was carried out by administering three injections of a total amount of 36 ml of 5% ethanolamine oleate.

However, the patient did not change his life-style and was admitted to the hospital with complaints of hematemesis four months later and died despite additional application of EIS. Pathologically, as shown in Fig. 6, a varix showed that significant dilatation and rupture occurred near the EC junction (Fig. 7). As shown in Fig. 6, the varix consisted of a significant dilatation of fine vessels in organized thrombi and of dilatation of the surrounding fine veins. Other variceal veins were obliterated by organized thrombi.

## Discussion

It has been only ten years since EIS was introduced to Japan as a medical treatment for esophageal varices. However, today a hemostasis rate of more than 90% is reported for emergency hemorrhagic cases in most hospitals. With these evaluations, EIS has come to be used for elective treatment and prophylactic treatment, and much concern has been aroused concerning the prevention of recurring varices and hemorrhage. Viewing the therapeutic effect of EIS pathologically, in cases of emergency hemorrhage, only thrombus formation should emerge on the ruptured bleeding varix. On the other hand, thrombus formation in all the varices of the

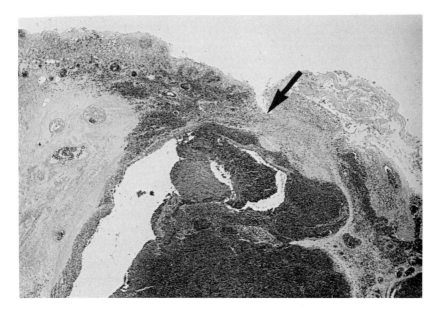

FIG. 7   Histological findings of ruptured varices of Case 11. An arrow indicates the bleeding point covered by fibrin thrombus.

gastric and esophageal walls seems to be nesessary for preventing hemorrhage and recurrence of varices.

To obtain this therapeutic effect, it is important in applying medical treatment and in judging its effect to understand how the angioarchitecture of the varices of the gastric and esophageal walls is made up. In the case of portal hypertension, blood flows into the veins of the gastric and esophageal walls through hepatofugal collaterals such as gastric coronary veins and short gastric veins. Esophageal varices mainly comprise gastric coronary veins [7]. We injected gelatin combined with barium from the gastric coronary veins of the gastric wall into about 25 cases of esophageal varices and prepared a transparent sample as shown in Fig. 2. This made the angioarchitecture and histological findings clear [8, 9].

Fig. 2 shows a representative case, and 'sudare-like' vessels can be seen running 2–3 cm from the esophago-cardiac junction on the esophageal side. These form a bundle varix with dilatation/meandering of the submucosa. This varix is generally composed of four veins. These pathological findings are also backed by endoscopical observations.

We have always observed the distribution of the thrombus formation after EIS keeping in mind the angioarchitecture of varices. As shown in the results, in Cases 2 and 8, thrombus formation only existed in two variceal veins and none was observed in the other two. If thrombus formation is insufficient, blood flow will greatly increase in varices without thrombus, leading to rapidly developing varices, and eventually leading to their rupture. It is pathologically questionable whether these cases may be called recurrence of varices or should rather be called recrudescence. In actual practice, however, these cases seem to be reported as a recurrence of varices. To prevent recurrence which should be called recrudescence in a strict pathological sense, it is important to repeat EIS until varices are fully eradicated by endoscopic observation. According to the literature [10–14], reports from the U.S. and Europe seem to show higher recurrence rates and rebleeding rates than those from Japan. This seems to show that medical treatment is being applied to achieve full eradication of varices in Japan. In order to prevent the recurrence of varices, Kitano et al. [12] attempt not only to bring about thrombogenesis in varices, but also to denude the area of varix occurrence by inducing ulcers with the depth of submucosa and lamina propria mucosa by repeated EIS.

Once thrombus formation occurs on all four variceal veins, thrombi cause complete intravenal obliteration and further sclerosis around the varices as they become organized. It is thought that recanalization or revarication will not easily occur in such conditions. It is considered that in many cases the blood flow of the gastric vein, which functions as collaterals to the stomach and esophagus, reduces while other collaterals develop to deter recurrence of the varix [13]. In 13 out of the 15 cases reported, thrombus formation was histologically sufficient and organized thrombi were noted in all of the variceal veins. In these cases, apart from one case no bleeding occurred from varices, and complication of malignant tumor was designated as the main cause of death. In the process, however, five cases developed atypical red-color sign, and intensification of telangiectasia was observed and additional EIS was carried out on these cases. Atypical red-color sign and telangiectasia were histologically composed of the dilatation of veins of the lamina propria mucosa and varices with organized thrombus in the submucosa. Although complete eradication of varices was observed once, Case 11 showed recurrence of varices and rupture/hemorrhage of varices due to excessive drinking after discharge from hospital and resulted in death. In Case 11, as clearly observed in the histological features (Fig. 6), varices comprise the dilatation of fine vessels in intravariceal organized thrombi together with the dilatation of surrounding veins, presenting evidence of real recurring varices. There was a case of recurring varices although it was rare even when varices were completely eradicated; regular observation by endoscopy is required.

## Summary

Pathological studies of the gastric and esophageal walls of the 15 cases of survival for longer than three months were carried out mainly on the distribution of intravarix organized thrombi. It was found as a result that what is important is to cause thrombi to form all over the varices of the gastric and esophageal walls, and then repeatedly carry out EIS until endoscopical esophageal varices are completely eradicated.

## References

1   Evans DMD, Jones DB, Cleary BK, Smith PM. Oesophageal varices treated by sclerotherapy: a histopathological study. Gut 1982; 23: 615 – 620.
2   Ayres SJ, Golf JS, Warren GH. Endoscopic sclerotherapy for bleeding esophageal varices: effects and complications. Ann Intern Med 1983; 98: 900 – 903.
3   Helpap B, Bollweg L. Morphological changes in the terminal oesophagus with varices, following sclerosis of the wall. Endoscopy 1981; 13: 229 – 233.
4   Matsumoto S. Clinicopathological study of sclerotherapy of esophageal varices: 1. A review of 26 autopsy cases. Gastroenterol Jpn 1986; 21: 99 – 105.
5   Matsumoto S, Arakawa M, Toyonaga A. Extent of thrombi following sclerotherapy of esophageal varices. Gastroenterol Jpn 1986; 21: 447 – 453.
6   Japanese research society for portal hypertension. The general rules for recording endoscopic findings on esophageal varices. Jpn J Surg 1980; 10: 84 – 87.
7   Takashi M, Igarashi M, Hino S, Musha H, Takayasu K, Arakawa M, Nakashima T, Ohnishi K, Okuda K. Esophageal varices: Correlation of left gastric venography and endoscopy in patients with portal hypertension. Radiology 1985; 155: 327 – 331.
8   Arakawa M, Noda T, Fukuda K, Kage M, Nakashima T, Sakisaka T, Nagata K, Eguchi T, Kawaguchi S, Toyonaga A, Yamana H. Clinicopathological studies of esophageal varices. The structure of blood vessels in the esophageal wall. Jpn J Gastroenterol 1983; 80: 2339 – 2346 (Jpn).
9   Noda T. Angioarchitectural study of esophageal varices. With special reference to variceal rupture. Virchows Arch (Pathol Anat) 1984; 404: 381 – 392.
10  Hennessy TPJ, Stephens RB, Keane FB. Acute and chronic management of esophageal varices by injection sclerotherapy. Surg Gynecol Obstet 1982; 154: 375 – 377.
11  Westaby D, Macdougall BRD, Williams R. Improved survival following injection sclerotherapy for esophageal varices: Final analysis of a controlled trial. Hepatology 1985; 5: 827 – 830.

12   Kitano S, Koyanagi N, Iso Y, Higashi H, Sugimachi K. Prevention of recurrence of esophageal varices after endoscopic injection sclerotherapy with ethanolamine oleate. Hepatology 1987; 7: 810 – 815.

13   Tanikawa K, Toyonaga A. Clinical evaluation of endoscopic injection sclerotherapy for esophageal varices. Chapter 6 of this volume.

14   Pitcher LP. Variceal sclerotherapy: The combination of thrombosclerosis and the intentional removal of the distal esophageal mucosa to treat variceal bleeding and to prevent variceal recurrence. Hepatology 1987; 7: 964 – 966.

© 1988 Elsevier Science Publishers B.V. (Biomedical Division)
*Treatment of esophageal varices*
*Y. Idezuki, editor*

Chapter 12

# Oesophageal transection for varices: rationale, indications, technique and results

R.A.J. Spence

*Belfast City Hospital, Lisburn Road, Belfast BT9 7AB, Northern Ireland*

## Introduction and background

The management of patients with bleeding oesophageal varices remains a difficult and challenging area. Although vasopressin [1], balloon tamponade [2] and acute injection sclerotherapy [3, 4] give initial control of variceal bleeding in 50 – 90% of patients further haemorrhage from varices is common if no further therapy is initiated. Although recent reports on the efficacy of somatostatin are encouraging [5] its role in the management of bleeding varices is still unclear. A porta-systemic shunt is the most effective way of preventing recurrent bleeding, but the high mortality in the emergency situation and the considerable incidence of postoperative encephalopathy, especially in Child's grade C patients, have made shunt surgery less acceptable for the majority of patients. Although the distal splenorenal shunt has produced more encouraging results, post-shunt encephalopathy has not been eradicated [6, 7].

The early promise of a medical therapy for portal hypertension using propranolol [8 – 10] has not been fulfilled when used in the British patient [11], although other drugs have been evaluated [12 – 14].

Chronic injection sclerotherapy is becoming increasingly popular, and encouraging results have been reported from Cape Town [15] and King's College Hospital [16, 17]. The latter group have noted an increase in survival, although Terblanche [15] and his group found no difference compared to a control group. The difference can be partly explained by the fact that the Cape Town patients were given injection sclerotherapy for episodes of rebleeding, while the King's patients received medical treatment only. However, both groups found a marked reduction in rebleeding compared to the control group. Chronic sclerotherapy requires multiple visits to hospital at weekly or monthly intervals (depending on the injection regimen) until the varices are eradicated and thereafter life-long endoscopy [18]. Hence, the idea of a local procedure on the dangerous collaterals in the distal oesophagus is attractive. Ideally this would prevent or markedly decrease the incidence of rebleeding and avoid encephalopathy.

## Rationale of 'direct attack' procedures

Chiles and his colleagues [19] were among the earliest workers to note that varices mostly bleed from the lower one-third of the oesophagus and this was confirmed by Orloff and Thomas in 1963 [20]. They found that variceal rupture tended to occur within 2 cm of the oesophago-gastric junction. Similarly Dagradi and his colleagues [21], Warren [22] and Paquet and Oberhammer [23] have all noted from their extensive experience that bleeding nearly always occurs within the distal 5 cm of the oesophagus. In addition Terblanche [24] has commented that pressure with the rigid oesophagoscope at the oesophago-gastric junction will control variceal bleeding immediately. Possible mechanisms proposed to account for this site of bleeding include acid reflux causing oesophagitis, the pressure changes which occur in the region of the cardia and the venous anatomy of the lower oesophagus.

In a previous study looking at oesophageal transection rings (transected immediately above the cardia) oesophagitis was rarely found in the absence of some other precipitating factor such as the presence of a Senstaken tube [25]. Further histological studies on the oesophageal transection rings from this vulnerable area have shown intra-epithelial channels lying in the epithelium and connected to the underlying submucosal vessels via the papillae [26]. These channels may correspond to the cherry-red spots of the Japanese literature [27].

Recent relook at the venous anatomy of the distal oesophagus using the modern technique of image analysis has shown there to be 3 zones. Zone 1 is the stomach, where the relative area occupied by veins in the lamina propria is 2.6% (normals) and 3.7% (varices). Zone 2 is the distal oesophagus and extends 2 − 5 cm. Here the mean area occupied by veins in the lamina propria is 19.8% (normals) and 32.8% (varices). Zone 3 is the remainder of the oesophagus and the area occupied by veins is 4.9% (normal) and 6.1% (varices). A reciprocal pattern is found in the submucosa. This anatomical work has indicated that the distal oesophagus (2 − 5 cm) is the vulnerable or dangerous area because of the proximity to the surface of the veins (lying mostly in the lamina propria) [28] (Fig. 1). Complementary anatomical studies have also been published from Cape Town [29]. In addition the description by McCormack et al. of a constant perforating vein in the distal oesophagus is a further indicator of the vulnerability of this area [30].

Although many direct attack surgical procedures have been advocated [31 − 34] mortality and morbidity have been significant. Tanner [35] suggested subcardiac porto-azygus disconnection, while Walker [36] described transection of the oesophageal mucosa and resuture with catgut. A combination of devascularization and oesophageal transection has been proposed by Suguira and Futagawa [37] and the results from this extensive procedure (with both thoracic and abdominal components) have been good in Japan [38]. However, there is little experience of this operation in the West.

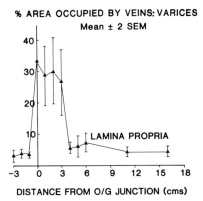

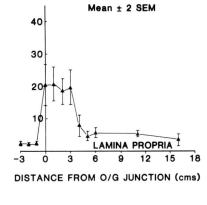

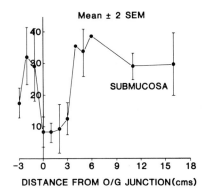

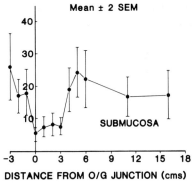

FIG. 1   Percent area occupied by veins. (From the British Journal of Surgery 1984, Vol. 71, pp. 739 – 744: with kind permission of the Editor and Publisher.)

In an attempt to avoid thoracotomy Boerema et al. [39] used a button anastomosis to resect 2 cm of the distal oesophagus but stricture at the anastomotic site was a problem [40]. Van Kemmel's [41] introduction of stapled oesophageal transection allows excision of a 1 cm ring of oesophagus, using an abdominal approach only. It therefore avoids the risk of thoracotomy and allows attack on the vulnerable area of the distal oesophagus, while preserving hepatic blood flow, and hence little risk of encephalopathy.

The current procedure of oesophageal transection and devascularization as practised in Belfast is described below.

## Technique of oesophageal transection and devascularization

The technique has been well described elsewhere [42] and is outlined below. Routine pre-operative preparation includes endoscopy to assess the degree of varices, routine liver function tests (and hepatitis screen), coagulation screen and correction of any metabolic or electrolytic abnormalities. Ascites is also treated pre-operatively.

*Technique*

The patient lies supine on the operating table and an upper midline incision is used. Occasionally a left subcostal incision is used if splenectomy for hypersplenism is considered. The lower oesophagus is identified and the phreno-oesophageal ligament is located. The pre-oesophageal peritoneum contains many vessels and these require diathermy before division. The ligament is pushed upwards to expose the oesophagus. Many large peri-oesophageal collateral veins run with the anterior vagus nerve and these are separated and ligated. Occasionally the anterior vagus may have to be sacrificed and this produces no post-operative sequelae. Liga-clips must not be used to control the veins as they may later be caught in the blade of the gun with distressing results!

The oesophagus is fully mobilized and the large collaterals running with the posterior vagus are freed from the nerve, ligated and divided. The anterior and posterior vagi are retracted on slings and a sloop is placed round the distal oesophagus. The perforating veins, usually 3 to the anterior collaterals and up to 6 to the posterior veins, are divided. Troublesome ooze may occur in patients with previous injection sclerotherapy or oesophagitis. The distal 5 – 6 cm of the oesophagus is cleared of all perforators, a concept supported by the anatomical studies noted above [28, 30].

The left gastric pedicle is then exposed and ligated. Although the pedicle can be approached in the gastrohepatic omentum, usually an approach through an opening in the gastro-colic omentum is easier. Several gastro-epiploic vessels require ligation and an opening into the lesser sac is made.

The mobilized stomach is retracted upwards and any adhesions in the lesser sac are divided until the left gastric pedicle is reached at the upper border of the pancreas. All the vessels in the pedicle are ligated en masse using a non-absorbable suture and tied in continuity. Usually two sutures are used.

An encircling No.0 linen suture is then placed around the now cleared oesophagus and loosely tied. A small anterior gastrotomy is made and one of the circular stapling guns is inserted through the gastrotomy with the head of the gun well lubricated. Earlier in the series the Russian SPTU gun was used but more recently the EEA gun has been used. The sizes of head of the latter are 25, 28, 31 mm in diameter. The sizer may be used to gauge the size of head required. The gun is advanced into the oesophagus for 5 – 6 cm and a gap in the head is opened up until the gap measures about 3 cm. The gun is then carefully positioned until the lowest part of the gap in the head lies immediately above the gastro-oesophageal junction. The previously placed linen ligature is now tied and this invaginates a full thickness of the oesophageal wall and the gap in the gun head is reduced to less than 2 mm, avoiding including the rubber sling. After firing the gun the gap in the head is re-opened and the gun is eased out of the anastomosis and withdrawn.

The ring of tissue in the gun is inspected to ensure the presence of a complete 'doughnut'. A nasogastric tube is directed carefully through the anastomosis into the stomach and the gastrotomy wound is closed in two layers using an absorbable suture. A drain is **not** used routinely.

Post-operatively the tube remains for 48 hours but fluids are generally withheld until 4 – 5 days after surgery. A routine niapam swallow is not performed unless there is cause for concern.

## Indications for transection/devascularization

The indications for the procedure will be discussed in detail later but until the results of ongoing controlled trials are available the procedure is used in our practice in mainly elective cases. Emergency sclerotherapy will control bleeding in 90% of cases in the acute episode [4], and the mortality of emergency transection is high (see later); only the rare failures of acute sclerotherapy should be considered for emergency transection. In the elective cases chronic sclerotherapy is probably the treatment of choice for Child's grade C patients in whom the mortality of transection is high. In Child's grade A the choice lies between chronic sclerotherapy, shunt (probably Warren) or transection. A shunt is probably best avoided in patients over 50 years of age, those with schistosomiasis and diabetes. Chronic sclerotherapy involves repeated visits to hospital and life-long endoscopic follow-up and, for those patients who do not wish this, or because of distance are unable to be available for regular endoscopy, transection is a reasonable alternative to chronic sclerotherapy in Child's grade A or B patients.

## Results of oesophageal transection/devascularization

The results of 110 consecutive transection/devascularization procedures are presented. The series began in 1976 and for the purposes of calculating cumulative survival and rebleeding rates the survival data on the first 100 patients are presented who have had sufficient long-term follow-up. All patients were considered unsuitable for shunt either because of acute bleeding, extra-hepatic block, age, diabetes or poor liver function. Ninety-six had intrahepatic disease and 14 had extrahepatic portal hypertension. Fifty were Child's grade A, 25 were Grade B and 35 were Grade C. Mean age in the series was 54 years with a range of 14 – 80 years. The cause of the intrahepatic portal hypertension is shown in Table 1. The commonest intrahepatic causes were alcoholic, cryptogenic and chronic active hepatitis. Twenty-six had emergency transection and the remainder had elective surgery. There were 59 males and 51 females in the series. Seven patients in the series underwent transection during the first admission for bleeding, while the majority underwent operation during the second or third admissions. Two patients had previous surgical treatment for varices – one patient had a portacaval shunt three years previously and had rebleeding and another patient had a conventional splenorenal shunt 4 years previously and also had rebleeding.

Pre-operatively, 36 had ascites, 14 had had previous encephalopathy, usually related to bleeding episodes, and 33 had hypersplenism. Furthermore 15 were diabetic, 8 had duodenal ulceration, 7 had gallstones, 5 had a hiatus hernia, 4 had gastritis and 2 had gastric ulcers. At surgery 3 patients were found to have a hepatoma.

TABLE 1   110 Consecutive oesophageal transections, 1976–1984

| Aetiology | No. of patients | Sex M | Sex F | Age (years) | Child's Class | Mortality Operative | Mortality Late | Rebleeding |
|---|---|---|---|---|---|---|---|---|
| **Extrahepatic** | 14 | 10 | 4 | 37 (14–58) | 14A | 0 | 0 | 4 |
| **Intrahepatic** | | | | | | | | |
| Alcoholic | 37 | | | | | | | |
| Cryptogenic | 28 | | | | | | | |
| Chronic active hepatitis | 16 | | | | | | | |
| Primary biliary | 8 | | | | 36A | 5 | 10 | 9 |
| Haemochromotosis | 1 | 49 | 47 | 57 (15–80) | 25B | 2 | 6 | 8 |
| Granulomatous | 1 | | | | 35C | 10 | 18 | 6 |
| Cystic fibrosis | 1 | | | | | | | |
| Partial nodular transformation | 1 | | | | | | | |
| Schistosomiasis | 2 | | | | | | | |
| Lupoid hepatitis | 1 | | | | | | | |
| Total | 110 | 59 | 51 | 54 (14–80) | 50A 25B 35C | 17 | 34 | 27 |

At the time of operation, in addition to transection and devascularization, 24 patients had splenectomy and 9 had splenic artery ligation. Eight had vagotomy and gastrojejeunostomy for peptic ulceration and 6 had cholecystectomy, 4 had hernia repair and one underwent liver resection for hepatoma.

The Russian gun was used on 61 patients in the earlier part of the series and the EEA gun for the remainder. The anterior vagus was sacrificed with its accompanying collaterals in 35 patients and the posterior in two.

## Results

### Dysphagia

Fourteen of the 93 patients who survived to leave hospital required dilatation and 35% overall had temporary dysphagia post-operatively. The average number of dilatations required was 1.9 with a maximum of 5 in one patient. Average duration of dysphagia was 5 – 9 months; there was no significant correlation between post-transection dysphagia and prior injection sclerotherapy, size of head used, or extent of peri-oesophageal devascularization.

Physiological studies following surgery have shown that the lower oesophageal sphincter pressure was less post-operatively and that there is poor relaxation of the sphincter after surgery [43]. These results may explain the temporary dysphagia after operation. Further studies using prolonged pH-monitoring have shown that there is greater reflux in this patient group compared to controls [44], although the difference is not very marked.

### Anastomotic leakage

Although two patients had oesophageal leaks none developed a leak from the anastomotic line. One patient leaked 2 cm above the transection line due to an unrecognized perforation following intra-operative dilatation from below of a pre-existing oesophageal stricture. He died subsequently from an empyema. A further patient leaked from the oesophagus also away from the anastomosis and his perforation was successfully repaired. One patient developed a leak from the gastrotomy incision and subsequently developed a subphrenic abscess. He made a satisfactory recovery following drainage.

### Postoperative encephalopathy

Only 6 of the 93 patients who survived to leave hospital have had subsequent bouts of encephalopathy. All 6 had had encephalopathic episodes before surgery.

### Recurrent haemorrhage

Three patients had recurrent bleeding within a few days of emergency transection: two bled from an unknown source and one subsequently died. The other bled from an erosion over a gastric varix and died 19 days after surgery. Of the 93 patients who left hospital alive, 27 patients have had recurrent bleeding in a follow-up extending from 6 months to 9 years. There have been 39 bleeding episodes in the 27 patients with 7 deaths. Recurrent varices have been shown to be the source of

130

bleeding in 11 patients with 2 deaths. Other causes of bleeding include Mallory-Weiss Syndrome, oesophagitis, peptic ulceration, duodenal erosions and gastritis. In addition in 6 patients the source of bleeding was unknown; of these 6, two died.

Cumulative rebleeding rate for the first 100 patients followed for more than 6 months is shown in Fig. 2 and Fig. 3 for all causes of rebleeding and for variceal haemorrhage only. Cumulative rebleeding was calculated using the survival programme of the Statistical Package for Social Services (SSPS) [45].

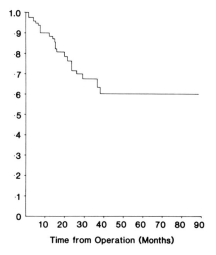

FIG. 2  Remission from bleeding: all causes (100 patients). (From Surgery, Gynaecology and Obstetrics, April 1985; with kind permission of the Editor and Publisher.)

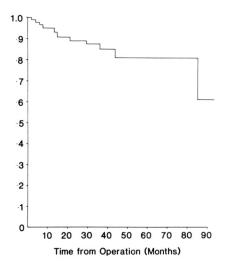

FIG. 3  Remission from variceal bleeding (100 patients). (From Surgery, Gynaecology and Obstetrics, April 1985: with kind permission of the Editor and Publisher.)

At one year from surgery 95% of all patients are free from variceal bleeding, and at 5 years 80% are still free of further variceal bleeding. At 7 years just over 60% are free of rebleeding from varices although numbers are small at this length of follow-up. The extrahepatic group had little rebleeding from varices in the series and over 90% have remained free of bleeding during the first 7 years of follow-up (Table 2).

When all causes of rebleeding are considered for the 100 patients, 60% have remained free of bleeding from any cause at five years. The yearly remission rates for all patients and for intra- and extra-hepatics separately are shown in Table 3.

*Mortality*

There were 17 post-operative deaths in the series − a hospital mortality of 15%. There were 7 deaths in the emergency transection group, giving an emergency mortality of 27% compared to a 12% mortality in the 84 patients undergoing elective surgery. There were no deaths in the extrahepatic group. Overall operative mortality in Child's grade A patients was 10%; in Child's grade B mortality was 8% and mortality in Child's grade C patients was 28.5%. Cause of hospital deaths were hepato-renal syndrome with multiple organ failure (12), septicaemia secondary to low grade peritonitis (2), respiratory failure (1), mediastinitis (after oesophageal leak) (1), and bleeding gastric varices.

*Other postoperative problems*

Twelve per cent of patients had postoperative chest infections, three developed wound infections and one patient developed an ascitic leak. One patient had acute glaucoma postoperatively, one had postoperative pancreatitis, one developed pleural effusions and one developed temporary foot drop.

TABLE 2   Remission from variceal haemorrhage (100 patients)

| Year | 1 | 2 | 3 | 4 | 5 | 6 | 7 |
|---|---|---|---|---|---|---|---|
| All patients (100) | 95.0% | 89.9% | 85.0% | 81.8% | 81.8% | 81.8% | 61.8% |
| Intrahepatics (88) | 95.6% | 83.2% | 83.2% | 79.4% | 79.4% | 79.4% | 79.4% |
| Extrahepatics (12) | 91.3% | 91.3% | 91.3% | 91.3% | 91.3% | 91.3% | 91.3% |

TABLE 3   Remission from bleeding − all causes (100 patients)

| Year | 1 | 2 | 3 | 4 | 5 | 6 | 7 |
|---|---|---|---|---|---|---|---|
| All patients (100) | 88.6% | 72.6% | 64.6% | 60.1% | 60.1% | 60.1% | 60.1% |
| Intrahepatics (88) | 88.2% | 69.1% | 61.7% | 58.8% | 58.8% | 58.8% | 58.8% |
| Extrahepatics (12) | 91.3% | 91.3% | 79.9% | 68.5% | 68.5% | 68.5% | 68.5% |

TABLE 4  Survival all 100 patients

|  | | 1 year | 2 year | 3 year | 4 year | 5 year | 6 year | 7 year | |
|---|---|---|---|---|---|---|---|---|---|
| All 100 patients | | 73.1% | 64.8% | 53.8% | 50.8% | 47.2% | 40.3% | 40.3% | |
| Intrahepatics | (88) | 69.5% | 60.0% | 47.4% | 44.0% | 40.1% | 31.9% | 31.9% | |
| Extrahepatics | (12) | 100.0% | 100.0% | 100.0% | 100.0% | 100.0% | 100.0% | 100.0% | P = 0.0023 |
| Child's grade A | (42) | 87.5% | 81.5% | 71.5% | 63.8% | 59.3% | 53.3% | 53.3% | |
| B | (24) | 78.9% | 74.6% | 62.4% | 62.4% | 62.4% | 62.4% | 62.4% | P = 0.0008 |
| C | (34) | 51.2% | 38.4% | 27.9% | 27.9% | 24.0% | 18.0% | – | |
| Intrahepatics by | | | | | | | | | |
| Child's grade A | (30) | 82.5% | 73.8% | 59.4% | 48.6% | 42.5% | 35.4% | 35.4% | |
| B | (24) | 78.9% | 74.6% | 62.4% | 62.4% | 62.4% | 62.4% | 62.4% | P = 0.0128 |
| C | (34) | 51.2% | 38.4% | 27.9% | 27.9% | 24.0% | 18.0% | – | |

*Survival*
Yearly cumulative survival figures were calculated using the SPSS programme and
comparison was made between groups using the Lee-Desu statistical method [46].
Survival has been calculated for the first 100 patients who have at least 6 months
of follow-up. Yearly cumulative survival figures for all 100 patients are shown in
Table 4 subdivided by Child's grade and into intra - and extra-hepatics. As expected,

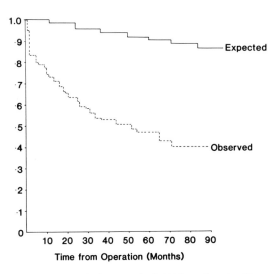

FIG. 4   Cumulative survival (100 patients). (From Surgery, Gynaecology and Obstetrics,
April 1985: with kind permission of the Editor and Publisher.)

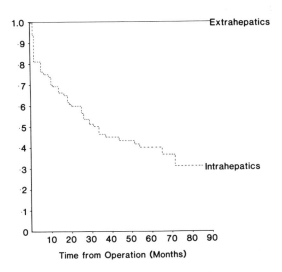

FIG. 5   Cumulative survival (100 patients). (From Surgery, Gynaecology and Obstetrics,
April 1985: with kind permission of the Editor and Publisher.)

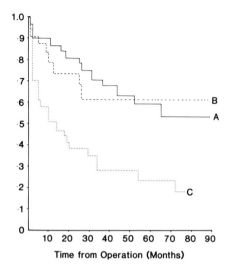

FIG. 6 Cumulative survival (100 patients). (From Surgery, Gynaecology and Obstetrics, April 1985: with kind permission of the Editor and Publisher.)

survival in the extra-hepatic group is better than for intra-hepatics and Child's grade C do significantly worse than Child's A and B patients.

Overall patient survival compared to an expected survival of subjects of similar age and sex is shown in Fig. 4. Survival for intra - and extra-hepatics and for Child's A, B and C is shown in Figs. 5 and 6 respectively.

The five year survival was 47.2% for all patients; prognosis was excellent in the extra-hepatic group, with no deaths, compared to 40.1% five-year survival in the intra-hepatic patients.

Five year survival of Child's grade A was 59.3%, Child's grade B was 62.4% and Child's grade C was significantly worse at 24% ($P = 0.008$). In the long-term there was no significant difference between diabetics and non-diabetics.

Causes of late deaths included liver failure (19), bleeding (7), carcinoma (3), respiratory failure (2), CVA (2) and DIC (1).

*Current status*
Of the 58 patients alive at the time of the review approximately 90% are well and free of jaundice, ascites and encephalopathy.

## Discussion

Although various medical therapies for bleeding oesophageal varices are being proposed and assessed, considerable controversy abounds. Somatostatin [5], propranolol [8, 11], nitroglycerine combined with vasopressin [47], isosorbide [48] and more recently metoclopropamide [49] all have their proponents but their effects are usually temporary and more definite therapy is required.

Endoscopic sclerotherapy can control variceal bleeding in up to 90% of patients [4, 50] but unless a further procedure is undertaken rebleeding is common. In the emergency situation endoscopy with early sclerotherapy, preceded if necessary by vasopressin, seems ideal in the light of current knowledge. There is little place for emergency transection in the acute situation in view of the high mortality, which approaches 30%. However, if several episodes of sclerotherapy are required to control bleeding the mortality rises progressively − after 3 or 4 injections overall mortality is 66% and reaches 89% when Child's grade A patients are excluded [51]. Therefore after failure to control bleeding with two injection episodes there may be a place for emergency urgent transection and devascularization. The mortality is less than in some series of emergency shunts and there is no problem of post-operative encephalopathy.

Following control of the acute episode some therapy must be given to control rebleeding. The place of long-term propranolol is still unclear [9, 11], but overall the evidence from the British studies is that it is probably of little benefit. The reasons for the varying results in different trials may relate to non-compliance of drug intake, continuation of alcohol abuse and the severity of underlying liver disease. There may be a role for propranolol in the congestive gastropathy of portal hypertension [52]. Repeated chronic sclerotherapy appears to reduce rebleeding although the effect on survival if control-group patients are also injected is less clear [15, 17]. However, this involves repeated endoscopy at weekly or three-weekly intervals until the varices are eradicated and life-long follow-up, and it is now recognized that the varices will recur as time goes by. This may not be acceptable to some patients and others may be non-compliant.

The role of shunting procedures is currently unclear in that despite efforts to make shunts more selective [53], and the recent modification of the Warren shunt to include spleno-pancreatic disconnection [54], they have not eliminated post-operative encephalopathy. In addition 6 prospective randomized trials have evaluated selective against total portacaval shunts and only three studies have shown lower encephalopathy in the selective shunt group [55].

Oesophageal transection and devascularization has produced no problem with post-operative encephalopathy and this is an attractive feature. The extensive transection and major devascularization technique of Suguira has produced superb results in Japan [56] with an elective mortality of 3.2% and a mortality in Childs's grade C of only 17%. These results can rarely be reproduced in the Western patient with the high proportion of alcoholics.

Sclerotherapy has been compared to portacaval shunt in actively bleeding patients of Child's grade C class. There was no difference in short-time survival (about 50%) but rebleeding from varices was greater in the sclerotherapy group [57]. A further study from Warren's group has compared sclerotherapy to the Warren shunt and also showed a higher rebleeding rate in the injected group, but the sclerotherapy group had improved survival. This study is important as it included all Child's classes [58].

However, a trial published from Durban [59] comparing oesophageal transection and sclerotherapy in high-risk patients has shown no rebleeding following transection, although follow-up is only up to 2 years. There was no difference in perioperative mortality (24% for sclerotherapy, 33% for transection). Rebleeding occurred after sclerotherapy and the authors advocated transection.

A more recent trial from Spain has suggested that transection is preferable to portacaval shunt in lower-risk patients and that sclerotherapy was preferable to transection in the high-risk group because of fewer complications [60].

From the data in the series reported herein it seems reasonable to agree with Teres and his colleagues [60] that patients who are Child's grade C should undergo a programme of chronic sclerotherapy because of the high mortality of shunting or transection procedures in the West. Patients who are Child's grade A or B are suitable for either transection or chronic sclerotherapy and this depends on the local geography and patients' compliance and wishes to some extent. Although it is to be expected that varices will probably recur after transection, this probably takes several years and ideally endoscopy should be performed at intervals 5 years after transection. Bleeds from these small recurrent varices are usually small and easily managed by sclerotherapy.

In Child's grade A patients there may still be a place for a selective shunt with splenopancreatic disconnection [54] but the recent trial from Warren's group shows good comparative results with sclerotherapy. The major advantage of transection is the absence of encephalopathy. In other patients (A or B) the choice lies between chronic sclerotherapy with life-long endoscopy and repeated injections until varices are eradicated, or elective oesophageal transection, which has a mortality of about 12% in the cold case. The answer lies in future long-term controlled trials of sclerotherapy versus transection and devascularization.

Although in our series 20% of patients rebled from varices by 5 years, a further 20% rebled from other causes such as 'gastritis' and 'gastric erosions'. It may be that the effects of portal hypertension are being re-directed from the oesophagus by the stapled ring to the stomach to form a portal hypertension gastropathy which if it gives rise to troublesome bleeding many only be amenable to a shunting procedure.

Finally oesophageal transection patients have a good quality of life, rarely become encephalopathic after surgery, and the procedure does not preclude other operations such as shunting or sclerotherapy, should that be neccessary in the future.

## References

1  Conn HO. Complications of portal hypertension. In: Gitnick GL, ed. Current Hepatology, Vol 2. New York: Wiley, 1982: 131 – 194.
2  Pitcher JL. Safety and effectiveness of the modified Sengstaken-Blakemore tube: a prospective study. Gastroenterology 1971; 61: 291 – 298.
3  Johnston GW, Rodgers HW. A review of 15 years experience in the use of sclerotherapy in the control of acute haemorrhage form oesophageal varices. Br J Surg 1973; 60: 797 – 800.
4  Spence RAJ, Anderson JR, Johnston GW. Twenty-five years of injection sclerotherapy for bleeding varices. Br J Surg 1985; 72: 195 – 198.

5   Jenkins SA, Baxter JN, Corbett W, Devitt P, Ware J, Shields R. A prospective randomised controlled clinical trial comparing somatostatin and vasopressin in controlling acute variceal haemorrhage. Br Med J 1985; 290: 275 – 278.

6   Langer B, Rotstein LE, Stone RM, Taylor BR, Patel SC, Blendis LM, Colapinto RF. A prospective randomised trial of the selective distal splenorenal shunt. Surg Gynaecol Obstet 1980; 150: 45 – 48.

7   Warren WD, Millikan WJ, Henderson JM, Wright L, Kutner M, Smith RB, Fulenwider JT, Salem AA, Galambos JT. Ten years portal hypertensive surgery at Emory. Results and new perspectives. Ann Surg 1982; 195: 530 – 554.

8   Lebrec D, Nouel O, Corbic M, Benhamou JP. Propranolol – a medical treatment for portal hypertension. Lancet 1980; ii: 180 – 182.

9   Lebrec D, Nouel O, Bernuau, J, Bouygue M, Rueff B, Benhamou JP. Propranolol in prevention of recurrent gastrointestinal bleeding in cirrhotic patients. Lancet 1981; i: 920 – 921.

10  Lebrec D, Poyrard T, Hillon P, Benhamou JP. Propranolol for prevention of recurrent gastrointestinal bleeding in patients with cirrhosis: a controlled study. New Engl J Med 1981; 305: 1371 – 1374.

11  Walt RP, Burroughs AK, Dunk AA, Jenkins W, Sherlock S. Propranolol for prevention of recurrent variceal bleeding in cirrhotic patients. Gut 1982; 23: A908 – 909.

12  Freeman JG, Barton JR, Rexord CO. Effects of vasodilators on portal pressure in patients with portal pressure. Gut 1983; 24: A971.

13  Dawson J, West R, Gertsch, P, Mosimanan F, Elias E. Endoscopic variceal pressure measurements: response to isosorbide clinitrate. Gut 1983; 24: A971.

14  Mills PR, Rae AP, Farah DA, Russell RI, Lorimer AR, Carter DC. Comparison of three adrenoreceptor blocking agents in patients with cirrhosis and portal hypertension. Gut 1984; 25: 73 – 78.

15  Terblanche, J, Bornman PC, Kahn D, Jonker MAT, Campbell JAH, Wright J, Kirsh R. Failure of repeated injection sclerotherapy to improve long term survival after oesophageal variceal bleeding. Lancet 1983; ii: 1328 – 1332.

16  Clark AW, Macdougal BRD, Westaby D, Mitchell KJ, Silk DBA, Strumin L, Dawson JL, Williams R. Prospective controlled trial of injection sclerotherapy in patients with cirrhosis and recent variceal haemorrhage. Lancet 1980; i: 552 – 554.

17  Macdougall BRD, Westaby D, Theodossi A, Dawson JL, Williams R. Increased long term survival in variceal haemorrhage using injection sclerotherapy: results of a controlled trial. Lancet 1982; i: 124 – 127.

18  Paquet KJ. Prophylactic endoscopic sclerosing treatment of the oesophageal wall in varices – a prospective controlled randomised trial. Endoscopy 1982; 14: 4 – 5.

19  Chiles NH, Baggenstoss AH, Butt HR, Olsen AM. Oesophageal varices: comparative incidence of ulceration and spontaneous rupture as cause of fatal haemorrhage. Gastroenterology 1953; 25: 565 – 573.

20  Orloff MJ, Thomas HS. Pathogenesis of oesophageal varix rupture. A study based on gross and microscopic examination of the oesophagus at the time of bleeding. Arch Surg 1963; 87: 301 – 307.

21  Dagradi AE, Arguello JF, Weingarten ZG. Failure of endoscopy to establish a source for upper gastrointestinal bleeding. Ann J Gastroenterol 1979; 72: 395 – 402.

22  Warren WD. Physiology and results of the selective distal splenorenal shunt. In: Najarian JS, Delaney JP, eds. Surgery of the liver, pancreas and biliary tract. New York: Stratton Intercontinental Medical Book Corp, 1975; 637 – 642.

23  Paquet KJ, Oberhammer E. Sclerotherapy of bleeding oesophageal varices by means of endoscopy. Endoscopy 1978; 10: 7 – 12.

138

24 Terblanche J. Treatment of oesophageal varices by injection sclerotherapy. In: Maclean LD, ed. Advances in Surgery, Vol. 15. London: Year Book Publishers, 1981: 257 – 291.

25 Spence RAJ, Sloan JM, Johnston GW. Oesophagitis in patients undergoing oesophageal transection for varices – a histological study. Br J Surg 1983; 70: 332 – 334.

26 Spence RAJ, Sloan JM, Johnston GW. Histologic factors of the oesophageal transection ring as clues to the pathogenesis of bleeding varices. Surg Gynaecol Obstet 1984; 159: 253 – 259.

27 Inokuchi K. The general rules for recording endoscopic findings on oesophageal varices. Jpn J Surg 1980; 10: 84 – 87.

28 Spence RAJ. The venous anatomy of the lower oesophagus in normal subjects and in patients with varices: an image analysis study. Br J Surg 1984; 71: 739 – 744.

29 Kitano S, Terblanche J, Kahn D, Bornman PC. Venous anatomy of the lower oesophagus in portal hypertension: practical implications. Br J Surg 1986; 73: 525 – 531.

30 McCormack TT, Rose JD, Smith PM, Johnston AG. Perforating veins and blood flow in oesophageal varices. Lancet 1985; ii: 1442 – 1444.

31 Phemister DB, Humphreys EM. Gastroesophageal resection and total gastrectomy in the treatment of bleeding varicose veins in Banti's syndrome. Ann Surg 1947; 126: 397 – 410.

32 Schafer PW, Kittle CF. Partial oesphagogastrectomy in treatment of oesphogastric varices. Arch Surg 1950; 61: 235 – 243.

33 Boerema I. Bleeding varices in the oesophagus in cirrhosis of the liver and Bantis syndrome. Arch Chir Neerl 1949; i: 253 – 260.

34 Crile G. Transoesophageal ligation of bleeding oesophageal varices: preliminary report of 7 cases. Arch Surg 1950; 61: 654 – 660.

35 Tanner NC. The late results of porto-azygos disconnection in the treatment of bleeding from oesophageal varices. Ann R Coll Surg Engl 1961; 28: 153 – 174.

36 Walker RM. Oesophageal transection for bleeding varices. Surg Gynaecol Obstet 1964; 118: 323 – 329.

37 Sugiura M, Futagawa S. A new technique for treating oesophageal varices. J Thorac Cardiovasc Surg 1973; 66: 677 – 685.

38 Sugiura M, Futagawa S. Further evaluation of the Sugiura procedure in the treatment of oesophageal varices. Arch Surg 1977; 112: 1317 – 1321.

39 Boerema I, Klopper PJ, Holscher AA. Transabdominal ligation – resection of the oesophagus in case of bleeding oesophageal varices. Surgery 1970; 67: 409 – 413.

40 Johnston GW, Kelly JM. Early experience with the Boerema button for bleeding oesophageal varices. Br J Surg 1976; 63: 117 – 121.

41 Van Kemmel M. Resection – anastomose de l'oesophage sus cardial pour rupture de varices oesophagiennes. Bilan d'une technique nouvelle. Nouv Press Med 1976; 5: 1123 – 1124.

42 Johnston GW. Gun transection for oesophageal varices. In: Cushieri A, Hennessy TPKJ, eds. Current operative surgery – General Surgery. Publ Bailliere-Tindall, 1985: 27 – 41.

43 Spence RAJ, Johnston GW, Parks TG. Oesophageal manometry in patients with varices and following oesophageal transection. Br J Surg 1985; 72: 96 – 98.

44 Spence RAJ, Johnston GW, Parks TG. Prolonged ambulatory pH monitoring in patients following oesophageal transection and in control subjects. Br J Surg 1985; 72: 99 – 101.

45 Hall CH, Nie NH. SPSS update 7 – 9. New procedures and facilities for releases 7 – 9. New York: McGraw-Hill, 1981: 205 – 219.

46  Breslow NE. A generalised Kruskal-Wallis test for comparing K samples subject to unequal patterns of censorship. Biometrika 1970; 57: 579 – 594.

47  Gimson AES, Westaby D, Hegarty J, Watson A, Williams R. A randomised trial of vasopressin and vasopressin plus nitroglycerine in the control of acute variceal haemorrhage. Hepatology 1986; 6: 410 – 413.

48  Merkel C, Finucci G, Zulin R, Bazzerla G, Bolognesi M, Sacerdoti D, Gatta A. Effects of isosorbide dinitrate on portal hypertension in alcoholic cirrhosis. J Hepatol 1987; 4: 174 – 180.

49  Hosking SW, Doss W, El-Zeing H, Barsoum MS, Johnston AG. Can metoclopramide arrest active bleeding from varices? A prospective controlled trial. Gut 1987; 28: A1380.

50  Terblanche J, Northover JMA, Bornman PC, et al. A prospective controlled trial of sclerotherapy in the long-term managment of patients after variceal bleeding. Surg Gynaecol Obstet 1979; 148: 323 – 333.

51  Bornman PC, Terblanche J, Kahn D, Jonker MAT, Kirsch RE. Limitations of multiple injection sclerotherapy sessions for acute variceal bleeding. South Afr Med J 1986; 70: 34 – 36.

52  Hosking SW, Kennedy HJ, Seddon I, Triger DR. The role of propranolol in congestive gastropathy of portal hypertension. Hepatology 1987; 7: 437 – 441.

53  Millikan WJ, Warren WD, Henderson JM, et al. The Emory prospective randomised trial: selective versus non selective shunt to control variceal bleeding. Ten year follow-up. Ann Surg 1985; 201: 712 – 722.

54  Warren WD, Millikan WJ, Henderson JM, et al. Splenopancreatic disconnection – improved selectivity of distal splenorenal shunt. Ann Surg 1986; 204: 346 – 355.

55  Henderson JM. Variceal bleeding: which shunt? Gastroenterology 1986; 91: 1021 – 1023.

56  Sugiura M, Futagawa S. Results of 636 oesophageal transections with paraoesphagogastric devascularisation in the treatment of oesophageal varices. J Vasc Surg 1984; i: 254 – 260.

57  Cello JP, Grendell JH, Crass RA, Weber TE, Trunkey DD. Endoscopic sclerotherapy versus portacaval shunt in patients with severe cirrhosis and acute variceal haemorrhage. New Engl J Med 1987; 316: 11 – 15.

58  Warren WD, Henderson JM, Millikan WJ, et al. Distal splenorenal shunt versus endoscopic sclerotherapy for long-term management of variceal bleeding. Ann Surg 1986; 203: 454 – 461.

59  Huizinga WKJ, Angorn IB, Baker LW. Oesophageal transection versus injection sclerotherapy in the management of bleeding oesophageal varices in patients at high risk. Surg Gynaecol Obstet 1985; 16: 539 – 546.

60  Teres J, Baroni R, Bordas JM, et al. Randomised trial of portacaval shunt, stapling transection and endoscopic sclerotherapy in uncontrolled variceal bleeding. Hepatology 1987; 4: 159 – 167.

© 1988 Elsevier Science Publishers B.V. (Biomedical Division)
*Treatment of esophageal varices*
*Y. Idezuki, editor*

Chapter 13

# Indications and results of portal-azygos disconnection surgeries (terminal esophago-proximal gastrectomy, proximal gastric transection and autosuture proximal gastrectomy) under endoscope assistance

SADAHIRO YAMAMOTO

*1st Department of Surgery, Aichi Medical University, Nagakute-cho, Aichi-ken 480-11, Japan*

## Summary

Devascularization and disconnection surgeries, i.e. terminal esophago-proximal gastrectomy, proximal gastric transection and autosuture proximal gastrectomy associated with extensive devascularization and splenectomy, were performed to eliminate any remnant esophageal varices under endoscopic assistance in 87 cases during the last 10 years.

Results of follow-up by scheduled endoscopy were studied in 72 cirrhotic cases who underwent therapeutic surgery. Survival rates did not show a significant difference compared with 'blind' surgery, and disappearance of the varices continued in 60%. The causes of recurrent varices, regardless of their grade, were assumed to be a further increase of portal vein pressure and a local factor of recanalization. The timing of recurrence and rebleeding could not be designated, although most recurrences occurred within 2 years after EAS.

To maintain the disappearance of the varices, additional sclerotherapy in the early stage of recurrence was recommended because the blood flow to the varices decreased remarkably with endoscopic assistance during surgery.

Because of severe post-shunt encephalopathy previously experienced in 154 end-to-side portocaval anastomoses and in some 30 classic splenorenal anastomoses, we have been performing terminal esophago-proximal gastrectomy and its modifications accompanied with extensive devascularization and splenectomy in more than 300 cases of esophageal varices [1].

During the last 10 years, endoscopic assistance during surgery (EAS) [2] was introduced to eradicate any remnant varices. This paper reports the indication and results of endoscope-assisted surgery.

## Materials and methods

Excluding personal experience in the previous institution, among the 336 cases of esophageal varices due to portal hypertension treated at the Aichi Medical School during the past 14 years, 175 cases received surgical treatment. Eighty-seven cases were operated upon under endoscopic observation and 72 of them were cirrhotic patients needing therapeutic surgery, i.e. classic terminal esophagoproximal gastrectomy (TEPG) in 20, proximal gastric transection (PGT) in 23 and EEA autosuture proximal gastrectomy (APGX) in 29 associated with extensive devascularization and splenectomy. Surgical indication and results in these cases, and especially the post-operative course of the varices after EAS, were analysed and compared with those of non-operative cases.

## Results

### 1: The indications for surgery

Table 1 shows surgical procedures in 175 cases, and the reason why the remaining 161 cases were ruled out from surgical treatment. It was clear that cases with encephalopathy, ascites and jaundice of Child's C criteria could not be candidates for surgery. In addition, in our cases liver cirrhosis was very closely related to viral hepatitis in origin and frequently revealed signs of an aggressive nature, and also associated with hepatocellular carcinoma. The complications of severe dysfunction of the multiple organ system, and also of both hepatic circulation and dye clearance, were frequently encountered. Prophylactic surgery was not indicated except for several cases for group study.

TABLE 1   Case distribution

| Surgery performed | | | Surgery not indicated | | |
|---|---|---|---|---|---|
| 1. Blind surgery | | 88 | 1. Poor risk | | 93 |
| PGD | 34 | | Encephalopathy | 3 | |
| TEPG | 26 | | Ascites | 6 | |
| PGT | 23 | | Jaundice | 11 | |
| Others | 5 | | Aggressive hepatitis | 17 | |
| | | | Complications of other organ system | 24 | |
| | | | Dysfunction in WHVP, ICG-R | 32 | |
| 2. Endoscope-assisted surgery | | 87 | | | |
| TEPG | 25 | | 2. Hepatoma | | 38 |
| PGT | 26 | | | | |
| A-PGX | 36 | | 3. Non-bleeder | | 30 |
| | Total | 175 | | | 161 |

PGD, proximal gastric devascularization; TEPG, terminal esophago-proximal gastrectomy; PGT, proximal gastric transection; A-PGX, autosuture proximal gastrectomy; WHVP, wedged hepatic vein pressure; ICG, indocyanine green retention.

## 2: On the results of EAS

Excluding non-cirrhotic patients and prophylactic surgery in cirrhotic patients, there were 72 cases of liver cirrhosis who underwent therapeutic EAS.

The features of the varices and the frequency, severity, timing and cause of the recurrent varices were analysed along with the survival rates.

Survival rates with EAS compared with those with portocaval anastomosis were far better, but almost the same as our previous results with TEPG under blind conditions because there was not much difference in case selection and surgical technique (Fig. 1).

The exact numbers of variceal recurrences, which we could not differentiate from remnants after previous blind surgeries, and their severity are shown in Table 2. Overall frequency was 37%, and 39% in cirrhotic therapeutic surgery. The rates were higher with PGT, which did not remove tissue continuity at the proximal

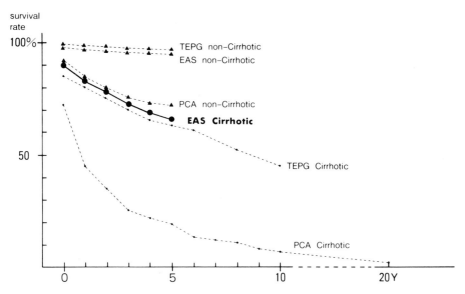

FIG. 1   Postoperative survival rate.

TABLE 2   Frequency of recurrent varices after EAS

|  | Overall | | Therapeutic cirrhosis | |
|---|---|---|---|---|
|  | Number | Recurrence | Number | Recurrence |
| TEPG | 25 | 9 | 20 | 7 |
| PGT | 26 | 12 | 23 | 11 |
| A-PGX | 36 | 11 | 29 | 10 |
| Total | 87 | 32 (37%) | 72 | 28 (39%) |

stomach, than those of both types of proximal gastrectomy. Eighteen cases (64%) among 28 recurrences reached their preoperative level of severity, although the blood flow within the recurrent varices diminished remarkably (Fig. 2).

Episodes of rebleeding from the recurrent varices occurred in 5 cases (Table 3), but were easily treated by sclerotherapy due presumably to the diminished blood flow. There were another 8 cases of rebleeding caused by small ulcerations at the site of the staple among two types of proximal gastrectomy. Four cases had recurrent varices but the other 4 had no recurrence. They were also treated successfully by endoscopic removal of the staple and cauterization.

Twenty cases (71%) out of 28 recurrences occurred within 2 years after the EAS (Fig. 3), but recurrence was not limited to within the early postoperative stage.

The causes of recurrence are listed in Table 4, and are suggested to be further increase of the portal vein pressure caused by atrophy, hepatoma or thrombosis, along with the local factor of recanalization of the vascular bed at the site of surgery in the proximal stomach.

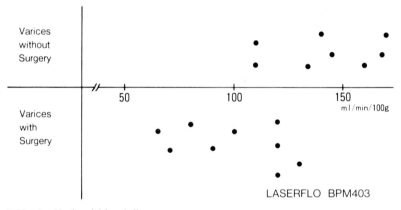

FIG. 2   Variceal blood flow.

TABLE 3   Severity of recurrent varices and rebleeding in cirrhosis after therapeutic surgery

|  |  | Rebleeding | |
|---|---|---|---|
|  |  | Varices | Staple ulcer |
| Disappeared | 44 |  | 4 |
| Recurrence | 28 |  |  |
| Less than before | 10 | 2 | 3 |
| Same as before | 18 | 3 | 1 |
| More than before | – | – | – |
| Total | 72 | 5 | 8 |

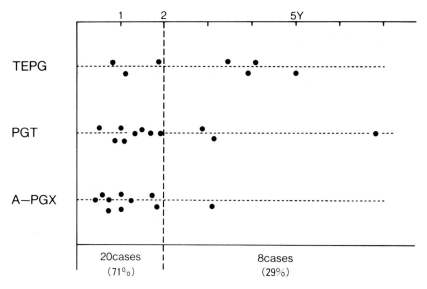

FIG. 3   Timing of recurrence in cirrhotics who underwent therapeutic surgery (28 cases).

TABLE 4   Causes of recurrence in cirrhosis after therapeutic surgery

| | |
|---|---|
| Atrophy of cirrhotic liver | 15 |
| Hepatoma | 5 |
| Portal vein thrombosis | 4 |
| Others | 4 |

## Discussion

Because our own experience of major portocaval shunts revealed discouraging results in survival rates and complications of disabling post-shunt encephalopathy, we had to abandon the procedure and turned to devascularization and disconnection surgeries (Fig. 4).

Terminal esophago-proximal gastrectomy (TEPG) with extensive devascularization and splenectomy improved the survival rate remarkably. However, the procedure could not eliminate remnant varices, and rebleeding from recurrent or remnant varices, and also we could not perform a precisely controlled study [1].

After carrying out TEPG 'blind' in 104 cases at the previous institution and in 26 cases at the present hospital along with almost 100 cases of modified surgery, we have introduced endoscopic assistance during the surgery (EAS) to eradicate any remnant esophageal varices [2].

After ensuring complete disappearance during surgery, we have followed up the

146

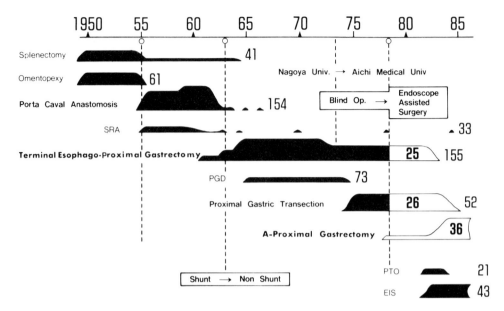

FIG. 4  Surgical treatment of esophageal varices in Nagoya.

technique by scheduled endoscopy without adding further treatment except when the recurrent varices bled. There was no significant difference in the survival rates between the blind surgery and EAS. But we could precisely determine the frequency, severity, timing and cause of recurrence by EAS for the first time.

Excluding non-cirrhotic cases and prophylactic surgery leading to a good outcome, the frequency of recurrent varices in 72 cirrhotic cases who underwent therapeutic surgery was close to 40%, the severity reached the preoperative level in two-thirds of them, and variceal rebleeding occurred in 5 cases. In spite of their endoscopic appearance, the blood flow of the recurrent varices diminished remarkably and additional sclerotherapy was quite successful. In cases of autosuture proximal gastrectomy and classic TEPG, we have experienced other episodes of bleeding from small ulcerative lesions caused by the staples in 8 cases. These results indicate the necessity for early and successful sclerotherapy on those recurrent varices, which are not avoidable in EAS which does not decrease portal vein pressure.

The frequency of recurrence was significantly lower in both types of proximal gastrectomy, which remove segmental tissue at the proximal stomach, but the complications in cases with autosuture proximal gastrectomy caused by the staples could be further improved.

The timing of recurrence could not be designated, but the cause of it was considered to be a further increase of portal vein pressure in the first place, and focal recanalization.

As described in the results, the indication for EAS was limited to cases with good or moderate risk and capable of rehabilitation. Permanent disappearance of the varices could be expected in 60% of EAS. In cases with recurrent varices, successful results from additional treatment by sclerotherapy could be expected because the main streams of blood flow to the varices had been devascularized by the previous EAS.

## References

1    Yamamoto S, Hidemura R, Sawada M, Takeshige K, Iwatsuki S. The late results of terminal esophago-proximal gastrectomy (TEPG) with extensive devascularization and splenectomy for bleeding esophageal varices in cirrhosis. Surgery 1976; 80: 106 – 114.
2    Yamamoto S, Takeshige K, Arakawa T. Endoscope assisted surgery for the treatment of bleeding esophageal varices. Jpn J Surg 1984; 14: 371 – 376.

© 1988 Elsevier Science Publishers B.V. (Biomedical Division)
Treatment of esophageal varices
Y. Idezuki, editor

Chapter 14

# Experience with non-shunting operation for esophageal varices, 1980 – 87

Mitsuo Sugiura, Shunji Futagawa, Masaki Fukasawa, Eiichi Kinoshita, Ryo Nakanishi and Yasuhiko Nishimura

*Second Department of Surgery, Juntendo University, Japan*

In Japan, the non-shunting operation is the primary surgical approach to the treatment of esophageal varices. However, in the West, total shunt and selective shunt are more common. Since the reports by Johnstone [1] (1973) and Terblanche [2] (1979) on sclerotherapy, this technique has become employed in an increasing number of institutions, including those in Japan, perhaps because of the ease with which this procedure can be performed by endoscopists. At the authors' institution this procedure has been employed since 1979 in order to improve the indications of treatment in inoperable cases or in cases of recurrence following the non-shunting operation, and remarkable effectiveness in the prevention of esophageal rebleeding has been obtained. This method has been employed not only as an independent modality but also in combination with the non-shunting operation.

Since we began employing sclerotherapy in 1979, there have been some changes in the indications for the non-shunting operation and this paper describes experience with this procedure over the past eight years.

### Indications for the non-shunting operation depending on the condition of the patient

In the past 8 years the authors have treated 369 cases of esophageal varices by non-shunting operation (Table 1) and 91 by sclerotherapy, totalling 460 cases. Of these, 210 (46%) belonged to the Child's A group [3], 138 (30%) belonged to the Child's B group and 112 (24%) to Child's C, and cases of severe hepatic dysfunction in which surgical intervention was absolutely contraindicated accounted for 24 cases, or 5.2% (Fig. 1). Classification into the various Child's groups depends in many cases on alcohol-related cirrhosis and therefore this classification is not necessarily the best with regard to the clinical situation in Japan. The nutritional items of the

Child classification do not agree well with the authors' cases and the serum albumin and albumin complement are relatively easy to correct rapidly. Concerning hepatic encephalopathy, cases showing abnormal EEG symptoms (i.e. other than normal or borderline) accounted for more than half of those treated. However, there is also a problem in terms of whether the cases had clinical symptoms of hepatic encephalopathy. Cases treated by emergency surgical procedures occasionally included cases of hepatic encephalopathy with hyperammonemia due to accumulation of blood in the gastroenteric tract, and good results were obtained in these cases.

Our experience suggests that cases of hyperammonemia due to accumulation of blood in the gastroenteric tract are not necessarily contraindications for emergency surgery.

However, apart from the nutritional condition, parameters such as serum bilirubin, serum albumin, ascites and hepatic encephalopathy are closely related to hepatic dysfunction and are therefore convenient to use clinically.

The indications for the non-shunting operation are shown in Table 2. For safety, in prophylactic procedures, serum total bilirubin should be 2.0 mg/dl or less. Great care is paid to the selection of indications in the Child C group, or cases with an indocyanine green excretion test K value (ICG-K) of 0.04 or less. The development of sclerotherapy has resulted in some changes in the indications for surgery, since

TABLE 1   The results of non-shunting operation (1980 – 1987)

|  | Cases | Operative death | Bleeding during one month | Bleeding after one month |
|---|---|---|---|---|
| Sugiura procedure | 308 | 11 (3.5%) | 2 (0.6%) | 9 (2.9%) |
| Hassab procedure | 33 | 5 (15.1%) | 0 | 1 (3%) |
| Transabdominal transection | 27 | 0 | 0 | 0 |
| Total gastrectomy/lower esophageal devascularization | 1 | 0 | 0 | 0 |

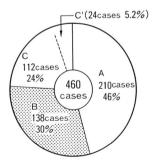

FIG. 1   Child's classification.

some cases can be treated with hemostasis followed by an elective surgical procedure; thus although originally a serum total bilirubin level of 5.0 mg/dl was considered an indication for an emergency procedure, now the level is considered to be 3.0 mg/dl or less.

In terms of the mortality rate and age, reviewing the results of the Sugiura procedure [4 – 6] (transthoracic esophageal transection with paraesophagogastric devascularization) performed in 780 cases over the past 20 years, the operative mortality tended to be greater in the age 60 and over group. However, in the third to sixth decades there was no significant relationship between age and operative mortality, instead there was a greater relationship with the degree of hepatic dysfunction of the primary lesion.

At the authors' institution, the rate of non-virus alcohol-related hepatic dysfunction was approximately 30% during the past 3 years. The rate of hepatic dysfunction cases related to both virus and alcohol was approximately 50%, therefore a close relationship between esophageal varices and alcohol intake is indicated. In cases of rupture of esophageal varices associated with alcohol-related hepatic dysfunction, it is possible to treat the patient initially by emergency hemostasis, followed by abstinence from alcohol and rest for 2 – 3 weeks, thereby obtaining significant improvement in the manifest jaundice. Depending on the individual case, the serum bilirubin can decrease from 5 – 6 mg/dl to 2 – 2.5 mg/dl following 2 – 3 weeks of such treatment. Such cases of jaundice on admission with alcohol-related hepatic dysfunction can become candidates for non-shunting operation after 2 – 3 months abstinence from alcohol.

Among the various hepatic function tests, the serum total bilirubin, as noted previously, is considered to be an important parameter, but the ICG exclusion is frequently regarded as important by many institutions in Japan. While the authors fully recognize the value of this test, it is nevertheless felt that a poor ICG-K or ICG-$R_{15}$ result does not necessarily mean that the non-shunting procedure is contraindicated. In other words the indications should be decided on a case-by-case basis. In particular, in the Child A or B groups the results of surgery can be good even in cases in which the ICG results were poor. However, in the Child C group of cases the ICG-$R_{15}$ test results can be regarded as the definitive parameter concerning the indications for surgery.

TABLE 2   Indication for the Sugiura procedure

| | |
|---|---|
| No restriction in age | |
| No severe hepatic failure | |
|   Ascites – medical control is not difficult | |
| In prophylactic op. | Total bilirubin < 2 mg/dl |
| | Albumin 3.0 g/dl < |
| | Red-color signs ( + ) |
| In elective op. | Total bilirubin < 3 mg/dl |
| | Albumin 2.7 g/dl < |
| In emergency op. | Total bilirubin < 3 mg/dl |
| | Albumin 2.5 g/dl < |

The results of the ICG excretion test were compared with the operative results and long-term results in cases of non-shunting operation. It was recognized that high operative mortality was observed in cases in which the results of the ICG excretion test were poor and the long-term survival rate was also recognized to be lower in such cases. In general, the ICG test shows the greatest correlation with other clinical tests.

Cases of ascites are treated by a sodium-limited diet of 6 g or less per day and use of diuretics. Cases of hypoalbuminemia are controlled by human plasma and so on. In emergency cases in which there is no ascites prior to rupture of esophageal varices and in which there is no sodium limitation, but in which the ascites develops after the rupture of the esophageal varices, the ascites can generally be easily controlled. If indicated, an emergency procedure should be carried out.

## Selection of the non-shunting procedure based on the site and the degree of severity of esophageal varices (Table 3)

In the cases of varices limited only to the stomach, the authors employ the Hassab procedure [7, 8], and, in cases of esophageal varices limited to the lower portion of the esophagus, the Hassab procedure, transabdominal esophageal transection or transthoracic esophageal transection is selected based on the condition of the patient and the varices. In order to obtain effective results in cases of severe esophageal varices we consider it necessary to perform a transthoracic (Sugiura) procedure. In cases in which thoracotomy is contraindicated or in patients aged 70 or more, combined therapy involving transabdominal esophageal transection and postoperative sclerotherapy is performed after informed consent has been obtained.

In cases of severe esophageal varices in which left thoracotomy was contraindicated, we originally performed transabdominal esophageal transection but, at present, if thoracotomy is indicated we perform right thoracotomy and then perform transthoracic esophageal transection. This is because we have frequently experienced cases of severe esophageal varices in which the effects of transabdominal transection were not satisfactory.

TABLE 3   Selection of nonshunting operation

| | |
|---|---|
| (i)   Gastric varices only | Hassab op. |
| (ii)   Esophageal varices | |
| Limited to lower esophagus | Hassab op<br>Transabd. Esoph. Trans.<br>Transthor. Esoph. Trans.<br>  (Sugiura procedure) |
| Severe | Transthor. Esoph. Trans.<br>  (Sugiura procedure) |
| Unable to open chest<br>Elderly cases (> 70 yrs.) | Transabd. Esoph. Trans. combined with sclerotherapy. |

In cases aged 70 or more a two-stage procedure can be performed if the patient is physically and mentally capable of withstanding the procedure. However, in such elderly cases, the invasiveness of a second procedure can be difficult to tolerate, and therefore in many cases combined therapy employing postoperative sclerotherapy is performed.

The indications for the non-shunting operation in cases of esophageal varices accompanied by hepatoma can be difficult to evaluate. In hepatoma accompanying severe esophageal varices, the Hassab procedure or endoscopic sclerotherapy is not sufficient. In many such cases massive hemorrhage due to esophageal variceal rupture can lead to a fatal outcome. The authors try to treat such cases whenever possible by esophageal transection and partial hepatectomy. However, the degree of invasiveness of partial hepatectomy plus esophageal transection is considerable. Even with partial hepatectomy, in cases with a tendency towards ascites there is the danger of infection spreading throughout the peritoneal cavity, and therefore great care must be exercised in such cases.

### Indications and timing of surgery (emergency, elective and prophylactic procedures)

Elective and prophylactic procedures depend greatly on the condition of the patient, the site and the degree of varices. There are great problems concerning which therapeutic strategy to adopt in emergency cases. The authors aggressively follow a policy of emergency transthoracic esophageal transection in Child A and B cases, while in Child C group cases emergency procedures are avoided and a Sengstaken-Blakemore tube is employed or endoscopic sclerotherapy is performed. Then, after the condition of the patient has improved, an elective procedure is performed. As is shown in Table 3, a variety of therapeutic strategies have been adopted over the past 8 years in 49 emergency cases.

In patients who are considered capable of tolerating the procedure, transthoracic esophageal transection (Sugiura procedure) is performed and, of 33 cases, operative mortality was observed in 4 cases (12%), gastroenteric tract bleeding within one month being seen in one case and late bleeding in 3 cases. Cases treated only by sclerotherapy consisted of 10 cases, 7 of whom (70%) died within one month. In this group rebleeding within one month was observed in 6 cases (60%). Of 3 cases treated by the Hassab procedure, there were 2 operative deaths (66%) and this group included cases accompanied by hepatoma.

Concerning surgical indications in emergency cases, cases in which ascites did not appear before or after bleeding are indicated for surgery. Also cases in which hepatic encephalopathy did not appear after bleeding or in cases in which they appeared after, but not before, bleeding are indicated for emergency surgery. In addition, cases without manifest jaundice after bleeding or cases in which even if there is mild jaundice after bleeding the serum total bilirubin count is below 2 mg/dl before the bleeding and below 3 mg/dl after the bleeding episode are indicated for emergency surgery. Cases in which prebleeding serum albumin is above 2.7 g/dl and in which the postbleeding value is over 2.5 g/dl are indicated for emergency surgery.

154

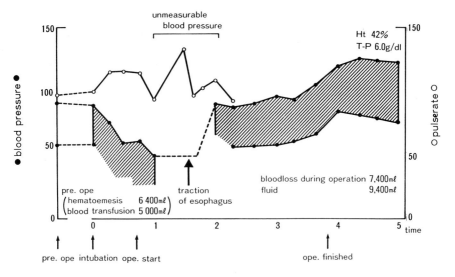

FIG. 2    Anesthesia record (54 male patients).

Examining the anesthetic charts of emergency cases of transthoracic esophageal transection, most cases showed good response once, after thoracotomy, traction of the esophagus by tape and transfusion was initiated, and the blood pressure also improved. At the end of the procedure, a normal blood pressure and hematocrit level was recognized. Rapid hemostasis can be performed in emergency cases by thoracotomy and traction of the lower esophagus (Fig. 2).

**Combined therapy employing non-shunting operation and sclerotherapy**

In cases in which thoracotomy is contraindicated, i.e. cases with a history of thoracoplasty of lung resection or bilateral mammary resection due to breast cancer or other abnormalities of respiratory function or the pleura, or in cases in which it is thought that the patient would be unable to undergo two highly invasive surgical procedures performed within a short time, a non-shunting operation followed by sclerotherapy is performed on the basis of the patient's informed consent. In the case of a non-shunting operation in which transabdominal esophageal transection has been performed, most of the cases have received this type of combined therapy. In cases of severe esophageal varices, many of the cases treated by transabdominal esophageal transection show residual varices. However, in the cases in which postoperative endoscopic sclerotherapy is performed, good results are obtained with a smaller number of injections than when sclerotherapy alone is performed.

In combined therapy, first of all the non-shunting operation is performed, then the endoscopic sclerotherapy is performed to treat residual varices. However, many internists raise the question of to what degree the non-shunting operation could be performed after having initially performed sclerotherapy. In other words, many internists tend to think that the non-shunting operation could be performed after having performed the sclerotherapy. This is a somewhat different standpoint from that of the surgeons who tend to think first of what cases the non-shunting operation is indicated in, and would postoperatively treat any possible residual varices by sclerotherapy.

The non-shunting operation was performed in 22 cases after sclerotherapy (Table 4). In terms of the type of operation performed, there were 12 cases of transthoracic esophageal transection, 2 cases of transabdominal esophageal transection and 8 cases of the Hassab procedure. Of the Hassab procedure cases, there was one case of death one month after intravasal sclerotherapy. The autopsy findings of this case showed a perforation of the abdominal esophagus and the formation of an abscess of approximately 2 cm in diameter, immediately adjacent to the abdominal esophagus. This in itself was not the cause of death and it was considered that in this case the actual sclerotherapy procedure itself (including the amount of sclerotherapeutic agent instilled) was also involved. In cases of transthoracic esophageal transection and transabdominal esophageal transection, if the intravasal method is performed with precision, then it is considered that there is no significant problem of cicatricial formation in the esophageal wall. It is thought that after a period of 2 months after the non-shunting procedure it is safe to perform the sclerotherapy procedure. In performing the paravasal injection method, the esophageal wall can develop necrosis or a similar condition relatively soon after performing the paravasal injections, and in such cases it would be extremely dangerous to perform the non-shunting procedure. In cases in which 9 months or more have elapsed the cicatricial formation in the esophageal wall generally is alleviated and from the experience of the authors the non-shunting operation can be performed with relative safety. Be that as it may, in cases of endoscopic sclerotherapy, the person performing the sclerotherapy and the person performing the non-shunting operation must have an extremely high level of expertise.

In the period before the appearance of endoscopic sclerotherapy, in cases in which following non-shunting operation esophageal varices recurred, those cases with a

TABLE 4   Non-shunting operations after sclerotherapy (22 cases; 19 cases after sclerotherapy in another hospital)

| Appearance of esophageal varices after sclerotherapy | Cases | Operative method | Cases |
| --- | --- | --- | --- |
| Disappeared | 4 | Hassab procedure | 4 |
| Appeared | 18 (5) (16 rebleeding) | Sugiura procedure | 12 (3)[b] |
|  |  | Transabdominal transection | 2 |
|  |  | Hassab procedure | 4 (2)[a] |

( ) emergency operation.
[a] Operative death 1.
[b] Operative death 2.

good hepatic function sometimes underwent a second operation. Some cases also underwent a second esophageal transection. In cases that had undergone esophageal transection with left thoracotomy, right thoracotomy was employed on the second procedure, and in cases of total gastrectomy, or resection of the cardia or interposition of the jejunum or transabdominal esophageal transection, this method could be performed with relative safety.

### Operative results of the non-shunting operation (Table 1)

In the past 8 years a total of 460 cases of non-shunting operation have been performed; of these a total of 308 cases consisted of the Sugiura procedure, among which there were 11 operative deaths (3.5%). There were 33 cases of the Hassab procedure, among which there were 5 operative deaths (15.1%). In addition there were 27 cases of transabdominal esophageal transection among which there was one case of operative mortality.

In terms of rerupture of esophageal varices, 2 cases treated by the Sugiura procedure were seen within one month postoperatively (0.6%) and late rebleeding was observed in 10 cases (2.9%). Of the 33 cases of the Hassab procedure, one-third were accompanied by hepatoma.

Incidences of bleeding following the Hassab procedure or transabdominal esophageal transection were very few. One of the reasons for that was that the cases of mild esophageal varices were selected for these procedures and in cases of recurrence or residual varices, sclerotherapy was immediately performed. Therefore combined therapy was performed in the majority of such cases.

Concerning survival in terms of the method of treatment, in Child's A and B groups the 8-year survival of cases treated by the Sugiura procedure was 81%, that of cases treated by the Hassab procedure was 58%, that of cases treated by transabdominal esophageal resection was 50% and the 5-year survival of cases treated by sclerotherapy was 37%.

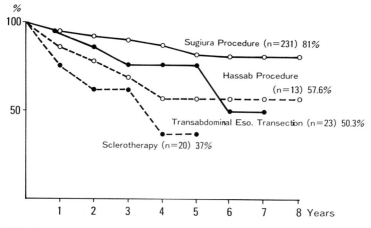

FIG. 3   Survival (cumulative survival rate) Child A and B groups.

In the Child C group the 5-year survival of cases treated by the Sugiura procedure was 55%, that of cases treated by transabdominal esophageal transection 33% and the 5-year survival of cases treated only by sclerotherapy was 38%. In cases accompanied by a high degree of hepatic dysfunction the 4-year survival was 9.6%. Even within the same Child C group classification, in those cases that could be treated by the Sugiura procedure good long-term survival could be obtained (Fig. 4).

## Cases of residual esophageal varices immediately after the Sugiura procedure

Cases treated by the Sugiura procedure during the past 8 years were examined by comparing the preoperative angiography findings and the degree of eradication of esophageal varices. The direction of blood flow in the coronary vein was evaluated on angiography of the superior mesenteric artery in terms of whether the blood flow was hepatofugal, hepatopetal, in both directions or whether the direction of the blood flow was unclear. In the preoperative angiography classification the hepatofugal flow group consisted of 130 cases (65%); the hepatopetal group consisted of 18 cases (9%), there were 30 cases with flow in both directions (15%), and in 22 cases (11%) the direction of the flow was unclear (Fig. 5).

The Sugiura procedure consists of a combination of intrathoracic and intraabdominal surgical manoeuvers. Examining the rate of eradication of esophageal varices by transthoracic esophageal transection, which is the intrathoracic surgical manoeuver, esophageal varices remained in 32.5% of cases of hepatofugal flow of the left gastric vein. However, in 90% of the other three types of blood flow group, complete eradication of the esophageal varices was recognized. In cases in which transabdominal transection procedures were additionally performed, 9% of cases of hepatofugal flow were observed to have mild residual varices. However, this tendency was not observed in the other 3 groups, varices being recognized to have disappeared in all cases (Fig. 6).

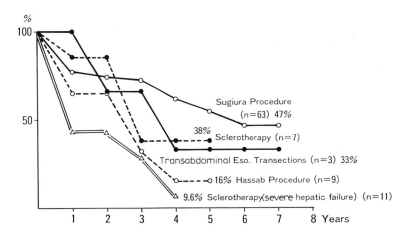

FIG. 4   Survival (cumulative survival rate) Child C group.

158

For the above reasons, in cases of hepatofugal flow in the left gastric vein thorough devascularization must be performed.

**Postoperative recurrence of esophageal varices in Sugiura procedure cases**

Concerning the long-term results following the Sugiura procedure, cases in which the esophageal varices were considered to be completely eradicated but in which recurrence was recognized were studied. In 15 cases, angiography was performed preoperatively and at the time of recurrence. These cases were evaluated in terms

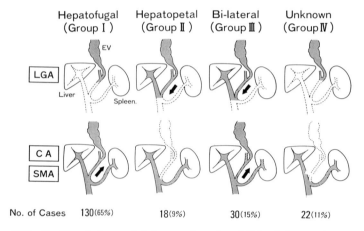

FIG. 5 Blood flow of left gastric vein. LGA, left gastric arteriography; CA, celiac arteriography; SMA, superior mesenteric arteriography.

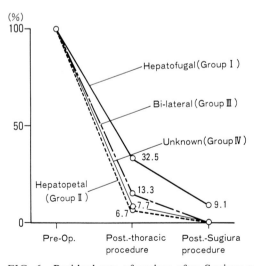

FIG. 6 Residual rate of varices after Sugiura procedure.

of the factors influencing recurrence. Cases of recurrence consisted of cases in which devascularization was considered to have been insufficient, in other words cases in which the left gastric vein or coronary vein remained, cases in which collaterals of these veins remained, or cases in which collaterals communicating with the ascending paraesophageal vein remained or in which small lace-like veins communicated from the gastric wall to beyond the site of esophageal transection. Considering these findings, it was considered possible to prevent recurrence in the former two types of cases by performing sufficient devascularization, but it is difficult to prevent recurrence after the non-shunting operation in the type of case with the small lace-like vessels extending from the gastric wall to the esophagus. This point will require further study.

## Conclusion

This paper examines the indications and results of non-shunting operations, primarily centered on the Sugiura procedure. In surgically treated Child A or B group cases (including emergency operations, elective operations and prophylactic operations) the procedure should be performed aggressively, while in Child C group cases the procedure should be performed selectively in those cases in which the procedure is considered indicated. In elderly patients or cases in which thoracotomy is considered to be contraindicated, transabdominal esophageal transection and sclerotherapy, i.e. combined therapy, should be considered.

## References

1    Johnston GW, Rodgers HW. A review of 15 years experience in the use of sclerotherapy in the control acute haemorrhage from oesophageal varices. Br J Surg 1973; 60: 797 – 800.
2    Terblanche J, Morthover JMA, Bornman P, Kahn D, Barbezat GO, Sellars SL, Saunders SJ. A prospective evaluation of injection sclerotherapy in the treatment of acute bleeding from esophageal varices. Surgery 1979; 85: 239 – 245.
3    Child CD III. The Liver and Portal Hypertension. Philadelphia and London: W.B. Saunders, 1964.
4    Sugiura M, Futagawa S. A new technique for treating esophageal varices. J Thorac Cardiovasc Surg 1973; 66: 677 – 685.
5    Sugiura M, Futagawa S. Further evaluation of the Sugiura procedure in the treatment of esophageal varices. Arch Surg 1977; 112: 1317 – 1321.
6    Sugiura M, Futagawa S. Esophageal transection with paraesophagogastric devascularizations (The Sugiura Procedure) in the treatment of esophageal varices. World J Surg 1984; 8: 673 – 682.
7    Hassab MA. Gastroesophageal decongestion and splenectomy. A method of prevention and treatment of bleeding from esophageal varices associated with bilharzial hepatic fibrosis. Preliminary report. J Intern College Surg 1964; 41: 232 – 248.
8    Hassab MA. Gastroesophageal decongestion and splenectomy in the treatment of esophageal varices in bilharzial cirrhosis. Further studies with a report on 355 operations. Surgery 1967; 61: 169 – 176.

© 1988 Elsevier Science Publishers B.V. (Biomedical Division)
Treatment of esophageal varices
Y. Idezuki, editor

Chapter 15

# Late results of 224 cases of esophageal transection for esophageal varices

SEIICHIRO KOBAYASHI AND KEN TAKASAKI

*Department of Surgery, The Institute of Gastroenterology, Tokyo Women's Medical College, 8-1 Kawada-cho Shinjuku-ku, Tokyo, Japan*

In 1972 we developed a method of transabdominal esophageal transection with subdiaphragmatic devascularization and splenectomy as a direct non-shunting interruption procedure using a stapler gun [1, 2]. The purpose of this procedure is to completely interrupt the vascular connection between the portal system and the azygos system at the level of the esophageal hiatus. This paper presents the results of the procedure.

## Transabdominal esophageal transection procedure

There are three upward collateral routes of portal outflow connecting with the esophageal varices; left gastric, short gastric and gastric wall vein. The transection procedure aims to block all three collateral routes. We usually use an upper midline incision of the abdomen without thoracotomy. After splenectomy, devascularization around the lower esophagus and upper portion of the stomach is performed. The left gastric artery and coronary vein are also devascularized. The stapler gun is introduced through anterior wall gastrotomy into the lower esophagus and transection is performed completely immediately above the esophagogastric junction.

## Indication for this procedure

The risk of variceal bleeding was judged by the endoscopic findings. Cases with endoscopic findings showing more severe than F2-grade varices with a red color sign [3], but in whom there is no jaundice (T. Bil. $\leq$ 2.5 mg/dl) and ascites having been controlled by medical treatment, are unhesitatingly considered as indicated for esophageal transection.

**Operated cases and results (Table 1)**

Until 1985 we experienced 224 cases of transabdominal esophageal transection. This operation was employed as an emergency procedure in 9 cases with uncontrolled variceal bleeding and electively in 154 cases of bleeding varices after temporary hemostasis and recovery of general condition. In 61 cases of varices, in which bleeding was considered likely, prophylactic operation was performed. Immediately before operation, 31.3% of cases were classified as Child's A, 50.0% as Child's B, and 18.7% as Child's C.

**Results**

The overall operative mortality was 4%, with operative deaths in 9 cases. In emergency cases, the operative mortality rate was 44.4%, with 4 deaths among 9 cases. In these 4 cases, control of bleeding by a Sengstaken-Blackemore tube was impossible, and they had all been evaluated as Child's C class before operation. In elective operation cases, the mortality rate was 1.3% (2 cases). Among prophylactic operation cases, the operative mortality rate was 4.9% (3 cases). Long-term results of cases operated between 1972 and 1985 were investigated (Fig. 1). Apart from the 9 operative death cases, 215 cases could be followed up. Five- and ten-year survival rates were studied. The five-year survival rate was 78.3%. The causes of deaths among this group were hepatic failure (9.9%), hepatoma (2.5%) and bleeding (6.2%). The ten-year survival rate was 46.3%. In this group the causes of deaths were hepatic failure (18.5%), hepatoma (14.8%) and bleeding (11%). Concerning

TABLE 1   Cases of transabdominal esophageal transection for esophageal varices

| Operation period | No. of cases | Child's classification | | Operative death | Mortality rate (%) |
|---|---|---|---|---|---|
| Emergency | 9 | A | 0 cases | 0 | |
| | | B | 3 | 0 | 4 (44.4%) |
| | | C | 6 | 4 | |
| Elective | 154 | A | 46 | 0 | |
| | | B | 82 | 2 | 2 (1.3) |
| | | C | 26 | 0 | |
| Prophylactic | 61 | A | 24 | 0 | |
| | | B | 27 | 1 | 3 (4.9) |
| | | C | 10 | 2 | |
| Total | 224 | A | 70 | 0 | |
| | | B | 112 | 3 | 9 (4.0) |
| | | C | 42 | 6 | |

the relationship between Child's classification and prognosis, Child's A and B group cases have a higher likelihood of long-term survival, but the prognosis of surgically treated Child's C group cases is poor. We have no experience of 3-year survival in Child's C group cases. To compare the postoperative course with the natural course of cirrhotic patients, the courses of 66 cases of liver cirrhosis with esophageal varices not treated surgically were studied (Fig. 2). The 5-year survival rate was 43.9%, and 31.8% cases succumbed due to variceal bleeding, suggesting that esophageal transection can reduce the risk of death due to bleeding to 1/5 (one-fifth) over a 5-year period. Upper GI tract bleeding after operation occurred in 25 cases, 18 of which succumbed due to bleeding. There were two types of GI tract bleeding, one from esophageal varices, the other from gastric erosion. Table 2 shows the relationship between the operative procedure and bleeding after operation. In some cases a modified procedure, the so-called limited devascularization procedure, and spleen-preserving operation was performed. However, in the group of cases undergoing the

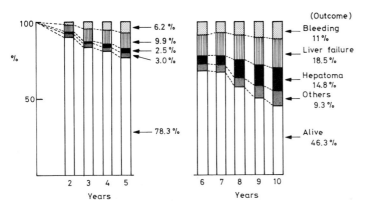

FIG. 1   Prognosis after esophageal transection (1972 – 1985, 215 cases).

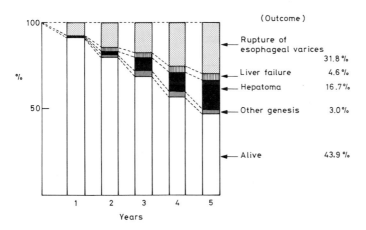

FIG. 2   Natural course of the cases of liver cirrhosis with esophageal varices (66 cases).

TABLE 2  Bleeding cases after operation

| Operation procedure | No. of cases | Bleeding cases (%) | Origin of bleeding | | Mortality (%) |
| --- | --- | --- | --- | --- | --- |
| | | | Varices | Gastric erosion | |
| Regular esophageal transection | 189 | 17 (9.0) | 14 | 3 | 14 (5.8) |
| (Modified) Limited devascularization | 5 | 2 (40.0) | 2 | | 1 (20.0) |
| (Modified) Spleen reservation | 21 | 6 (28.6) | 2 | 4 | 3 (14.3) |
| Total | 215 | 25 (11.6) | 18 | 7 | 18 (8.3) |

modified operation there were many instances of rebleeding. In cases undergoing the standard procedure, rebleeding after operation occurred in only 9% and the mortality rate was 5.8%, so this modified procedure is no longer used. As further treatment for re-bleeding cases, we employed several methods to control bleeding; reoperation (transthoracic esophageal devascularization), transcatheter embolization of the proper esophageal artery, transportal obliteration of recurrent varices (PTO) and endoscopic injection sclerotherapy (EIS). We reached the conclusion that EIS is a more effective treatment for post-operative rebleeding cases. EIS is considered to be more effective when used in post-operative cases than as the first therapeutic modality. Recently, we have selected EIS as the first treatment of choice for re-bleeding. We treated 26 cases of recurrent esophageal varices by EIS, including 11 cases of re-bleeding and 15 cases of non-bleeding. Varices disappeared easily after only 2 – 4 injections in 8 of the 11 cases of bleeding and in 14 of the 15 non-bleeding cases.

## Discussion

There are two kinds of procedure for the direct non-shunting interruption of esophageal varices, the transthoracoabdominal approach (Sugiura procedure) [4, 5] and the transabdominal approach [1, 2]. These two procedures differ in the extent of devascularization, i.e. whether there is devascularization or not around the mid-lower esophageal portion. In our transabdominal procedure, the esophageal artery is not dissected but the transthoracic procedure is a method aimed at devascularizing around the lower esophagus with dissection of the esophageal artery. The relationship of hyperdynamic state of the esophageal arteries to the esophageal varices is not evident. The reason for this is that, after our operative procedure, even if the esophageal artery is not dissected, esophageal varices are well decompressed. Sometimes we can recognize remaining variceal venous dilatation, which is easily reduced by a slight increase of intraluminal pressure, and we call these 'dead varices'. We developed our transabdominal esophageal transection procedure using an auto-suture device in 1972. Up to now, we have been improving the operative technique and the auto-suture device instrument for increased simplicity and safety. Consequently, the operation time has been shortened to less than 2 hours, the blood loss has been decreased to under 1000 ml (average 500 – 600 ml), so no blood transfusion is usually required. The risk of bleeding of esophageal varices can be evaluated by endoscopic findings [3]. In our study, 22% of cases of F1 grade varices had episodes of bleeding, about half of F2 and 64% in F3. And 63% of R-C sign (+) cases had a history of bleeding, but only 17% of R-C sign (−) cases had a history of bleeding. Based on the above data, we prefer operative treatment for F2-grade cases with R-C sign (+). Concerning prophylactic operation [6], it is necessary to select the indications with great care in cases in good condition with varices which are thought likely to bleed, especially when the patients wish to undergo the operation to eliminate bleeding. The risk involved in operation has decreased due to the improvement in operative procedure and preoperative and postoperative care. Now, we perform the operation in most cases, if there is no jaundice and ascites is well controlled by medical treatment. In emergency bleeding cases, it is well known that operative mortality is high, thus operation should be avoided, if possible [7]. Hemostasis with Sengstaken-Blackemore tube or EIS, in addition to liver-supporting treatment, is important, and then after at least one month the surgical operation is performed. With bleeding, hepatic function will decrease temporarily; however, usually within three weeks all cases recover. The ten-year survival rate of our operated cases is poor, because many cases died due to liver insufficiency and hepatoma. In Japan, more than 60% of liver cirrhosis originates from HB virus or non-A non-B virus and hepatic function steadily decreases after operation. Among these cases, the incidence of recurrent esophageal varices is high. It is therefore necessary to follow-up cases closely after they are discharged.

**Acknowledgement**

The authors wish to thank Associate Professor Patrick Barron of St. Marianna University, School of Medicine, for his review of the manuscript.

## References

1   Takasaki T, Kobayashi S, et al. Treatment of esophageal varices: our method of esophageal transection by using a suture device. Chir Gastroent 1976; 10: 136 – 143.
2   Takasaki T, Kobayashi S, et al. Transabdominal esophageal transection by using a suture device in cases of esophageal varices. Intern Surg 1977; 62: 426 – 428.
3   Japanese Research Society for Portal Hypertension. The general rules for recording endoscopic findings on esophageal varices. Jpn J Surg 1980; 10: 84 – 87.
4   Sugiura M, Futagawa S. A new technique for treating esophageal varices. J Thorac Cardiovasc Surg 1973; 66: 677 – 685.
5   Sugiura M, Futagawa S, et al. Further evaluation of Sugiura procedure in the treatment of esophageal varices. Arch Surg 1977; 112: 1317 – 1321.
6   Inokuchi K. Prophylactic portal nondecompression surgery in patients with esophageal varices. Ann Surg 1984; 200: 61 – 65.
7   Inokuchi K. Present status of surgical treatment of esophageal varices in Japan: a nation-wide survey of 3588 patients. World J Surg 1985; 9: 171 – 180.

© 1988 Elsevier Science Publishers B.V. (Biomedical Division)
Treatment of esophageal varices
Y. Idezuki, editor

Chapter 16

# Indications and results of transabdominal esophageal transection for esophageal varices

KAORU UMEYAMA, TAKAFUMI YAMASHITA, KAZUHIKO YOSHIKAWA AND TETSURO ISHIKAWA

First Department of Surgery, Osaka City University, Medical School, 1-5-7 Asahi-machi, Abeno-ku, Osaka, 545 Japan

## Introduction

The surgical treatment of portal hypertension complicated by esophageal varices, may be classified into portasystemic shunting operations and direct operations.

Portal decompression is a popular operation in Europe and America, but systemic portal encephalopathy and late hepatic failure occur in a significant proportion of patients. In Japan direct operations, such as transthoracic or transabdominal esophageal transection are mainly used for controlling variceal bleeding. This is because of the high possibility of postoperative encephalopathy and late hepatic failure after the shunting operation [1 – 3], furthermore, post-necrotic liver cirrhosis is very common in Japan.

We have performed transabdominal esophageal transection for esophageal varices since 1968. In this paper, we discuss our operative technique and report our results and indications.

## Patients and Methods

From February 1968 to December 1985, we performed transabdominal esophageal transection on 139 patients using our own technique. This procedure was used in 102 cases with liver cirrhosis, 30 with idiopathic portal hypertension and seven with extrahepatic portal obstruction. The average age was 47.0 years and ranged from 14 to 73 years: 96 patients were male and 44 female. Preoperative liver function was classified according to Child's method, grade A was found in 81, grade B in 48 and grade C in 10 patients. Twenty patients had an emergency operation within 24 h of hemorrhage, 106 had an elective operation and 13 had a prophylactic procedure.

**Operative Technique**

An upper midline incision with left lateral extension provided good exposure. Splenectomy with devascularization of the greater curvature was started after portal venography and manometry. Devascularization of the lesser curvature was done from the angle to the E-C junction and the left gastric artery was ligated and divided. The abdominal esophagus and cardia were devascularized from the lesser to the greater curvature and this procedure was followed to about 8 cm oral site from E-C junction. Then, the vagal nerve and para-esophageal vessels were ligated and divided. The esophagus was completely transected at the level of the 2 cm oral site from E-C junction and the mucosa was anastomosed with interrupted sutures of 3-0 Dexon, followed by pyloroplasty. Recently, we have used the EEA stapler in 36 cases for transection, which shortened the operative time by at least one hour (Fig. 1).

**Results**

*Operative mortality*
Seventeen of 139 patients died postoperatively within 30 days of surgery (13.2%). Six of the 17 patients with liver cirrhosis died after emergency operation. The overall postoperative mortality for the emergency operation was 30.0%. Eleven patients with liver cirrhosis died after elective operation and no patients died after prophylactic operation. Therefore, mortality rates for the elective and prophylactic operation were low, 10.4 and 0%, respectively.

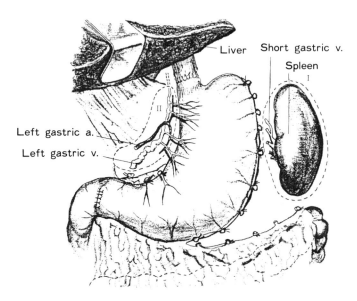

FIG. 1   Diagram illustrating our operative technique: transabdominal esophageal transection with para-esophagogastric devascularization.

There were no operative deaths in patients with idiopathic portal hypertension or extrahepatic portal obstruction. Anastomosis leakage was the main cause of operative death. Six of 17 patients died of this complication. Four patients died of hepatic failure, two died of variceal bleeding and five died of other causes, such as postoperative bleeding, renal failure, mesenteric thrombosis and so forth.

The operative mortality in patients with grade C (Child's classification) liver function was high, the rate was 40.0%, but the rates in grades B and A were 20.8 and 3.7% (Table 1).

Therefore we determined the indication for transabdominal esophageal transection on the basis of patient's liver function as shown in Table 2. Using these criteria, we performed the operation safely and the operative mortality decreased remarkably. Only two of 41 (4.9%) patients died from surgery in the last six years.

*Improvement and disappearance of esophageal varices*
The effectiveness of the operation for esophageal varices was assessed by X-ray examination 6 months postoperatively. Complete disappearance of the varices was seen in 68 of 92 patients who had elective and prophylactic operation. The rate of disappearance was 73.9%.

Recently, endoscopic examination has been used more frequently and 77 patients have been assessed by this method 6 months after operation. In 54 of these (70.1%) the varices disappeared completely, while in 16 there was incomplete disappearance.

On the other hand, the red-colour (R-C) sign completely disappeared in 72 of 77 (93.5%) patients.

TABLE 1   Causes of operative death and Child's classification

| Child's classification | Liver failure | Leakage | Variceal bleeding | Others | Total (%) |
|---|---|---|---|---|---|
| A | – | 2 | – | 1 | 3/81 ( 3.7) |
| B | 3 | 4 | – | 3 | 10/48 (20.8) |
| C | 1 | – | 2 | 1 | 4/10 (40.0) |
| Total | 4 | 6 | 2 | 5 | 17/139 (12.2) |

TABLE 2   Our criteria for transabdominal esophageal transection

| | |
|---|---|
| **1.** Serum albumin | $> 3.0$ g/dl |
| **2.** Total bilirubin | $< 2.0$ mg/dl |
| **3.** Wedged pressure of hepatic vein | $< 300$ mmH$_2$O |
| **4.** ICG (15 min) | $< 40\%$ |
| **5.** Ascites | None or controllable |

*Post-transection bleeding*
Further bleeding from the gastrointestinal tract after transabdominal esophageal transection was seen in 11 of 77 patients followed up by endoscopy. Of these, eight had liver cirrhosis and three had idiopathic portal hypertension. Seven of 11 (9.1%) patients with hemorrhage bled from esophageal varices and the rest of them bled from gastric lesions such as hemorrhagic gastritis and gastric ulcer. Bleeding from recurrent varices was observed in three of seven patients and residual varices in four patients.

Three of five patients with liver cirrhosis who had variceal rebleeding died. In the other two, transthoracic esophageal transection in one and endoscopic sclerotherapy in the other stopped further bleeding.

Two patients with idiopathic portal hypertension had variceal bleeding. One patient successfully underwent transthoracic esophageal transection, the other patients who had no bleeding episode had conservative treatment (Table 3).

*Five and ten years survival*
The survival curves for patients are shown in Fig. 2.

The prognosis was good in patients with grade A liver function, with a 5-year survival of 73.3% and a 10-year survival of 62.1%. Survival rate in patients with grade B was 74.7% at 5 years and 46% at 10 years.

However, the prognosis in patients with grade C was not as good, with a 5-year survival of 41.7%. But, there were no cases of encephalopathy in our series.

TABLE 3   Further bleeding cases from gastrointestinal tract after operation

| | Esophageal varices | | | | | Gastric lesion | | | | |
|---|---|---|---|---|---|---|---|---|---|---|
| Years after operation: | > 1 | 1 – 3 | 3 – 5 | 5 – 7 | 7 < | > 1 | 1 – 3 | 3 – 5 | 5 – 7 | 7 < |
| Cirrhosis of the liver (*n* = 60) | – | 1[a] | 2(1)[b] | 1 | 1 | – | 1 | 1 | – | 1 |
| Idiopathic portal hypertension (*n* = 17) | 1 | – | 1(1)[b] | – | – | – | – | – | 1 | – |
| Extrahepatic portal obstruction (*n* = 0) | – | – | – | – | – | – | – | – | – | – |
| Total (*n* = 77) | 1 | 1[a] | 3(2)[b] | 1 | 1 | – | 1 | 1 | 1 | 1 |

[a] Sclerotherapy.
[b] Transthoracic esophageal transection.

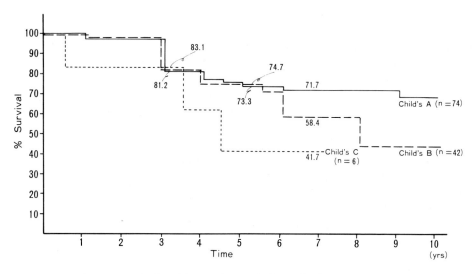

FIG. 2   Survival rate calculated by Kaplan-Meier's method.

## Discussion

Portacaval shunt operation for the treatment of portal hypertension provides good decompression of the varices, but is accompanied by various degrees of encephalo-pathy.

In Japan, extensive shunt operations have been largely abandoned on account of the frequent incidence of severe portal-systemic encephalopathy and have been replaced either by procedures attacking the varices directly or selective shunt pro-cedures which keep the portal pressure above a certain level. In 1967 Warren et al. [4], and in 1968 Inokuchi [5] designed their selective shunt operations in order to preserve intestinal portal venous perfusion of the liver while allowing continued hepatopedal portal perfusion with a significantly decreased incidence of encephalo-pathy.

However, recent reports have documented the occurrence of encephalopathy and the occlusion of shunt after this surgery [6 – 8].

We have performed transabdominal esophageal transection for esophageal varices since 1968 in order to attain hepatic protection, although non-shunting operations have an associated high incidence of recurrent bleeding. Our method in-cludes splenectomy, which even now remains controversial. Splenectomy seems to be an essential procedure in order to produce complete devascularization of the greater curvature and prevention of hypersplenism which is a frequent complica-tion.

Seventeen of 139 patients died postoperatively within 30 days of surgery and the overall postoperative mortality was 12.2%. But our postoperative mortality for emergency operation was 30.0%. The operative mortality for emergency shunting and non-shunting procedures is reported to be high ranging from 20 to 40% [9 – 11].

Our operative mortality was similar to those of other institutes. It seems our procedure may not be suitable for emergency operation because of the high mortality.

It is difficult to compare the results because the risks and the degree of liver damage differ among patients. Child's classification correlates well with surgical results, which were good in grades A and B and poor in grade C.

Operative mortality for the patients with grade C in our series was poor, the rate was 40%, though Sugiura and Futagawa [12] reported good results with an operative mortality rate of 17.2% in patients with grade C.

We have determined the indication for transabdominal esophageal transection from the analysis of the data on liver function from patients who died from surgery (Table 2).

According to our criteria, most the patients with grade C, including those with active hemorrhage are not candidates for our procedure. Some researchers who performed non-shunting operations in Japan described the same criteria for surgery as we have determined.

Using our criteria, we have performed the operation safely and operative mortality has decreased remarkably. Only two of 41 (4.9%) patients in our series died from surgery in the last 6 years.

For the treatment of the patients with grade C and with acute bleeding, we have performed endoscopic injection sclerotherapy with good results since 1979 [13].

The rate of disappearance of varices after a direct operation, such as simple esophageal transection or esophageal transection with devascularization, has been reported to be between 71 and 98% by X-ray assessment [9, 11] and this was 73.9% in our series. However, we observed complete disappearance of red-colour sign (R-C sign) in 72 of 77 (93.5%) patients.

The R-C sign, which is a very important sign for the surgeon, indicates likelihood of bleeding and is seen as a change of reddish colour seen immediately beneath the submucosa. It is considered, especially in Japan, that varices with this sign are an indication for treatment, and are useful in the assessment of surgical efficacy. Recently, we have used endoscopy during operation in order to confirm the disappearance of this sign.

The incidence of rebleeding after elective shunt operations was reported to be 15% by McDermott et al [14] and 21.1% by Sedgwick et al. [15]. In contrast, after immediate elective surgery, it was reported to be 1.5% by Sugiura and Futagawa [12] for transthoracic esophageal transection, splenectomy and devascularization, 6% by Hirashima et al. [16] for transabdominal esophageal mucosal transection and 14.1% by Yamamoto et al. [17] for terminal esophagoproximal gastrectomy. In our series, 11 out of 77 (14.3%) patients had rebleeding; four patients bled from gastric lesions and seven from esophageal varices, the true rebleeding rate from esophageal varices was, therefore, 9.1%. In the other reports, this factor was not detailed. Koyama et al. [11] found that the incidence of esophageal varices was 6%, with most of them recurring within 1 year, and he emphasized that all of these rebleeders received only esophageal transection or esophageal transection and splenectomy without devascularization. In our series with devascularization, the rate of rebleeding within 1 year was 1.3%. We suggest that varices devascularize from pre-existing vessels near the thoracic esophagus which have many shunts to the esophagus, the azygos system and the intercostal vein because two patients with rebleeding were successfully treated by transthoracic esophageal transection.

In our study, the prognosis after transabdominal esophageal transection was good in patients with grade A (Child's classification) liver function, with a 5-year survival of 73.3% and a 10-year survival of 62.1%. However, the prognosis in patients with grade C was not as good: a 5-year survival of 41.7% and no cases who survived to 10 years after surgery. It was difficult to compare our results with previous reports because of the differences in the degrees of risk and liver damage. The most important factor determining the clinical results was the underlying liver function.

## Summary

The results of transabdominal esophageal transection in 139 patients with esophageal varices and the indications for undertaking this operation are reported. This procedure was done in 102 patients with liver cirrhosis, 30 with idiopathic portal hypertension and seven with extrahepatic portal obstruction. Preoperative liver function was classified according to Child's method; grade A was found in 81, grade B in 48 and grade C in 10 patients. The operative mortality in our series was 12.2% and the mortality rate for emergency operation was higher than that for elective and prophylactic operation but, in the last 6 years, the mortality has decreased to 4.9% since we began using our criteria as an indication for the surgery.

Complete disappearance of esophageal varices judged by endoscopic examination, was 70.1%, and that judged by the R-C sign was 93.5%.

Post-transection rebleeding was observed in 11 of 77 (14.3%) patients during the follow-up period but seven of these bled from esophageal varices and the rest bled from gastric lesions. The 5-year survival rate was 73.5% in the patients with grade A, 74% in grade B and 41.7% in grade C. We consider that our procedure is suitable for esophageal varices, except for patients with grade C and active hemorrhage.

## References

1  Mikkelsen WP, Turrill FL, Pattison AC. Portacaval shunt in cirrhosis of the liver: clinical and hemodynamic aspects. Am J Surg 1962; 104: 204 – 215

2  Coon HO, Lindermuth WW. Prophylactic portacaval anastomosis in cirrhotic patients with esophageal varices. A progress report of a continuing study. New Engl J Med 1965; 272: 1255 – 1263

3  Voorkes AB, Price JBJr, Britton RC. Portasystemic shunting procedures for portal hypertension: Twenty-six years experience in adults with cirrhosis of the liver. Am J Surg 1970; 119: 501 – 505

4  Warren MD, Zeppa R, Fomon JJ. Selective trans-splenic decompression of gastroesophageal varices by distal splenorenal shunt. Ann Surg 1967; 166: 437 – 455

5  Inokuchi K. A selective portacaval shunt. Letter to the editor. Lancet 1968; ii: 51 – 52

6  Kobayashi M, Inokuchi K, Saku M, Nagasue N. Transition and evaluation of selective shunting operation (Japanese). Gekachiryo 1977; 37: 289 – 299

7  Maillard JN, Flamant YM, Hay JM. Selectivity of the distal splenorenal shunt. Surgery 1979; 86: 663 – 671

8    Belghiti J, Grenier P, Nouel O, Nahum H, Fekete F. Long-term loss of Warren's shunt selectivity. Arch Surg 1981; 116: 1121 – 1124

9    Sugiura M, Futagawa S. A new technique for treating esophageal varices. J Thorac Cardiovasc Surg 1973; 66: 677 – 685.

10   Langer B, Patel SC, Stone RM, Colapinto RF, Phillips MJ, Fisher MM. Selection of operation in patients with bleeding esophageal varices. CMA J 1978; 118: 369 – 372.

11   Koyama K, Takagi Y, Ouchi K, Sato T. Results of esophageal transection for esophageal varices: Experience in 100 cases. Am J Surg 1980; 139: 204 – 209.

12   Sugiura M, Futagawa S. Further evaluation of the Sugiura procedure in the treatment of esophageal varices. Arch Surg 1977; 112: 1317 – 1321.

13   Yoshikawa K, Sowa M, Asai T, et al. An evaluation and indication of endoscopic injection sclerotherapy for esophageal varices (Japanese). Jpn J Gastroenterol Surg 1987; 20: 1623 – 1630.

14   McDermott WV, Palazzi H, Nardi GL, Mondet A. Elective portal systemic shunt: an analysis of 237 cases. New Engl J Med 1961; 264: 419 – 427.

15   Sedgwick CE, Paulantgas JD, Miller WH. Portasystemic shunt in 102 patients with portal hypertension. New Engl J Med 1966; 274: 1290 – 1293.

16   Hirashima R, Hara T, Takeuchi H, et al. Transabdominal esophageal mucosal transection for the control of esophageal varices. Surg Gynecol Obstet 1980; 151: 36 – 40.

17   Yamamoto S, Hidemura R, Sawada M, Takeshige K, Iwatsuki S. The late results of terminal esophagoproximal gastrectomy (TEPG) with extensive devascularization and splenectomy for bleeding esophageal varices in cirrhosis. Surgery 1976; 80: 106 – 114.

© 1988 Elsevier Science Publishers B.V. (Biomedical Division)
Treatment of esophageal varices
Y. Idezuki, editor

Chapter 17

# Indications and results of non-shunting operations for esophageal varices

Y. Idezuki, K. Sanjo, H. Koyama, H. Sakamoto and N. Kokudo

*Second Department of Surgery, University of Tokyo Faculty of Medicine, Tokyo, Japan*

During the last two decades, non-shunting operations have been most widely performed as the operation of choice for bleeding esophageal varices in most of the surgical institutions in Japan. Eighty-seven percent of operations performed in Japan for esophageal varices during the last 10 years were non-shunting operations [1]. Among the non-shunting operations for esophageal varices, esophageal transection has been the most popular operation. Esophageal transection in Japan was started in our department in 1964 [2] modifying Walker's transthoracic esophageal transection [3], and this was then developed into the Sugiura procedure in 1967 [4], (this is more popularly known as the University of Tokyo method in our country). The essential elements of this procedure are extensive devascularization of the distal esophagus and the proximal half of the stomach and transection of the esophagus.

Our experiences of these operations over the last two decades are summarized and reported here.

## Materials and Methods

From January 1964 to September 1987, non-shunting operations were performed in 509 patients with esophagogastric varices in our department. Original diseases causing esophageal varices in these patients were liver cirrhosis (362 patients), idiopathic portal hypertension (102), extrahepatic portal obstruction (38), schistosomiasis (4) and other diseases (3). Three hundred and forty-seven patients were male and 162 were female. Mean age of the patients was 46.3 ± 13.3 years (range 1 − 74 years).

Transthoracoabdominal esophageal transection was performed in 287 patients, of which 127 operations were one stage operation and 160 were performed in two stages. Transthoracic esophageal transection was performed in 125 patients (31 Walker's transection, 94 esophageal transection with devascularization of distal esophagus). Transabdominal esophageal transection was performed in 42 patients. Hassab's operation was performed in 43 patients and three patients were treated with other direct operations (proximal gastrectomy, etc.) (Table 1). Type of operation and method of approach were decided by evaluating the patient risk and by ascertaining the development of portal collaterals (presence and absence of gastric varices, etc.).

Transection of the esophagus was performed approximately 3 cm above the esophagocardiac junction irrespective of the methods of approach, however the extent of devascularization of the esophagus and the stomach differed by the method of approaches. In transthoracic esophageal transection, approximately 16 cm of the distal esophagus is devascularized but devascularization of the stomach is limited only to 2 – 3 cm of the cardia below the esophagocardiac junction (Fig. 1). With the transthoracoabdominal approach, devascularization is performed most extensively, approximately 15 cm of the distal esophagus and proximal half of the stomach is completely devascularized (Fig. 2). Since both the thoracic and abdominal cavities are opened, operative risk to the patient is very great and cannot be tolerated by

TABLE 1   Operative mortality of non-shunting operations (Jan. 1949 – Sept. 1987, 2nd Dept. of Surg., Univ. of Tokyo)

| Operation | Disease | | | | | |
| --- | --- | --- | --- | --- | --- | --- |
| | Liver cirrhosis | Idiopathic portal hypertension | Extra-hepatic portal obstruction | Schistosomiasis | Others | Total |
| Univ. of Tokyo method (1 stage) | 77 (3) | 36 | 14 | 0 | 0 | 127 (3) |
| Univ. of Tokyo method (2 stages) | 127 (4) | 24 | 5 | 3 | 1 | 160 (4) |
| Walker's op. | 16 (1) | 13 | 2 | 0 | 0 | 31 (1) |
| Transthoracic esophageal transection | 77 (15) | 11 | 6 | 0 | 0 | 94 (15) |
| Transabdominal esophageal transection | 31 (0) | 7 | 3 | 0 | 1 | 42 (0) |
| Hassab's op. | 31 (2) | 11 | 0 | 0 | 1 | 43 (2) |
| Others | 3 (1) | 0 | 8 | 1 | 0 | 12 (1) |
| Total | 362 (26) | 102 (0) | 38 (0) | 4 (0) | 3 (0) | 509 (26) |

(Operative deaths given in parentheses.)

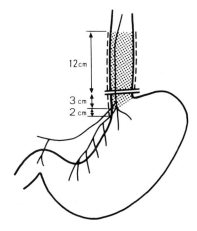

FIG. 1 Transthoracic esophageal transection.

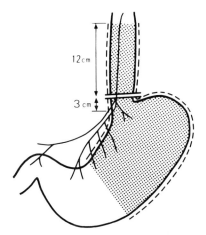

FIG. 2 Thoracoabdominal esophageal transection (University of Tokyo method, Sugiura procedure).

most of the patients in Child's C category. Using the abdominal approach, the proximal half of the stomach is devascularized, but the extent of esophageal devascularization is limited to the distal 10 cm of the esophagus above the esophagocardiac junction. Recently, we have been using EEA autosuture in abdominal approach in order to shorten the duration of the operation. In transabdominal transection the vagal nerves are divided during the devascularization of the esophagus, and pyloroplasty is routinely performed (Fig. 3).

Since transthoracic esophageal transection is the least agressive procedure of the three, it has been performed mainly in emergency cases and in patients with severe liver damage (Child's C). Hassab's operation was performed when varices were limited to the cardia and esophageal varices were absent.

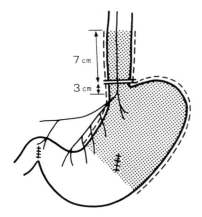

FIG. 3   Transabdominal esophageal transection.

## Results

Overall mortality of non-shunting operations was 5.1% (26/509). Operative mortality of transthoracic esophageal transection was 15.9% and higher compared to other operations. Operative mortality of this operation in cirrhotic patients was even higher, reaching 19.5%. These high operative mortalities reflect that this operation has often been performed as an emergency operation at the time of bleeding and in patients with severe liver damage (Child's C).

Operative mortalities and causes of late deaths of the patients with liver cirrhosis, idiopathic portal hypertension and extrahepatic portal obstruction according to the timing of operation are listed in Table 2 and those according to the severity of liver disease (Child's classification) are listed in Table 3. Operative mortality was only observed in patients with liver cirrhosis. No operative deaths occurred in patients with idiopathic portal hypertension or extrahepatic portal block. In emergency operations for patients with liver cirrhosis, operative mortality was even higher, and 14 out of 60 patients (23.3%) died within 1 month after emergency operation. The operative mortality of elective and prophylactic operations was around 4% even in cirrhotic patients. Operative mortality was not observed in Child's A patients, very low in Child's B but rather high (17.1%) in Child's C liver cirrhosis patients.

Among the 476 patients who survived the operation, 222 patients were already dead at the time of this summary, of which 189 patients were those with liver cirrhosis. Main causes of late deaths were liver failure, hepatic cell carcinoma and recurrent bleeding. Eighty-nine patients died of hepatic deterioration, 65 of development of hepatic cell carcinoma in postnecrotic cirrhosis, 33 of recurrent bleeding, and 35 from other causes. The late deaths from recurrent bleeding occurred in 6.9% of patients who survived the operation. Liver failures have been the most common cause of late deaths, but in recent years hepatoma as a cause of death in cirrhotic patients has been increasing and is an important problem in Japan.

The overall cumulative survival rate of the patients at 5 and 10 years were 66.2

TABLE 2  Results of non-shunting operations (Jan. 1964 – Sept. 1987, 2nd Dept. of Surg., Univ. of Tokyo)

| Disease | Operation | No. of cases | Operative death (%) | Late death | | | |
|---|---|---|---|---|---|---|---|
| | | | | Hepatoma | Liver failure | Bleeding | Others |
| Liver cirrhosis | Emergency | 60 | 14 (23.3) | 12 | 10 | 2 | 2 |
| | Elective | 183 | 7 (3.8) | 32 | 46 | 15 | 11 |
| | Prophylactic | 119 | 5 (4.2) | 19 | 24 | 8 | 8 |
| Idiopathic portal hypertension | Emergency | 13 | 0 (0) | 0 | 2 | 1 | 2 |
| | Elective | 51 | 0 (0) | 1 | 3 | 5 | 3 |
| | Prophylactic | 38 | 0 (0) | 1 | 4 | 0 | 7 |
| Extrahepatic portal obstruction | Emergency | 5 | 0 (0) | 0 | 0 | 1 | 0 |
| | Elective | 26 | 0 (0) | 0 | 0 | 1 | 2 |
| | Prophylactic | 7 | 0 (0) | 0 | 0 | 0 | 0 |
| Total | | 502 | 26 (5.1) | 65 | 89 | 33 | 35 |

TABLE 3  Results of non-shunting operations (Jan. 1964 – Sept. 1987, 2nd Dept. of Surg., Univ. of Tokyo)

| Disease | Classification | No. of cases | Operative death (%) | Late death | | | |
|---|---|---|---|---|---|---|---|
| | | | | Hepatoma | Liver failure | Bleeding | Others |
| Liver cirrhosis | A | 69 | 0 (0) | 12 | 15 | 2 | 3 |
| | B | 164 | 4 (2.4) | 24 | 32 | 13 | 9 |
| | C | 129 | 22 (17.1) | 27 | 33 | 10 | 9 |
| Idiopathic portal hypertension | A | 67 | 0 (0) | 1 | 5 | 4 | 6 |
| | B | 30 | 0 (0) | 1 | 2 | 1 | 5 |
| | C | 5 | 0 (0) | 0 | 2 | 1 | 1 |
| Extrahepatic portal obstruction | A | 36 | 0 (0) | 0 | 0 | 2 | 2 |
| | B | 2 | 0 (0) | 0 | 0 | 0 | 0 |
| | C | 0 | 0 (0) | 0 | 0 | 0 | 0 |
| Total | | 502 | 26 (5.1) | 65 | 89 | 33 | 35 |

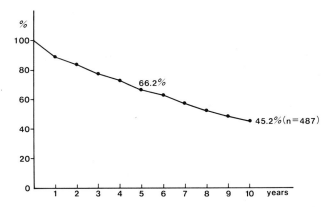

FIG. 4   Overall cumulative survival rate of non-shunting operations (2nd Dept. of Surgery, Univ. of Tokyo, 1964 – 1987).

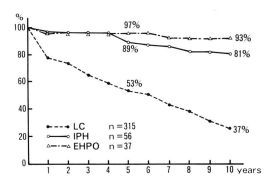

FIG. 5   Cumulative survival rate of non-shunting operations by type of diseases (2nd Dept. of Surgery, Univ. of Tokyo, 1964 – 1987).

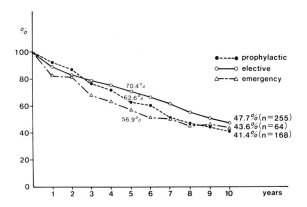

FIG. 6   Cumulative survival rate of non-shunting operations by timing of operation (2nd Dept. of Surgery, Univ. of Tokyo, 1964 – 1987).

182

and 45.2%, respectively (Fig. 4). The cumulative survival rates differed among the diseases. In idiopathic portal hypertension and extrahepatic portal block, survival rates at 5 years were 89 and 97%, respectively, and at 10 years 81 and 93%, respectively. However, in liver cirrhosis, survival rate was 53% at 5 years and 37% at 10 years (Fig. 5).

There was no significant difference in 5 or 10 year survival rates whether the operation was performed at emergency or electively or prophylactically (Fig. 6). However, the survival rates of patients differed with the severity of liver damage. Child's A patients had the best prognosis, survival rate at 10 years being 72.4%, whereas the survival rate in Child's C patients was only 8.9% at 10 years (Fig. 7).

The cumulative survival rates of patients according to the type of operation are shown in Fig. 8. Transthoracic esophageal transection and Hassab's operation had poorer results compared to transabdominal transection or the University of Tokyo

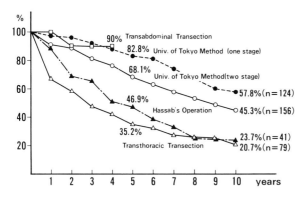

FIG. 7   Cumulative survival rate of non-shunting operations by Child's classification (2nd Dept. of Surgery, Univ. of Tokyo, 1964 – 1987).

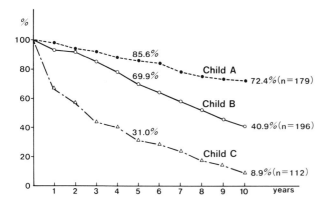

FIG. 8   Cumulative survival rate of non-shunting operations by method of operation (2nd Dept. of Surgery, Univ. of Tokyo, 1964 – 1987).

method (thoracoabdominal transection). We feel that this is mainly because the former two procedures were used in patients with more advanced liver failure in whom thoracoabdominal transection cannot be tolerated.

## Discussion

Our overall results with esophageal transection over the last two decades have been satisfactory, and much better than those with portal decompression operations which had been performed in our department until the introduction of esophageal transection in 1964 [5]. However, our experiences clearly have revealed that the results in Child's C patients and those in emergency cases have been so unsatisfactory that we now feel emergency operations during bleeding should be avoided whenever possible and operations of any type in Child's C patients may not be justifiable. Satisfactory results with non-shunting operations have been reported from other institutions in Japan [6, 7] and this is in contrast with the reports from other western countries [9 – 11] where the results of similar operations have been less satisfactory having much higher operative mortalities and morbidities and poor prognosis. It has been suggested that the discrepancies in results reported from Japan and other western countries may originate from the differences of etiology of the liver cirrhosis, namely the nature of the hepatic diseases per se.

It is interesting to note that the long-term results of operations have not been affected by the timing of operation. There have been no significant differences in the late results, whether the operation was performed at emergency, electively or prophylactically, once surgery was tolerated by the patient.

As expected, long-term results were affected by the nature of the original diseases of the liver and the severity of hepatic deterioration. Survival rates of the patients with idiopathic portal hypertension and extra portal block have been much better than those with cirrhosis. Although 6.9% of the patients who survived the operation (33/476) died from recurrent bleeding, more of the patients died of hepatic failure and development of hepatic cell carcinoma, inevitable consequences of the advancement of postnecrotic cirrhosis.

Esophageal transection was performed using three different approaches in our hands, namely, transthoracically, thoracoabdominally and transabdominally. Devascularization of the esophagus and the stomach is most extensive and complete in thoracoabdominal approach, however this is the most drastic procedure and it has not been tolerated in most of the Child's C patients and in many of the Child's B patients. Moreover, in patients with moderate to severe liver failure, this operation should often be performed in two stages in order to avoid the operative risks for the patients.

More recently, transabdominal approach using EEA autosuture for esophageal transection is routinely used in our department. Devascularization of the esophagus is less extensive compared to the thoracoabdominal approach and limited to approximately 10 cm of the distal esophagus. However, varices have disappeared completely in 80% of patients with this transabdominal transection. This operation offers less risk to the patients and can be performed in one stage, which is an important advantage in patients with moderate to severe liver damage. Recent development of endoscopic sclerotherapy is remarkable, and the varices if remaining after transabdominal transection may be successfully treated by adjutant sclerotherapy.

Transthoracic transection is a less aggressive operation for the patient and often has been tolerated even in Child's C patients, however, the extent of gastric devascularization is limited by this approach, and disappearance of esophageal varices was not complete in 50% of the patients. This operation has often been performed as an emergency procedure to control bleeding, but it has been necessary in many of the cases to add transabdominal gastric devascularization after the patient recovered from the emergency operation.

Treatment of esophageal varices has been controversial and still is. Our experiences have clearly shown that esophageal transection with extensive devascularization of distal esophagus and proximal stomach is a satisfactory operation for esophagogastric varices, however the method of treatment and ways of approach should be carefully selected for each patient by evaluating the patients conditions from many angles (Table 4).

Emergency operations of any kind should be avoided since we now have other effective means to control massive bleeding successfully (endoscopic balloon tamponade [12], endoscopic sclerotherapy, etc.). Also, operations on Child's C patients should be avoided since the results in these patients have been unsatisfactory. Endoscopic sclerotherapy may be the treatment of choice for this category of patients.

TABLE 4   Indications for esophageal transection

Age: 70 years old
History: variceal bleeding

Endoscopic findings: R-C sign (+), $F_{2-3}$, $C_B$

Clinical findings:
  ascites (−)
  encephalopathy (−)
  cachexia (−)

Laboratory findings:
| | |
|---|---|
| Albumin, | 2.8 g /dl < |
| Total bilirubin, | 3.5 mg/dl > |
| S − GOT, | 200 U > |
| S-GPT, | 200 U > |
| Antipyrin clearance, | 0.10 ml/min/kg < |
| Aminopyrin clearance, | 0.40 ml/min/kg < |
| Prothrombin time, | 50% < |
| Hepaplastin test, | 50% < |
| ICG 15, | 40% > |
| K-ICG | 0.04 $min^{-1}$ < |

No severe complications in other organs

In Child's A and B patients, with a history of bleeding from varices, transabdominal esophageal transection using EEA is the operation of choice. Sugiura's procedure (thoracoabdominal approach) may be performed in Child's A patients, but it should be limited only to the cases where transabdominal transection using EEA have not provided sufficient effect on the esophageal varices; less than 20% of the cases of transabdominal transection in our hands.

## References

1   Japanese Research Society for Portal Hypertension. National surgery of treatment of esophageal varices in Japan. 1983 (in Japanese).
2   Idezuki Y, Sugiura M, Sakamoto K, et al. Rational for transthoracic esophageal transection for bleeding esophageal varices. Dis Chest 1967; 52: 621 – 631.
3   Walker RM. Transection operation for portal hypertension. Thorax 1960; 15: 218 – 224.
4   Sugiura M, Futagawa S. A new technique for treating esophageal varices. J Thorac Cardiovasc Surg 1973; 66: 677 – 685.
5   Kimoto S. Operations for portal hypertension and their late results. J Jpn Surg Soc 1966; 67: 1743 – 1754 (in Japanese).
6   Yamamoto S, Hidemura R, et al. The late results of terminal esophagoproximal gastrectomy (TEPG) with extensive devascularization and splenectomy for bleeding esophageal varices in cirrhosis. Surgery 1976; 80: 106 – 114.
7   Hirashima T, Hara T, Takeuchi H, et al. Transabdominal esophageal mucosal transection for the control of esophageal varices. Surg Gynecol Obstet 1980; 151: 36 – 40.
8   Johnston GW. Treatment of bleeding varices by esophageal transection with SPTU gun. Ann Roy Coll Surg Eng 1977; 59: 404 – 408.
9   Wexler MJ. Treatment of bleeding esophageal varices by transabdominal esophageal transection with the EEA stapling instrument. Surgery 1980; 88: 406 – 416.
10  Cooperman M, Fabri PJ, Martin EW, et al. EEA esophageal stapling for control of bleeding esophageal varices. Am J Surg 1980; 140: 821 – 824.
11  Kuzmak LI. Use of EEA stapler in transection of esophagus in severe hemorrhage from esophageal varices. Am J Surg 1981; 141: 387 – 390.
12  Idezuki Y. Endoscopic balloon tamponade. In: Burroughs AK, ed. Methodology and reviews of clinical trials in portal hypertension. Amsterdam: Excerpta Medica, 1987: 125 – 128.

© 1988 Elsevier Science Publishers B.V. (Biomedical Division)
Treatment of esophageal varices
Y. Idezuki, editor

Chapter 18

# Indications and results of non-shunting operations: experience in 190 cases

KIYOAKI OUCHI[1], TOSHIO SATO[1] AND KENJI KOYAMA[2]

[1]1st Department of Surgery, Tohoku University School of Medicine, and [2]1st Department of Surgery, Akita University School of Medicine, Japan

## Introduction

Sugiura and Futagawa [1] described a rational concept of local non-shunt therapy for variceal hemorrhage by a combined two-stage procedure of extensive devascularization of the abdominal and thoracic esophagus, esophageal transection and splenectomy. After transthoracic esophageal transection, splenectomy and proximal gastric devascularization are carried out as the second stage operation 3 or 4 weeks later. Although a low operative mortality rate and low incidences of recurrent hemorrhage and encephalopathy of this operative procedure have been reported in Japan [2, 3], these operative results have not been reproduced by many investigators outside Japan [4, 5]. However, the most recent reports advocated the excellent results of this operative procedure [6]. The surgical results in our series of 190 patients who were subjected to Sugiura's non-shunt operation are reported herein and selection criteria for this operative treatment are discussed.

## Material and methods

Since 1969 to the present, 14 patients with extrahepatic portal occlusion (EHO), 52 with idiopathic portal hypertension (IPH) and 124 with liver cirrhosis have been subjected to the non-shunting operation in the First Department of Surgery, Tohoku University School of Medicine. Among the cirrhotic patients, 36 were of alcoholic origin and the remaining 88 non-alcoholic. Diagnosis was made

Reprint requests: Kiyoaki Ouchi, M.D., 1st Department of Surgery, Tohoku University School of Medicine, 1-1 Seiryocho, Sendai 980, Japan.

histologically and by angiographic examination. Operations performed were esophageal transection and splenectomy with devascularization (the Sugiura procedure) in 112 patients, esophageal transection and splenectomy (with or without ligation of the left gastric vein) in 41, and esophageal transection alone in 37.

In liver cirrhosis, 71 patients underwent the complete operation, that is, esophageal transection and splenectomy with devascularization. Eighteen patients underwent esophageal transection and splenectomy with or without ligation of the left gastric vein. Esophageal transection alone, however, was carried out in 35 patients who did not undergo the second-stage operation due to early postoperative death, progressive liver dysfunction or the appearance of or an increase in ascites. Twenty-one patients had emergency operations within 24 h after hemorrhage, 82 had elective operations, and 21 had prophylactic operations.

Frequencies of operative mortality and late mortality patients related to certain values of various preoperative factors were retrospectively analysed, and statistical comparisons were made using the $\chi^2$ method. Child's classification, plasma disappearance rate of indocyanine green (ICG k), albumin, prothrombin time and GOT were selected. ICG k was obtained after i.v. injection of 0.5 mg/kg of ICG. According to established criteria for operative treatment using those factors, patients selected were subjected to esophageal transection.

## Results

### Operative results

Of 14 patients with EHO, none died in the 30-day postoperative period and one died of burns in the follow-up period (Table 1). Of 52 patients with IPH, two died during the 30-day postoperative period of cerebral hemorrhage and bleeding from gastric varices after emergency esophageal transection. Three other patients died during the follow-up period due to a traffic accident, rectal cancer and an unknown cause. Of 124 patients with liver cirrhosis, in contrast, 12 died within the 30-day postoperative period and 52 died during the follow-up period. The cumulative five-year survival rate, including operative mortality, was 100% in EHO, 90.2% in IPH and 63.0%

TABLE 1   Results of esophageal transection in liver disease

|                 | No. of cases | No. of operative deaths | No. of late deaths |
|-----------------|--------------|-------------------------|--------------------|
| EHO             | 14           | 0                       | 1 ( 7)             |
| IPH             | 52           | 2 ( 4)                  | 3 ( 6)             |
| Liver cirrhosis | 124          | 12 (10)                 | 52 (42)            |
| Total           | 190          | 14 ( 7)                 | 56 (29)            |

EHO, extrahepatic portal occlusion; IPH, idiopathic portal hypertension. Numbers in parentheses are percentages.

in liver cirrhosis (Fig. 1). In the liver cirrhosis group, eight patients died after esophageal transection within the 30-day postoperative period, six due to progressive liver failure, and two due to acute gastric ulcer (Table 2). Operative deaths after splenectomy and devascularization were found in four patients (liver failure in one, acute gastric ulcer in one and renal failure in two). Post-transection bleeding was encountered in 8 patients. The incidence of rebleeding was low in patients subjected to esophageal transection and splenectomy with devascularization compared with those subjected to esophageal transection alone or esophageal transection with splenectomy. Bleeding was controlled by esophageal retransection through a right thoracotomy in two patients and endoscopic sclerotherapy in one patient. One patient, who already had esophageal transection, underwent emergency splenectomy with devascularization. The other four patients died from hepatic coma shortly after the onset of bleeding. Postoperative hepatic encephalopathy was found in only four patients, and all cases were transient and controlled by the administration of a branched-chain enriched amino acids solution and Lactulose®.

As shown in Table 3, the operative mortality rate for emergency operations was 24%, and only 6% in elective operations ($P < 0.05$). Two out of 21 patients (9%)

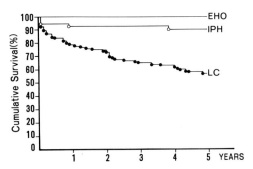

FIG. 1  Survival curves for 14 patients with extrahepatic portal occlusion (EHO), 52 with idiopathic portal hypertension (IPH), and 124 with liver cirrhosis (LC). Cumulative survival rates were obtained by use of the Kaplan-Meier method.

TABLE 2  Operative results according to types of operation: liver cirrhosis

|  | No. of cases | No. of operative deaths | No. of late deaths | No. of rebleedings | No. of encephalopathies |
|---|---|---|---|---|---|
| ET-SPDV | 71 | 4 ( 6) | 25 (35) | 3 ( 4) | 2 (3) |
| ET-SP(CL) | 18 | 0 | 10 (56) | 2 (11) | 1 (5) |
| ET alone | 35 | 8 (23) | 17 (49) | 3 ( 9) | 1 (3) |
| Total | 124 | 12 (10) | 52 (42) | 8 ( 7) | 4 (3) |

ET, esophageal transection; SP, splenectomy; DV, devascularization; CL, ligation of the coronary vein. Numbers in parentheses are percentages.

who were subjected to prophylactic operation died within the 30-day postoperative period. Late deaths were found in 62% of emergency cases and 37% of elective cases, and this difference was statistically significant ($P < 0.05$). Liver failure was the most frequent cause of death in both early and late postoperative periods. Four patients died of rebleeding from esophageal varices.

*Factors influencing survival of cirrhotic patients*
The operative mortality rate was significantly higher in Child's group C than in group A ($P < 0.01$) and B ($P < 0.05$), as shown in Fig. 2. In addition, among the

TABLE 3   Operative results according to urgency of operation: liver cirrhosis

|  | No. of cases | No. of operative deaths | No. of late deaths | Causes of death | | | |
|---|---|---|---|---|---|---|---|
|  |  |  |  | Liver failure | Hepatoma | Rebleeding | Others |
| Emergency | 21 | 5 (24) | 13 (62) | 12 | 3 |  | 3 |
| Elective | 82 | 5 ( 6) | 30 (37) | 18 | 4 | 4 | 9 |
| Prophylactic | 21 | 2 ( 9) | 9 (45) | 8 | 2 |  | 1 |
| Total | 124 | 12 (10) | 52 (42) | 38 | 9 | 4 | 13 |

Numbers in parentheses are percentages.

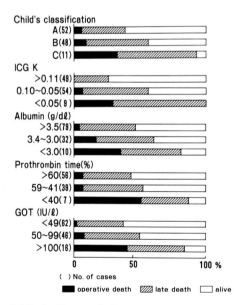

FIG. 2   Factors influencing survival of patients with liver cirrhosis. ICG k, plasma disappearance rate of indocyanine green; GOT, glutamine-oxaloacetic transaminase.

patients who tolerated the operation, late deaths were more frequently found in Child's group C than in group A ($P < 0.05$). Operative deaths were more frequent in patients whose ICG k values were less than 0.05 than in those whose ICG k values were greater than 0.11 ($P < 0.001$) and from 0.051 to 0.10 ($P < 0.05$). Furthermore, the incidence of late deaths increased with the reduction of ICG k ($P < 0.05$ between the patients with ICG k less than 0.05 and those with ICG k from 0.10 to 0.05, $P < 0.001$ between the patients with ICG k less than 0.05 and those with ICG k greater than 0.11, $P < 0.01$ between the patients with ICG k from 0.051 to 0.10 and those with ICG k greater than 0.11). With respect to the serum albumin level, patients who showed a value less than 3.0 g/dl had higher operative and late mortality rates than those who showed a value greater than 3.5 g/dl ($P < 0.01$ and $P < 0.05$, respectively). The operative mortality rate of the patients whose prothrombin time (PT) was less than 40% was significantly higher than those whose PT was greater than 60% and from 41 to 60% (both $P$ values less than 0.001). But there were no differences in the incidence of late deaths among these three groups of patients. Operative deaths were more frequent in patients with serum GOT values greater than 100 IU/l than in those with GOT values below 49 IU/l ($P < 0.001$) and those whose GOT values were between 50 and 99 IU/l ($P < 0.01$). However, the incidence of late deaths was not different among those three groups.

## Discussion

There is little doubt that endoscopic sclerotherapy is an important therapeutic advance in the treatment of esophageal varices. However, although sclerotherapy significantly reduces the incidence of life-threatening bleeding, patients require lifelong follow-up and repeated injections to prevent recurrence of bleeding. In addition, Terblanche [7] has not shown an improved survival of patients treated with sclerotherapy.

Regarding the surgical treatment of esophageal varices, selective and nonselective shunting and non-shunting procedures are all presently used with varying success. The selective distal splenorenal shunt (DSRS) of Warren has been considered to be superior to the nonselective shunts [8, 9]. After reviewing the 10-year follow-up of the Emory experiences, Millikan et al. [10] concluded that there was less rebleeding and encephalopathy after DSRS compared to nonselective shunts. However, improved survival was not confirmed in alcoholics and postoperative encephalopathy occurred in 27% of the patients, a high frequency, although significantly lower than the 75% of the nonselective shunts. Harley et al. [11] have failed to demonstrate the superiority of DSRS over the portacaval shunt (PCS) in patients with alcoholic liver disease with respect to postoperative encephalopathy (39% after DSRS, 32% after PCS) or five-year survival (43% after DSRS, 31% after PCS). Furthermore, they also had a 27% variceal rebleeding rate after DSRS.

Disappointment with shunt procedures has given rise in recent years to an acute search for non-shunting operations. We have been performing esophageal transection and devascularization with splenectomy. Operative results are strongly influenced by the hepatic function. Patients with EHO or IPH who have normal or near normal hepatic function have less mortality and morbidity than liver cirrhosis [12]. In our patients with liver cirrhosis, the operative mortality rate was 10% and the five-year survival rate was 63%. Recurrent variceal bleeding was seen in 7%, and postoperative encephalopathy in 4% of the patients. The operative mortality and frequency of rebleeding and encephalopathy have been low with this operative procedure. Sugiura and Futagawa [3] also reported a low rebleeding rate 1.5%, in their operative results.

The complete operation (esophageal transection, splenectomy and devascularization) showed the best results with respect to the disappereance of esophageal varices [2]. Esophageal transection with splenectomy or esophageal transection alone was not sufficient for the complete disappearance of varices. The incomplete operation produced a rebleeding rate of approximately 10%. Devascularization plays, therefore, an important role in the complete disappearance of varices. In the two-stage operation, the indication and timing for the second-stage operation, splenectomy with devascularization, are determined on the basis of the postoperative condition of the patient.

Selection criteria for the indication of esophageal transection which we have been using are listed in Table 4. Among various easily obtainable preoperative parameters, Child's classification, ICG k and serum albumin are considered to be important factors in determining not only early but also late mortality of patients after esophageal transection. Prothrombin time and GOT are only valuable for determining the early operative mortality. The operative mortality for emergency operation was 24%, which was higher than that for elective and prophylactic operations. Most patients with acutely bleeding esophageal varices have deteriorated liver function, and it is not always possible to obtain sufficient preoperative data to determine if they are suitable for operative treatment. After the introduction of injection sclerotherapy in 1980, we have never performed emergency esophageal transection. We believe that sclerotherapy is the procedure of choice in patients whose variceal bleeding continues after medical treatment. Following the initial control of bleeding the elective operation must be considered in selected patients.

Sclerotherapy is also valuable for patients whose hepatic function is judged to be not an indication for surgery. We also consider that the indication for prophylactic operation should be much stricter than for elective operation. Recently we have been applying a scoring system obtained from a combination of four prognostic factors

TABLE 4 Indication for esophageal transection

|  | Elective operation | Prophylactic operation |
|---|---|---|
| ICG k | > 0.05 | > 0.07 |
| Albumin (g/dl) | $\geq$ 3.0 | $\geq$ 3.5 |
| PT (%) | > 40 | > 60 |
| GOT (IU/l) | < 100 | < 100 |
| Ascites | none or controllable | none or controllable |
| Encephalopathy | none or controllable | none |

to predict the two-year survival and to determine the operative indication for the Sugiura procedure more precisely [13]. Based on the low operative mortality rate and the efficacy in eliminating rebleeding from varices and encephalopathy, we believe that esophageal transection and splenectomy with devascularization is the best procedure currently available.

## References

1   Sugiura M, Futagawa S. A new technique for treating esophageal varices. J Thorac Cardiovasc Surg 1973; 66: 677 – 685.
2   Koyama K, Takagi Y, Ouchi K, Sato T. Results of esophageal transection for esophageal varices: experience in 100 cases. Am J Surg 1980; 139: 204 – 209.
3   Sugiura M, Futagawa S. Esophageal transection with paraesophagogastric devascularizations (the Sugiura procedure) in the treatment of esophageal varices. World J Surg 1984; 8: 673 – 679.
4   Joffe SN. Non-shunting procedures for control of variceal bleeding. Semin Liver Dis 1983; 3: 235 – 250.
5   Durtschi MB, Carrico CJ, Johansen KH. Esophageal transection fails to salvage high-risk cirrhotic patients with variceal bleeding. Am J Surg 1985; 150: 18 – 23.
6   Abouna GM, Baissony H, Al-Nakib BM, Menkarios AT, Silva OSG. The place of Sugiura operation for portal hypertension and bleeding esophageal varices. Surgery 1987; 101: 91 – 98.
7   Terblanche J. The long-term management of patients after an oesophageal variceal bled: the role of sclerotherapy. Br J Surg 1985; 72: 88 – 90.
8   Rikkers LF, Rudman D, Galambos JT, Fulenwider JT, Millikan WJ, Kutner M, Smith RB, Salamn AA, Jones PJ, Warren WD. A randomized, controlled trial of the distal splenorenal shunt. Ann Surg 1978; 188: 271 – 282.
9   Zeppa R, Hutson DG, Levi JU, Livingstone AS. Factors influencing survival after distal splenorenal shunt. World J Surg 1984; 5: 733 – 738.
10  Millikan WJ, Warren WD, Henderson JM, Smith RB, Salam AA, Galambos JT, Kutner MH, Keen JH. The Emory prospective randomized trial: selective versus nonselective shunt to control variceal bleeding. Ann Surg 1985; 201: 712 – 723.
11  Harley HAJ, Morgan T, Redeker AG, Reynolds TB, Villamil F, Weiner JM, Yellin A. Results of a randomized trial of end-to-side portacaval shunt and distal splenorenal shunt in alcoholic liver disease and variceal bleeding. Gastroenterology 1986; 91: 802 – 809.
12  Ouchi K, Koyama K, Sato T. Differential diagnosis of idiopathic portal hypertension. In: Okuda K, Omata M, eds. Idiopathic portal hypertension. Tokyo: University of Tokyo Press, 1982; 363 – 373.
13  Ouchi K, Abe M, Sato T. Prediction of outcome following Sugiura's procedure in patients with liver cirrhosis: a multiple linear regression analysis and scoring system. Dig Surg 1987; 4: 93 – 97.

© 1988 Elsevier Science Publishers B.V. (Biomedical Division)
*Treatment of esophageal varices*
*Y. Idezuki, editor*

Chapter 19

# The role of non-shunting surgery in the treatment of esophageal varices in comparison to injection sclerotherapy

KEISUKE YOSHIDA, KAZUHIRO TSUKADA AND TERUKAZU MUTO

*1st Department of Surgery, Niigata University School of Medicine, Asahimachi 1, Niigata 951, Japan*

In our department, esophageal transection as described by Sugiura [1] has been employed as the first choice of treatment of varices since 1972. However, recent advances in endoscopic injection sclerotherapy have contributed significantly in extending the possibility of bleeding control to severely ill patients. Under these circumstances, it is necessary to select the indications for these multiple therapeutic approaches.

In order to assess the role of operative and endoscopic treatment for esophageal varices, results of both direct interrupting surgery and injection sclerotherapy in liver cirrhosis were reviewed. The preliminary result of the prospective comparative study is also presented.

## Patients and Methods

Table 1 shows our total experience on the management of esophageal varices from 1955 until June 1987.

*Retrospective study*
In the retrospective study, long-term survival rate and postoperative rebleeding rate were determined in 74 cirrhotic patients who underwent direct interrupting surgery and 43 patients who had injection sclerotherapy. All patients had at least one episode of variceal hemorrhage. Patients who had hepatocellular carcinoma at the time of initial treatment were excluded.

Our first choice operative procedure is esophageal transection with both thoracic and abdominal devascularization which is usually performed in two stages for cirrhotic patients. Some of those patients who had previous upper abdominal surgery

TABLE 1   Total experience in the treatment of esophageal varices

| Procedures | No. of cases |
|---|---|
| Shunt surgery | 16 |
| Non-shunting surgery | 212 |
|   Esophageal transection | 165 |
|   Proximal gastrection | 22 |
|   Hassab's op. | 22 |
|   Others | 3 |
| Injection sclerotherapy | 115 |
| Total | 343 |

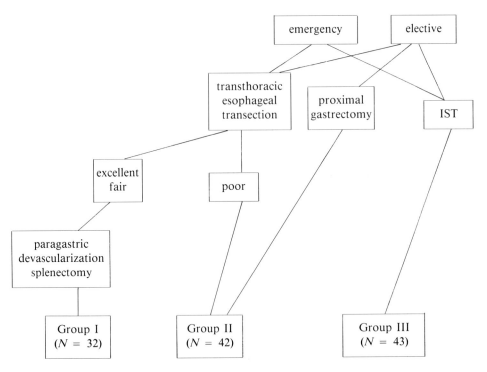

FIG. 1   Study groups according to the therapeutic approaches. IST, injection sclerotherapy.

(splenectomy or others), or who showed unfavorable recovery from the first thoracic operation, underwent only transthoracic esophageal transection. Some patients refused the second abdominal operation. For those patients who were not suitable for thoracotomy or refused two-staged operations, abdominal procedures including proximal gastrectomy ($n = 9$), transabdominal esophageal transection or gastric transection ($n = 1$) were employed. The surgical patients were, therefore, divided into two subgroups (Fig. 1). Group 1 consisted of patients who underwent typical Sugiura's procedure ($n = 32$). Patients who underwent either thoracic or abdominal procedure only were classified as Group II.

Consequently, Group II included relatively high risk patients and devascularization in this group was less complete than in Group I. Patients who had sclerotherapy were classified as Group III. As the routine technique of sclerotherapy, intravasal injection of 5% ethanolamine oleate was employed (Table 2). Age and sex distribution and status of hepatic functional reserve (Child's classification) are described in Table 3.

Survival and rebleeding rates after the initial treatment were estimated by the life table method. Statistical analysis was performed by the generalized Wilcoxon test. Early deaths within 30 days were included in the calculation of survival rate. In the

TABLE 2  Method of injection sclerotherapy

5% ethanolamine oleatae
1 – 5 ml/injection
1 – 2 injections for every varix
↓
7 – 10 days
evaluation endoscopy
↓
supplementary treatment
(repeat until eradication)
↓
follow up at every 3 months

TABLE 3  Age, sex distribution and Child's classification in the study groups

| Group | Type of treatment | No. of cases | M/F | Age (M ± SD) | Child A | B | C |
|-------|-------------------|--------------|------|--------------|---------|----|----|
| I | Surgery | 32 | 26/6 | 46.8 ± 12.5 | 15 | 14 | 3 |
| II | Surgery | 42 | 37/5 | 54.6 ± 9.3 | 8 | 18 | 16 |
| III | IST | 43 | 30/13 | 54.8 ± 11.8 | 9 | 19 | 15 |

IST, injection sclerotherapy

sclerotherapy group, early rebleeding before accomplishment of eradication was counted as the rebleeding. Rebleeding rate was estimated in those patients who survived longer than 30 days after the initial treatment.

*Prospective study*

To examine the usefulness of injection sclerotherapy in patients with good hepatic functional reserve, 23 consecutive patients with cirrhosis and bleeding esophageal varices were randomly divided into two therapeutic groups, surgical and endoscopic. All were treated electively and the state of their hepatic function corresponded to Child's class A or B (Table 4). Among 11 surgical patients, nine underwent esophageal transection with thoracoabdominal devascularization, while the other two underwent the thoracic procedure only. Clinical results were estimated in the same manner as stated above.

## Results

*Retrospective study*

Eight patients out of 32 in Group I, 21 out of 42 in Group II and 26 out of 44 in Group III were treated as emergency. As the emergency procedure, transthoracic esophageal transection was performed in 27 patients with an operative mortality rate of 22.2% (proximal gastrectomy and gastric transection were each performed in one patient and the latter resulted in operative death), even though initial control of

TABLE 4   Elective treatment of patients studied in the prospective randomized study

| Surgery | | | I S T | | |
|---|---|---|---|---|---|
| No. | Case | Child | No. | Case | Child |
| | age sex | | | age sex | |
| 1. | 36 m | B | 1. | 47 f | B |
| 2. | 52 m | A | 2. | 44 m | A |
| 3. | 59 m | B | 3. | 54 f | B |
| 4. | 46 f | B | 4. | 64 m | B |
| 5. | 41 m | B | 5. | 48 m | B |
| 6. | 55 m | A | 6. | 72 f | B |
| 7. | 44 m | A | 7. | 58 m | A |
| 8. | 58 m | A | 8. | 48 m | A |
| 9. | 40 m | A | 9. | 40 f | B |
| 10. | 36 m | A | 10. | 59 m | B |
| 11. | 46 f | B | 11. | 63 f | A |
| | | | 12. | 37 m | A |

hemorrhage was accomplished in all. Operative mortality in Child's C patients was 26.7% after emergency transthoracic esophageal transection. On the other hand, rate of early death within 30 days after emergency sclerotherapy was 14.6% and initial hemostasis was obtained in 92%.

In the elective situation, there was no early death in the sclerotherapy group while 4.4% died within 30 days postoperatively. The cumulative 5-year rebleeding rate in Groups I, II and III was 3.6, 20.1 and 28.6%, respectively (Fig. 2). Control of bleeding seemed most excellent in Group I. However, the difference was statistically not significant. In Group III, two thirds of bleeding episodes occurred during the first 6 months after the initial injection. After the end of the first year, incidence of hemorrhage decreased markedly (Fig. 2). Cumulative survival rate also seemed most excellent in Group I (Fig. 2). As the background of the patients was not uniform in each group, cumulative survival rate was compared between all surgical

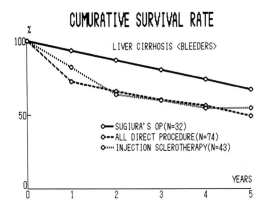

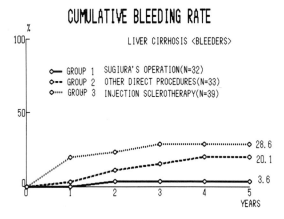

FIG. 2 Postoperative survival and rebleeding rates in the three study groups.

patients (Groups I + II) and Group III based on Child's classification. In Child's class A and B, there was no apparent difference, while in Child's class C the results of sclerotherapy seemed slightly more favorable than those of surgery. The difference was statistically not significant (Fig. 3).

The preliminary results of our prospective study indicated the same tendency shown by the retrospective one, that is, almost the same survival curves in both groups and better bleeding control in the surgical group (Fig. 4).

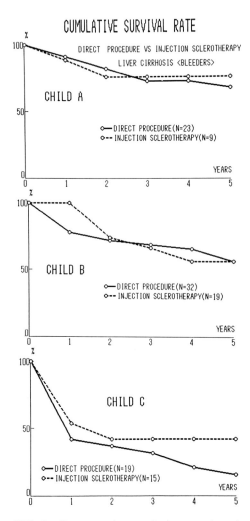

FIG. 3   Postoperative survival curves based on Child's classification.

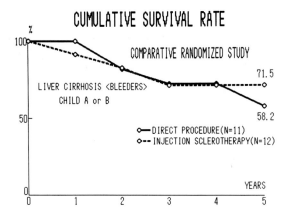

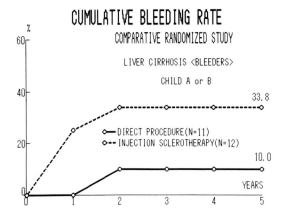

FIG. 4   Preliminary results of prospective study.

## Discussion

Reliability of direct interrupting surgery as the hemostatic procedure for bleeding esophageal varices is already well established [2 – 5]. As shown by the results of our retrospective study, variceal hemorrhage was most effectively controlled by Sugiura's esophageal transection if it was performed faithfully to Sugiura's original description [1], including both intrathoracic and abdominal devascularization. However, as it was a considerably major surgery for cirrhotic patients, two-staged operations were often necessary. Sometimes, abdominal devascularization had to be abandoned because of unfavorable postoperative course after the first thoracic procedure. In these cases, control of variceal hemorrhage remained unsatisfactory.

Endoscopic injection sclerotherapy is becoming more and more widely employed as a non-surgical approach to bleeding esophageal varices in Japan. Even though it is less hazardous and more easily tolerable for severely ill patients, controversies in results of recent randomized trials [6 – 8] indicate that true efficacy of this approach has to be established through further investigations.

In the series of our retrospective study, esophageal transection with thoracoabdominal devascularization showed the best results both in bleeding control and postoperative survival. Obviously, there was a distinct bias in the selection of patients into these groups. In Group I, a great majority of patients had already tolerated the first stage operation and, consequently, the ratio of Child's class C patients in this group was significantly lower than in the other two groups. Accordingly, the difference in survival rates might only be a reflection of the difference in the severity of liver disease among these groups. In fact, when the survival rates were compared between surgically and endoscopically treated patients based on Child's classification, no distinct difference was found between all three classes.

Regarding the control of rebleeding, the status of the hepatic function seemed not to be a major determinant factor. Rebleeding rate in Group II did not change even after patients in Child's class C were excluded (cumulative 5-year rebleeding rate in Child's A and B was 22.6% in Group II). The incidence of rebleeding after direct interrupting surgery tended to increase as postoperative time increased, while early rebleeding was more significant after sclerotherapy. Cumulative 5-year rebleeding rate of 3.6% in Group I was really excellent and could be attributed to more extended devascularization even if candidates for this procedure are somewhat limited to those patients with relatively favorable hepatic functional reserve.

In the management of emergency cases, results of sclerotherapy were considered satisfactory. As the estimation of hepatic functional reserve during acute bleeding is quite difficult, it is obviously desirable to reserve surgical treatment for the elective situation after the initial control of bleeding by sclerotherapy, if possible. Esophageal transection was performed in two cases without difficulty 2 months after sclerotherapy. When emergency sclerotherapy was not successful, the supplementary effect of Hassab's gastroesophageal devascularization was satisfactory.

The results of our retrospective study were not conclusive by any means as our series was too small and the follow-up period was not long enough. At least in terms of survival, results of both surgical and endoscopic treatment seemed almost equivalent. Preliminary results of the prospective study also showed the same tendency. This may imply that the patients' hepatic functional reserve is a more im-

TABLE 5   Current policy for the selection of the initial therapeutic approach

| Indication | Child's classification | | |
|---|---|---|---|
| | A | B | C |
| Prophylactic | ET | ET | IST |
| Elective | ET | ET | IST |
| Emergency | IST | IST | IST |
| Post-op. recurrence | IST | IST | IST |

ET, esophageal transection; IST, injection sclerotherapy

portant prognostic factor. However, direct attack surgery is thought to retain an important role in the management of bleeding varices in patients who can tolerate esophageal transection with extended devascularization without much difficulty, as high incidence of early rebleeding still remains a basic problem in sclerotherapy. To clarify the role of these two therapeutic modalities more exactly, further well-documented prospective studies are essential. As the conclusion of this study, our current policy in selecting primary approach to esophageal varices is summarized in Table 5. At present, in addition to comparative studies, it is essential to make every effort to improve the reliability of both modalities.

**Summary**

In order to assess the role of non-shunting surgery for bleeding esophageal varices, the results of direct interrupting operation and injection sclerotherapy for cirrhotic patients with bleeding varices are reviewed.

Operative mortality rate following emergency esophageal transection was 22.2% ($n = 27$), while 14.6% died within 30 days after emergency sclerotherapy. Cumulative 5-year survival rates including operative death in the surgical patients ($n = 74$) were 68.0% in Child's classification A ($n = 23$), 56.3% in Child's B ($n = 32$), and 15.8% in Child's C while those for the sclerotherapy patients ($n = 43$) were 76.2 ($n = 9$), 56.2 ($n = 19$) and 41.9% ($n = 15$), respectively. Cumulative 5-year rebleeding rates were 3.6% following esophageal transection with thoracoabdominal devascularization (Sugiura's procedure) and 28.6% after sclerotherapy.

At present, non-shunting surgery is considered advantageous for those patients who have relatively favorable hepatic functional reserve and can tolerate complete devascularization without difficulty. Sclerotherapy seems preferable in emergency situations and for Child's C patients.

**References**

1    Sugiura M, Futagawa S. A new technique for treating esophageal varices. J Thorac Cardiovasc Surg 1973; 66: 677 – 685.

2    Takano Y, Yoshida K, Honma K, Abe Y, Muto T. Esophageal transection combined with splenectomy and paraesophago-gastric devascularization for esophageal varices. Chir Gastroenterol 1978; 13: 21 – 27.

3    Johnston GW. Treatment of bleeding varices by oesophageal transection with the SPTU gun. Ann R Coll Surg Engl 1977; 59: 404 – 408.

4    Sugiura M, Futagawa S. Esophageal transection with paraesophago gastric devascularization (the Sugiura procedure) in the treatment of esophageal varices. World J Surg 1984; 8: 673 – 679.

5    Abouna GM, Baissony H, Menkarios A. The role of Sugiura operation for portal hypertension and bleeding varices. Surgery 1987; 101: 91 – 98.

6    Westaby D, MacDougall B, Williams R. Improved survival following injection sclerotherapy for esophageal varices: final analysis of a controlled trial. Hepatology 1985; 5: 827 – 830.

7    Korula J, Balart LA, Radvan G, et al. A prospective, randomized controlled trial of chronic esophageal variceal sclerotherapy. Hepatology 1985; 5: 584 – 589.

8    Soderlund C, Ihre T. Endoscopic sclerotherapy v. conservative management of bleeding esophageal varices: a 5-year prospective controlled trial of emergency and long term treatment. Acta Chir Scand 1985; 151: 449 – 456.

© 1988 Elsevier Science Publishers B.V. (Biomedical Division)
*Treatment of esophageal varices*
*Y. Idezuki, editor*

Chapter 20

# Selective variceal decompression by the distal splenorenal shunt: an Emory perspective 20 years later

J. Michael Henderson, William J. Millikan, Jr. and W. Dean Warren

*The Department of Surgery, Emory University School of Medicine, 1364 Clifton Road, N.E., Atlanta, GA 30322, U.S.A.*

Emory has made major contributions to the improvement in the management of patients with variceal bleeding over the past 15 years. The single greatest factor in this has been the evolution and study of selective variceal decompression by the distal splenorenal shunt (Fig. 1). This new operative method, which was originally presented by Drs Warren, Zeppa and Foman [1] in Miami in 1966 applied a pathophysiologic approach to the problem of variceal bleeding. Emory entered this arena in the early 1970s, beginning the first prospective randomized study conducted to compare selective and total shunts for variceal bleeding. However, the story is more complex than just an iteration of clinical trials. Rather, it tells of the evolution of a management method, with improvements in surgical technique, measurement of hemodynamic and metabolic consequences and finally careful follow-up of all patients. It has been the requirement to study the patients and quantitatively measure the effects of therapy that sets this work apart.

In this review we shall trace this progress through the format of a critical reappraisal of the most pertinent papers from Emory in each of the above main areas. The many participants who have been involved in this effort from Emory over the 15 years can be recognized from the title pages of the cardinal papers interspersed through the text. Finally, we shall comment on how far these papers are supported or refuted by comments on other data in the literature.

## 1. The beginning

*The initial paper on the distal splenorenal shunt was presented at the American Surgical Association in 1966, and published in the Annals of Surgery 1967 [1].*

This paper [1], one of the most cited papers in Index Medicus, is a surgical classic, marking the introduction of a new operative approach to an old problem. It traces

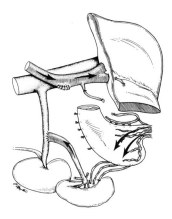

FIG. 1   Distal splenorenal shunt. Varices are decompressed via the short gastric veins, spleen, splenic vein to the left renal vein. Portal hypertension is maintained in the superior mesenteric and portal veins to maintan portal flow to the liver.

the reasoning that led to selective variceal decompression, gives experimental data in support of the concept, and presents the first patient data.

The paper starts by presenting the four main questions which gave cause for concern at that time.

**1.** What are the long-term results of portacaval shunt? Randomized studies [2 – 5] had clearly shown that while variceal bleeding could be prevented by total decompression of portal hypertension, survival was not improved. The accelerated rate of liver failure in portacaval shunt patients completely offset the advantage in bleeding control.

**2.** Would other major operative procedures accelerate hepatic failure comparably? Data at that time showed that non-shunt procedures did not accelerate liver failure [6]. In addition it was appreciated that total portal diversion was not entirely benign for the normal liver as reported by Mikkelsen et al. [7]. In 17 patients with idiopathic portal hypertension and good initial liver function, 10 developed encephalopathy and five died in hepatic coma after portacaval shunt.

**3.** Should 'non-shunting procedures' be used routinely? The advantage of maintaining hepatic function by this operative method was more than offset by a rebleeding rate of 40% [6]. This ineffectiveness reduced widespread application.

**4.** Should splanchnic hypertension be completely decompressed? The main advantage documented for complete splanchnic decompression was improvement in ascites. A disadvantage which had been documented was an accelerated ammonia absorption following successful total shunt in patients with portal hypertension [8]. This factor may play a role in encephalopathy.

The summation and discussion of these questions led to the following conclusion: "Ideally, an operation should allow continued perfusion of hepatic parenchyma by portal blood flow from the intenstine and yet decompress the venous system in the gastroesophageal area.''

Experimental dog studies supported the concept that the spleen may serve as an outflow tract for the fundus of the stomach under conditions of venous hypertension. Reversal of flow in the short gastric veins was documented by xenon studies from the gastric fundus to the spleen following distal splenorenal shunt. Shunt patency was documented for at least 3 months in these studies. Feasibility was demonstrated.

The clinical data in this initial paper encompassed both the operative technique and case reports. We shall return to the operative method in the next section when we examine its overall evolution. Six patients were presented in this initial paper. DSRS was achieved in four of these patients, while the other two had devascularization procedures. Two of the DSRS patients died from postoperative complications, but had patent shunts. The other two shunt patients had patent distal splenorenal shunts with bleeding control, good prograde portal flow in one, to-fro portal flow in the portal vein in the other, and well maintained protein tolerance.

The specific objectives of distal splenorenal shunt as stated in this original publication were:

(1) selective reduction of pressure and volume of flow through gastroesophageal veins;
(2) maintain portal venous perfusion of the liver;
(3) maintain continual venous hypertension in the intestinal bed.

These three objectives had formed a basis for much subsequent work. It must be remembered that at the time when this paper was first presented it was not known (i) if variceal bleeding would be effectively controlled or (ii) if portal flow to the liver could be maintained *at all* in the presence of a shunt adequate to prevent gastroesophageal variceal bleeding.

Let us trace the evolution from this beginning.

## 2. The operative technique

*The method of DSRS was summarized and illustrated in a paper in Contemporary Surgery 1981 [9].*

### Technical principles

The evolution in operative technique of DSRS has at all times kept in focus the originally stated goals of, first, providing adequate transsplenic variceal decompression to control bleeding and, second, maximing portal flow to the liver to maintain hepatocyte function.

This paper embodies the main points in operative technique and illustrates the basic operative steps of DSRS. These are shown in Fig. 2. The venous anatomy is converted from A to J, creating a low pressure transsplenic drainage route, but maintaining a high pressure splanchnic/hepatic axis.

208

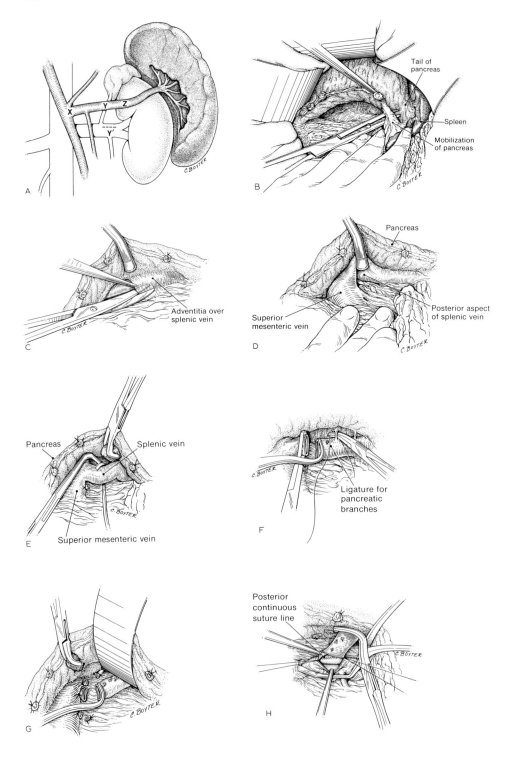

Tail of
pancreas

Spleen

Mobilization
of pancreas

A

B

Adventitia over
splenic vein

C

Pancreas

Superior
mesenteric vein

Posterior aspect
of splenic vein

D

Pancreas          Splenic vein

Superior mesenteric vein

E

Ligature for
pancreatic
branches

F

G

Posterior
continuous
suture line

H

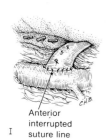

Anterior
interrupted
suture line
I

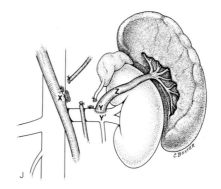

FIG. 2   The principle operative steps of DSRS. Steps A – J are described in the text.

The principle technical points of emphasis are the following:

**1.** The pancreas is approached through the lesser sac, with the additional take-down of the splenic flexure to improve access to the retropancreatic plane. This latter move has the extra advantage of dividing a major collateral pathway which develops to the inferior ramus of the splenic vein. This approach differs from the original method of pancreatic mobilization which was done below the mesocolon. We now only utilize the infra-mesocolic approach in patients in whom the lesser sac is obliterated from previous surgery or pancreatitis.

**2.** Mobilization of the pancreas. The most common error in performing DSRS is failure to adequately mobilize the pancreas. The whole gland should be mobilized along its inferior border from the superior mesenteric vein to the splenic hilus. It is rotated cephalad to allow dissection of the splenic vein out of the pancreas. Failure of adequate mobilization leads to improper and incomplete dissection of the splenic vein.

**3.** Dissection of the splenic vein (C – G). The main principles of this phase are: first, dissect the vein on the vein; second, dissect the posterior surface before the anterior surface; third, control the splenic and superior mesenteric vein junction. Finally, it is important to dissect sufficient vein from the pancreas to make certain it comes down to the renal vein without kinking. Current modification (see below) extends this dissection out to the splenic hilus. The key to the whole procedure lies in accurate identification and ligation of the pancreatic perforating veins as they enter the splenic vein. The above principles help in achieving this goal.

**4.** The anastomosis. This should be performed without tension or kinking of the splenic vein. Typically, the anastomosis lies just in front of the ligated adrenal vein on the left renal vein. The posterior wall is sewn with a continuous suture, while interrupted sutures complete the anterior wall. This avoids a pursestring effect and allows the anastomosis to enlarge.

**5.** Portal-splenic disconnection. This final phase of the operative procedure, while initially recognized as important, has undergone considerable modification in the past few years in an attempt to better achieve its purpose. First, the coronary

210

venous system is disconnected by identifying and ligating the coronary vein, both as it leaves the portal (or splenic) vein, and also in its suprapancreatic portion as it approaches the lesser curvature of the stomach. Second, the pancreatic tributaries which remain connected to the splenic vein will enlarge over time (see below) and open a major portaprival pathway. This pancreatic siphon (Fig. 3) is a major venous bridge between the high pressure portal and low pressure splenic veins. Complete disconnection of the splenic vein from the pancreas can prevent this problem and is a currently recommended component of the disconnection phase (Fig. 4). Finally, major pathways from the portal to splenic vein can develop along the mesocolon. These, on study, have been found to have a single final common pathway through the splenocolic ligament into the inferior ramus of the splenic vein. Taking down

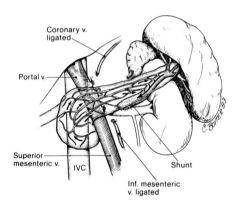

FIG. 3  The pancreatic siphon. Following standard DSRS major venous channels form from the high pressure portal vein to low pressure splenic vein. In this way *all* pancreatic venous drainage is to the shunt.

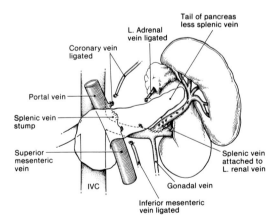

FIG. 4  DSRS with splenopancreatic disconnection. This modification improves the selectivity of variceal decompression.

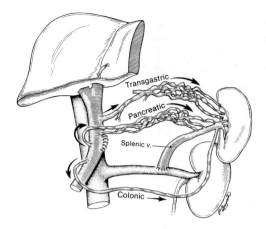

FIG. 5 Collateral pathways which develop from the high pressure portal vein to low pressure splenic vein after DSRS.

the splenic flexure of the colon at surgery effectively disconnects this pathway. These three major collateral routes are illustrated in Fig. 5.

*Comment*

The two distinct phases of the operation are the shunt itself, and the isolation of the low pressure variceal drainage from maintained portal hypertension. Figures 6 and 7 illustrate angiographically these two phases, with the conversion of the splenic vein to the variceal outflow track to the cava, and the maintenance of prograde portal flow to the liver. What changes have occurred over time with each of these phases?

The shunt has been found to control bleeding in most experience in over 90% of patients [10]. Failure to control bleeding is usually secondary to a technical failure. What lessons have been learned? First, shunt occlusion, if it is going to occur, happens early. For this reason we advocate catheterization of all shunts at 1 week with pressure measurement in the splenic vein, left renal vein and inferior vena cava. Unexpected shunt occlusion at this time may be surgically corrected. Late thrombosis, in a shunt demonstrated to have been open at one week, is exceedingly uncommon (< 1%). Rebleeding from varices may occasionally be seen in patients with a patent DSRS (5 – 10%), with the first post-operative month being the high risk time for this complication [11]. The postulated mechanism is an initially inadequate outflow track for the varices, which may occur as renal vein hypertension (renal vein to cava gradient > 10 mmHg) or possibly an inadequate short gastric outflow. Management of bleeding after DSRS should initially document shunt patency by angiography, and then treat the patient expectantly, with blood transfusion, pitressin and sclerotherapy if necessary. The pressure gradient will resolve over 4 – 6 weeks as alternative pathways open and perioperative edema subsides.

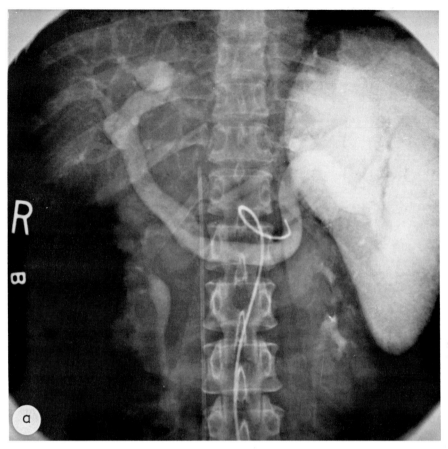

FIG. 6 (a) Venous phase of splenic arteriogram in a patient with portal hypertension prior to DSRS. The splenic vein is clearly visualized with contrast passing into the portal vein and liver. (b) The same study after DSRS shows contrast passing into the left renal vein and inferior vena cava.

An alternative operative method which circumvents the problem of renal vein hypertension is direct splenocaval anastomosis. This may be particularly useful in (a) patients with a very large spleen, in whom the enormous extra flow into the left renal vein might be anticipated to give increased venous pressure and (b) in patients with abnormal left renal vein, particularly retro-aortic, in whom the renal vein may not be an adequate outflow tract. Technically, this variant requires anastomosis to the infra renal inferior vena cava in a manner similar to that already described.

Alternative methods of performing DSRS have been advocated [12 – 14]. The common denominator to most of these is an attempt to minimize dissection of the splenic vein from the pancreas. While a shunt *can* be achieved by such alternatives, we believe most of them represent inadequate operations within the overall purposes because they fall short of an adequate disconnection of the shunt from the portal system.

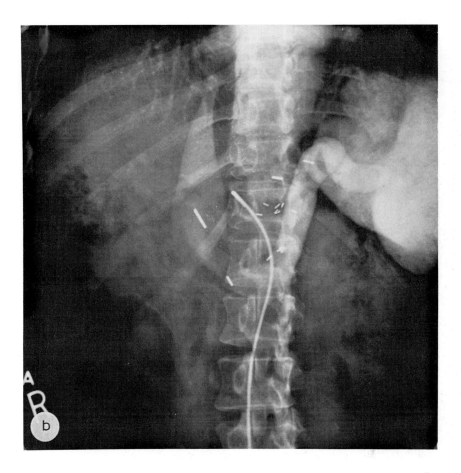

Disconnection of the gastro/splenic/shunt pathway from the splanchnic/hepatic axis is the operative area of greatest controversy and change. The Emory group's stance is clear: every effort should be made to maximize and maintain prograde portal flow. This is best achieved by an aggressive interruption of the major venous bridges which tend to develop from the high pressure portal vein to low pressure splenic vein after DSRS (Fig. 4). The major steps of coronary, pancreatic and colonic disconnection have already been outlined.

Support for this aggressive surgical approach comes from Dr. Inockuchi and his group [15]. Their demonstration of 'portal malcirculation' after standard DSRS, led to their introduction of a 'splenic hilar, renal shunt' which has now been modified to an entire pancreatic disconnection similar to that described. Improved maintenance of portal perfusion, and lessening of portaprival collaterals has been shown. In this setting, portal hypertension is required to maintain a sufficient head of pressure to perfuse the cirrhotic liver.

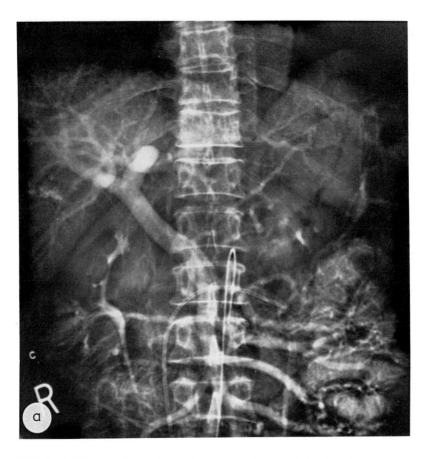

FIG. 7 (a) Venous phase of superior mesenteric artery injection clearly shows prograde portal venous flow. A small coronary vein is also visualized. (b) The same study after DSRS shows the ideal maintenance of prograde portal flow with no collateral formation.

Dissent as to the necessity [16] or feasibility [17] of such separation of high and low pressure systems can be found in the literature. While some collateralization is inevitable, some pathways (e.g., the pancreatic) are more associated with loss of portal flow. This is addressed further in Section 7. If one accepts the premise, and data, that maintaining portal flow is good for the liver, then why accept second best rather than go for improvement?

Continued careful studies, by angiography and quantitative assessment, are ongoing in patients being treated by the evolving operative methods. Early data has shown improved maintenance of portal flow using the newer methods [18]. Continued study and follow up is required to demonstrate whether or not this will lead to improved survival.

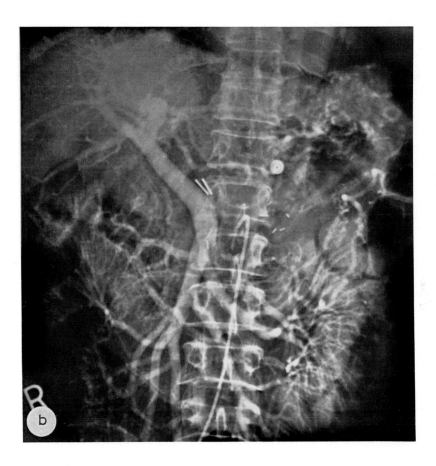

## CLINICAL EXPERIENCE WITH DSRS

### 3. Experience from non-randomized series

*The first 10 years of DSRS at Emory provided data on 348 DSRSs. This was presented at the Southern Surgical Association in 1981 and published in Annals of Surgery 1982 [19].*

This paper reports the largest consecutive series of DSRS in the literature, and summarizes the first 10 years of the Emory experience. Over that time the first prospective randomized trial was initiated, and 55 patients were entered into a study comparing DSRS to total shunt: this is presented in more detail below. Apart from this randomized study a further 322 DSRS and 128 total shunts were performed for variceal bleeding.

The patient groups undergoing DSRS and total shunts in this overall experience were not comparable. A higher proportion of emergency operations for uncontrolled variceal bleeding were total portal systemic shunts. This can be appreciated from the overall survival curves of this paper (Fig. 8) which shows the much higher im-

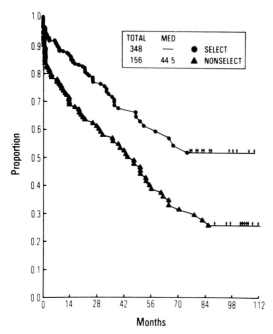

FIG. 8   Survival analysis of all DSRS (●) and total shunts (▲) at Emory 1971 – 1981.

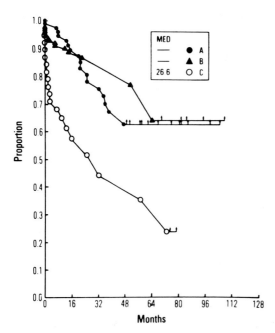

FIG. 9   Survival by Child's class for DSRS. Child's A and B have similar survival, which is significantly ($P < 0.01$) better than Child's C patients.

mediate mortality of the total shunt group. However, even when survival is analysed, excluding operative mortality, the divergence of the DSRS and total shunt curves
can be appreciated. The focus of this paper is on DSRS, so let us emphasize the pertinent lessons learned from this 10 year experience as regards this procedure.

The overall operative mortality for the 348 DSRSs was 4.1% and the 5 year survival was 59%. However, two important facets of that survival pattern were observed which differed markedly from that previously seen for total shunts. First, the
long-term survival of Child's Class A and B patients was identical, both being
significantly better than Child's C patients (Fig. 9). Second, patients with non-
alcoholic liver disease had significantly ($P < 0.05$) improved survival compared to
those with alcoholic cirrhosis (Fig. 10).

Bleeding control was > 90%, with an angiographic documented early shunt
patency rate of 93%. Late shunt occlusion was extremely rare, and was only
documented in two patients. Portal perfusion was retained in 93% of patients at
7 – 10 days follow-up angiography, but was not systematically examined in this
population at late follow-up.

Finally, the importance of maintained portal flow in preventing encephalopathy
was emphasized in this report, with an illustrative case report of how restoration of
portal flow can reverse encephalopathy.

### Comment

How far are the principle observations of this major review supported by other data
in the literature?

Over the past 20 years at least 30 centers have now reported data on the DSRS
[20]. The pertinent points are summarized in Table 1. Not every paper has reported
all the listed parameters, but the following generalizations hold. (a) Good to

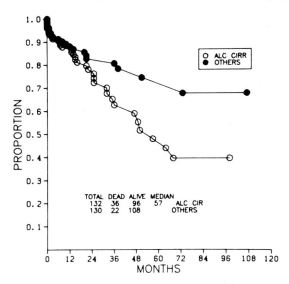

FIG. 10   Survival analysis after DSRS for nonalcoholic (●) and alcoholic (○) liver disease.
Survival is significantly ($P < 0.05$) improved for non-alcoholic patients.

moderate risk patients have been operated on with an acceptable mortality and good bleeding control. **(b)** Long-term survival has governed more by severity of liver disease than by the operation. **(c)** Quality of life is significantly improved in most reports compared to what the authors had previously found with total shunts. Encephalopathy rates were low and, if present, this complication was usually relatively easily controlled.

The specific observation of the improved survival in patients with non-alcoholic compared to alcoholic cirrhosis has not been uniformly seen in other series. First, the original report of this advantage to non-alcoholics came from Zeppa et al. [21] in 1979 when the Miami group reported 85% 5 year survival in non-alcoholic patients after DSRS. This was initially ascribed to the particularly good risk, stable post-hepatitic patients seen by that group, but the observation in the current group of patients, 30% of whom required steroids for chronic hepatitis, suggests a real phenomenon. However, three other papers [22 – 24] which have analysed this variable have not found significant differences. In two of these reports [23, 24] the small number of patients may well have contributed to this, while in the third report [22] from the Mayo Clinic the survival in patients with alcoholic cirrhosis (60% at 5 years) approaches the survival we achieved in non-alcoholic disease. Our assessment at this time is that survival after DSRS in patients with non-alcoholic liver disease is significantly better than for those with alcoholic cirrhosis.

Bleeding control has been good in all other non-randomized reported series with > 90% control. We would emphasize the greatest risk time for rebleeding is in the first postoperative month, a time when technical failure or initial inadequate decompression may play a role. A paper from Michigan [11] recently reemphasized this point, and again affirmed the importance of early accurate angiographic assessment of the DSRS.

The question of maintained portal flow after DSRS is the most controversial issue, and will be addressed fully below in the section on hemodynamics. However, as a brief aside, the importance of prograde flow as the dominant factor in preventing hepatic encephalopathy in some patients is emphasized in the current paper. The Miami group [25] have also pointed out that encephalopathy after DSRS should be fully evaluated, which should include angiography. A correctable cause such as

TABLE 1   Summary of reported worldwide experience with DSRS from 30 centers

| | |
|---|---|
| Number of patients | > 1000 |
| Etiology | 60% alcoholic cirrhosis |
| | 40% non-alcoholic etiology |
| Child's class | A = 46% |
| | B = 40% |
| | C = 14% |
| Operative mortality | 9% (range 1 – 19%) |
| Survival rates | 3 year, 60 – 75% |
| | 5 year, 50 – 60% |
| Shunt patency | 90% |
| Encephalopathy | 10% (range 0 – 18%) |

a large collateral pathway may be found which can be embolized angiographically or interrupted surgically. Other reports of operative [25] and radiologic [26] intervention to restore portal perfusion in patients with encephalopathy have had dramatic success in some cases [26], but must be tempered with the risk of major intervention in others [25].

## EXPERIENCE WITH RANDOMIZED TRIALS

### 4. DSRS versus total Shunts

*The final report of Emory's prospective randomized study, comparing DSRS to total portal systemic shunt, was presented at the Southern Surgical Association in 1984, and published in Annals of Surgery 1985 [28].*

This paper reports the ten year follow-up to the first Emory randomized study for the management of variceal bleeding [28]. This study compared DSRS to total portal systemic shunt, either mesocaval or mesorenal. It is the third major paper on this trial, with earlier reports appearing in 1976 [29] and 1978 [30]. This study entered 55 patients with variceal bleeding secondary to cirrhosis between 1971 and 1975. All patients were Child's class A or B and 73% had alcoholic cirrhosis. DSRS was done in 26 patients and total shunt in 29 patients. The outcome and status of all patients entered was known over the ten years of follow-up. This group has been extensively studied on a longitudinal basis with respect to survival, bleeding control, hemodynamics, quantitative hepatic function and encephalopathy.

The first of these parameters to show a significant improvement in the DSRS group was hepatic encephalopathy. In the initial report of this trial [29] only one of 22 at risk patients in the DSRS group, as opposed to 10 of 24 in the total shunt group, had developed encephalopathy. This was significant ($P < 0.005$) and was the major factor leading to cessation of patient entry into that trial with only 55 patients entered. Improved maintenance of hepatic function was also documented at that in-

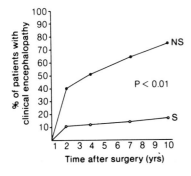

FIG. 11   Encephalopathy after total shunt (NS) continues to increase over time, and is significantly ($P < 0.01$) more common than after DSRS (S).

itial report [29], with better urea synthesis rate in the DSRS group. This significantly lower incidence of encephalopathy was been maintained in the DSRS group at all time points of evaluation (Fig. 11).

Late occlusion of mesocaval and mesorenal shunts was an unanticipated occurrence, which in the latter years has complicated the analysis of this study. These operative procedures were chosen at the initation of this study because of prevailing opinion at that time that they were the best 'total shunt' alternative. The documented occlusion rate of nine such shunts in this study (31%) is in keeping with our larger experience [31]. These shunt occlusions have been associated with variceal rebleeding in four patients, leading to the death of two of these patients. Equally important, in terms of data analysis, has been the associated restoration of prograde portal perfusion which has been documented in four patients with shunt occlusion. This has had a profound effect on hepatic function at later follow-up. When analysed by the originally randomized groups there was no significant difference in quantitative function at late follow-up but, as shown in Table 2 there was a significant advantage to DSRS at all time intervals when analysis is based on patients with patent shunts.

Portal perfusion has been well maintained in the DSRS group: 14 of 16 patients at 1 – 2 years, nine of 12 at 4 years, nine of 11 at 7 years and six of eight at 10 years. A possible factor contributing to this high percentage maintaining portal flow is the increased survival of non-alcoholics (five of eight randomized patients at 10 years) in the DSRS group. This variable is discussed in more detail in Section 7. In contrast, all patients with patent total shunts have had no prograde portal flow at any time point.

The disappointing feature of this study is that, despite the significant advantages of DSRS as outlined above, there has been no significant difference in survival between the two groups at any time interval (Fig. 12).

*Comment*

This study is one of six prospective randomized clinical trials which has evaluated

TABLE 2  Quantitative liver function in randomized study of DSRS versus total shunt

| | GEC (mg/min) | | |
| --- | --- | --- | --- |
| | 3 – 4 Years | 7 Years | 10 Years |
| 1. Selective (patent) | 321 ± 86(12)[a] | 345 ± 87(10) | 316 ± 91 (8) |
| 2. Non-selective (patent) | 256 ± 68(12) | 253 ± 64(4) | 259 ± 50(4) |
| 3. Non-selective (occluded) | 315 ± 82(2) | 367 ± 143(4) | 312 ± 67(4) |
| 1 vs. 2 | < 0.05 | < 0.05 | < 0.05 |
| 1 vs. 3 | > 0.1 | > 0.1 | > 0.1 |
| 2 vs. 3 | > 0.1 | > 0.1 | > 0.1 |

[a] No. of patients studied.

DSRS versus total portalsystemic shunts in the past 12 years [32 – 36]. The consistent finding in all studies is that survival was not improved in the DSRS groups. While this is a clearcut endpoint, and presents the most definitive data, it must be viewed in the light of the patients entered into study. The practicing physician must ask himself the question, were the patients in this study recognizably similar to his own? Data from one study population cannot be applied to another. Thus, in the context of the current randomized studies, 87% of the patients entered had alcoholic cirrhosis and, as we have already shown, survival patterns vary by disease etiology. Standard DSRS has not shown improved survival in randomized study compared to total shunts in patients with variceal bleeding secondary to *alcoholic* cirrhosis. No conclusions can be drawn in non-alcoholic populations because of insufficient data.

The data on encephalopathy and quality of survival in these studies is conflicting. Three of the studies have shown a significantly lower encephalopathy rate in the DSRS group [28, 32, 33] while the other three have shown no significant difference [34 – 36]. These discrepancies may arise for several reasons. First, what is the natural history for occurrence of encephalopathy in the population studied? For example, in one study [36] the high incidence of encephalopathy (39%) in the DSRS group may be largely due to a 100% alcoholic population with a high rate of returning to drinking. Such a population may develop encephalopathy due to progression of their liver disease regardless of any shunt. Second, how good was the surgery, and were the pathophysiologic goals achieved? In the context of DSRS, two of the studies [35, 36] present data which suggests an inadequate portal splenic disconnection was performed. Large portaprival collaterals can contribute to encephalopathy after DSRS. Full investigation of patients who develop encephalopathy, including angiography, should be done as a correctable cause may be found [25, 37].

Bleeding control has been similar in five of these studies, with an overall 9.4% rebleeding rate, and this is similar to the larger reported non-randomized series. One study [36], however, showed a 30% variceal rebleeding rate, which is somewhat at variance with the other reports. This study does perhaps, however, emphasize the importance of adequate training in the overall management of these patients, and also in the specifics of surgical training for shunt operations. An excessively high rebleeding rate suggests technical failure [37].

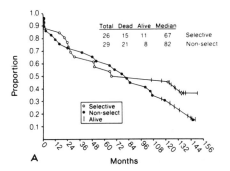

FIG. 12   Survival analysis of the Emory prospective trial of DSRS (○) versus total shunts (●) shows no significant difference in survival at any time point.

222

## 5. DSRS versus endoscopy sclerotherapy

*The initial report of Emory's prospective randomized study, comparing DSRS and endoscopic variceal sclerosis, was presented at Southern Surgical Association in 1985, and published in Annals of Surgery 1986 [38].*

This paper reports the preliminary results of a prospective randomized trial comparing DSRS and endoscopic variceal sclerosis in the management of patients with cirrhosis and variceal bleeding [38]. The entry of 71 patients between 1981 and 1985 shows an exact 10 year time lag from the initial randomized trial to which the DSRS was submitted. The conduct of this trial emphasizes two important points. First, the commitment of the Emory portal hypertension group to conduct such studies. Prospective randomized clinical trials, carefully designed and conducted, offer the best method for testing management methods. Second, it reflects the change in world opinion as to optimum management methods for variceal bleeding. The resurgence of interest in sclerotherapy had brought this widely applicable therapy to the fore by the early 1980s, such that the most pertinent question in prevention of recurrent variceal bleeding was the comparative roles of DSRS or sclerosis. This study addresses this question.

Seventy-one patients were entered following stabilization of their acute variceal bleed. All had full evaluation prior to randomization. Forty patients were Child's Class A or B, and 31 Child's C. Forty-three patients had alcoholic cirrhosis and 28 non-alcoholic cirrhosis. Thirty-five patients were randomized to DSRS and 36 to sclerosis. Surgery was by the methods described and was done within one week of randomization in all but one patient, who developed non-A/non-B hepatitis and died without being shunted. Sclerosis was done by two gastroenterologists using the flexible endoscope, a combination of intra- and para-variceal injection, with initial and subsequent sessions one week apart, then monthly to obliteration, with follow-up sessions as clinically indicated. No patients have been lost to follow-up.

Figure 13 shows the survival curves at median follow-up of 26 months. The 2 year survival of the sclerosis group (84%) is significantly ($P < 0.01$) better than the

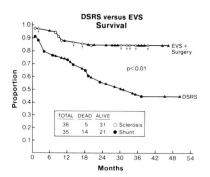

FIG. 13  Survival analysis for DSRS (●) and sclerotherapy (○) shows significantly ($P < 0.01$) improved survival at 2 years in the sclerotherapy group *provided* surgical salvage is achieved for the 30% who fail sclerosis.

DSRS group (59%). It should be noted that the 31 patients in the sclerosis group survivors include eight patients who failed sclerosis treatment and required surgical intervention to stop bleeding. It, therefore, is a composite survival of sclerosis plus surgery for failures of that therapy.

Rebleeding occurred significantly ($P < 0.05$) more frequently in the sclerosis group (19 of 36:53%) compared to the DSRS group (1 of 35:3%), but only 11 of 36 patients (31%) failed sclerosis because of uncontrolled rebleeding. These patients required surgery, which was achieved with good salvage (8 of 11). Figure 14 shows the curves when analysed by failure of therapy, and there is no significant difference in these curves. Obviously, the crux lies in defining 'failure of sclerotherapy', which in this study was defined as the inability to control recurrent portal hypertensive gastroesophageal bleeding despite repeated attempts. This decision required the concurrence of the sclerosing gastroenterologist and hepatologist who believed that the patient's life was threatened by withholding surgical therapy. The number or severity of rebleeding episodes per se did not define failure.

Other data collected during this study shows important differences between these therapies. First, portal perfusion was significantly ($P < 0.05$) better maintained in the sclerosis (93%) compared to the DSRS group (53%). Quantitative hepatocyte function, measured by the galactose elimination capacity, was significantly ($P <$

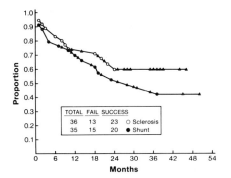

FIG. 14   Plot of failure of therapy for sclerosis (○) and DSRS (●) shows no difference by randomized study. However, the majority of sclerosis failures had rebleeding (11 patients) requiring surgery while the majority of DSRS failures died (14 patients).

TABLE 3   Quantitative liver function at 1 year in randomized DSRS versus sclerosis study

|  | n | GEC (mg/min) | |
|---|---|---|---|
|  |  | Pre-randomization | 1 year |
| DSRS | 17 | 323 ± 110 | 287 ± 78 |
| EVS | 21 | 306 ± 66 | 356 ± 82[a] |

[a] $P < 0.01$.

0.05) improved at 1 year in 21 patients in the sclerosis group successfully treated by that therapy. Furthermore, galactose elimination capacity (GEC) was significantly ($P < 0.01$) better maintained in the sclerosis group compared to the DSRS group (Table 3).

Liver volume showed a similar and significant ($P < 0.05$) reduction in both groups at 1 year, and probably reflects the natural history of cirrhosis in these patients. The hemodynamic parameters of cardiac output and effective liver blood flow showed no change in either group and no significantly different pattern between groups at 1 year. The conclusions from this study at this preliminary report are thus:

(1) survival can be significantly improved in patients with cirrhosis and variceal bleeding managed by sclerotherpy, provided surgical back-up is available for uncontrolled bleeding;

(2) the rebleeding rate through sclerosis is 53% at 2 years, with 31% failing that therapy because of uncontrolled bleeding;

(3) hepatic function is significantly better maintained in patients successfully managed by sclerosis compared to those managed by DSRS.

*Comment*

The place of sclerotherapy in the overall management of patients with variceal bleeding is the most pertinent issue in this whole field at this time. The current paper is the first major contribution in defining the relative roles of sclerosis and DSRS in elective management. To put this in perspective let us briefly review and define the current role of sclerotherapy as indicated by other studies.

Sclerosis of varices was first introduced in 1939 [39], but did not gain much acceptance at that time because of the re-introduction of portal systemic shunts shortly thereafter [40]. It was the prevailing opinion at the time that shunts would control bleeding, and thus take care of the problem. It took time for the fact to be recognized that such operations simply altered the mode of death from bleeding to hepatic failure, and did not improve survival [2 – 4]. In the past 5 years over 500 papers have been published in the medical literature on sclerotherapy of varices [41]. The floodgates have opened, but from this abundance of publications what does the 'good' data show?

Sclerosis has the advantages of wide applicability and relative simplicity. Passage of an endoscope, visualization of varices and injection of sclerosant can be performed by most gastroenterologists or hepatologists. Thus a clear definition of its role, with benefits and limitations clearly defined, is of paramount importance in improving the worldwide management of patients with variceal bleeding.

Acute variceal bleeding can be stopped by sclerosis. The cessation of bleeding, with the visible evidence through the endoscope as a column of blood which stops flowing, is a dramatic sight which anyone with an interest in this problem should see. While instinct tells us that this action should be in the patient's best interest, data is hard to come by. Only one randomized study [42] has shown that survival is improved by emergent sclerotherapy for active bleeding. Other studies [43, 44] have shown a decreased frequency of rebleeding, but not improved survival. This points to the influence of other factors, particularly the underlying liver disease, in determining outcome.

Prevention of recurrent bleeding by sclerotherapy has been shown to significantly improve survival when compared to standard medical therapy. The report from King's College in London was the first prospective randomized trial of any therapy for the prevention of recurrent variceal bleeding to show a significant improvement in survival in a treatment limb [45, 46]. Two other important facts emerged from this trial. First, the rebleeding rate was 55%, most occurring prior to variceal obliteration. Second, the complication rate was 42%, with esophageal ulcers and stricture most common. A further study in schistosomiasis showed improved survival in the sclerosis group [47]. However, Terblanche and co-workers [48] found no difference in survival in their randomized study.

Two clinical trials have addressed the role of acute followed by chronic sclerosis, with randomization at the time of admission for acute bleeding. Cello and his associates [49] compared sclerotherapy and emergency portacaval shunt in Child's C patients with alcoholic cirrhosis and variceal bleeding. Survival, which was poor, was not significantly different between groups. The Copenhagen combined study [50] compared sclerosis to standard medical management and, while showing an improved long-term survival in the sclerosis group, showed similar early rebleeding and mortality.

Where does the current trial fit into this broader picture? First, it clearly shows that, at 2 years, survival can be significantly improved in cirrhotic patients initially treated with sclerotherapy and in whom surgical 'salvage' is available for the one third in whom bleeding is not controlled. The survival curve in the current study for the sclerosis group (84% at 2 years) is the best survival achieved in any such study, and this is a population with 44% Child's Class C patients.

A second major finding in this study, which has not previously been reported is that hepatic function can improve significantly in patients having sclerotherapy. In the context of overall patient management two factors, bleeding control and hepatic failure, must be balanced. Sclerosis while having a significant rebleeding rate gives improvement in that balance by lessening the risk of hepatic failure. The important question raised by the current study, and not yet defined, is what constitutes a sclerosis failure? If this could be clearly defined, the data presented indicates that sclerosis should be initial management of this patient population, backed up by DSRS for sclerosis failures.

## 6. DSRS in portal vein thrombosis

*The pathophysiology of portal vein thrombosis, and rationale for DSRS, was presented at the American Surgical Association in 1980 and published in Annals of Surgery 1980 [51].*

This paper addresses the pathophysiology of noncirrhotic portal vein thrombosis, and the rationale behind DSRS being the optimum treatment method for patients with this problem who have had variceal bleeding [51].

Portal hypertension and variceal bleeding in this population had long been recognized to have a better prognosis than bleeding in patients with cirrhosis. A normal liver, with good function, was recognized as the key differentiating factor.

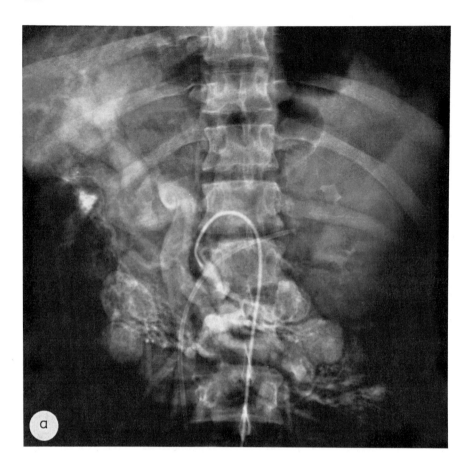

However, controversy existed over the role of total portal systemic shunts in this population. The advocates of total decompression reasoned that **(a)** this population was already deprived of portal flow by their portal vein thrombosis, and **(b)** they did not develop encephalopathy after such procedures. Data refuting these two contentions is presented in this paper.

Radiologic findings were presented in four patients with this diagnosis before and after DSRS. In all patients cavernous transformation of the portal vein clearly results in perfusion of intrahepatic portal veins in all patients pre- and postoperatively. Figure 15 shows this observation in one of these patients on both pre- and post-DSRS study. As pointed out in this paper, the importance of these hepatopetal portal collateral veins was recognized in Pawlow's classic paper of 1893 [52]. In his discussion of the Eck fistula animal, he clearly points out the critical factors. First, animals who did well after an Eck fistula had regained portal flow to the liver. Second, this flow was delivered by a collateral venous network of previously undescribed veins. Third, these collaterals only developed when the anastomosis was closed, or almost closed, and the obstructed high pressure portal vein formed collaterals to normal low pressure hepatic sinusoids. These observations of Pawlow

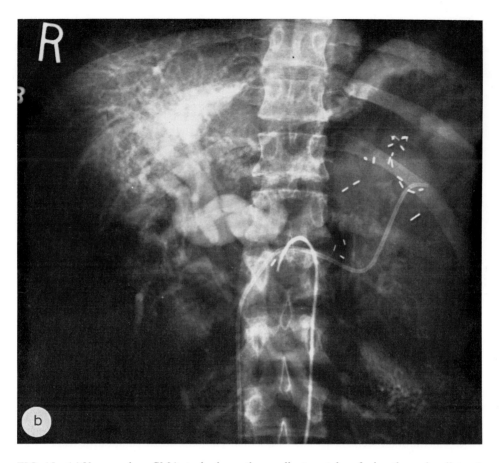

FIG. 15 (a) Venous phase SMA study shows the excellent portal perfusion through collateral varices prior to DSRS in a patient with a normal liver and portal vein thrombosis. (b) The pattern is unchanged after DSRS.

apply directly to the problem of non-cirrhotic portal vein thrombosis in man.

The two other patients presented in this paper had undergone total shunts, one central splenorenal and one cavo-mesenteric, 21 and 8 years previously. In neither patient was there any angiographic evidence of continued prograde portal perfusion through cavernous transformation. The first patient, whose liver had been deprived of portal flow for 21 years had severe incapacitating encephalopathy. She could tolerate no more than 10−20 g of protein per day. Fasting ammonia levels consistently ran 140 $\mu$g/dl, with post-prandial levels up to 500 $\mu$g/dl. EEG showed the classic changes of a metabolic encephalopathy. Ligation of her splenorenal shunt resulted in restoration of prograde portal perfusion. After an initial withdrawal-like syndrome, her mental state improved dramatically. Protein tolerance increased to 100 g/day, and fasting ammonia fell to 50 $\mu$g/dl. Her EEG improved, but did not return entirely to normal. This case clearly demonstrated that encephalopathy *can* develop in such patients, with a normal liver and in the absence of cirrhosis. Further, it showed that portal perfusion was the vital factor in this complication. As a single case it makes a potent argument for attempting to maintain portal flow in such patients.

*Comment*

Since the publication of the above paper, we have subsequently reviewed a series of 32 patients which was our total experience with such patients up to 1984 [53]. Fifteen of these patients had undergone splenectomy prior to referral and emphasize a major management error in this population. In most cases splenectomy had been performed for splenomegaly and hypersplenism, and this error had deprived these patients of their chance of definitive therapy. This subset had a significantly greater risk of rebleeding from varices despite further surgery (devascularization) and/or sclerosis. In contrast, 13 of the 17 patients referred with their spleen 'in situ' had DSRS with only a single transient rebleeding episode in one patient. DSRS will not only prevent recurrent variceal bleeding, but will also result in significant reduction in spleen size [53] and improvement in platelet count [53, 54]. The thrombocytopenia seen in these patients is more alarming to the physician than dangerous to the patient, and therapy *must* be directed at complete patient management rather than a single hematologic index.

Further data in this paper [53] documents a reduced, but stable, liver volume in this population. In addition, quantitative liver function is normal per unit liver size, as are hemodynamic parameters. An additional observation is that, at angiography, these patients do not develop major collateral pathways to their splenic vein and shunt like patients with cirrhosis, but appear to continue to favor collateral formation to the liver.

Published data from other centers [55 – 57] has also documented the efficacy of DSRS in the management of such patients. They are ideal candidates for DSRS: bleeding is controlled and, with a normal liver, they have a normal life expectancy.

Schistosomiasis is a major health problem in some parts of the world which makes it the commonest cause of variceal bleeding in such endemic areas. While Emory has no direct experience with such patients, participation of Faculty and training of Fellows has introduced DSRS into the treatment options in the Middle East and China. Since the pathology in this disease is a portal hypertension from a presinusoidal block with preservation of normal lobular architecture and hepatocellular function, it seemed appropriate to make a brief comment on DSRS in this population at this point.

A recent review from Egypt [58] of 60 patients with schistosomal hepatic fibrosis, not complicated by cirrhosis, shows excellent results. All patients were followed to a median follow-up of 37 months. DSRS was done with 1.7% operative mortality, 93% patency and 7% rebleeding rates. Encephalopathy was found in only three patients (5%), and was only severe in one patient. The five year survival of 88% indicates the excellence of this procedure for such patients.

A randomized study [59] from Brazil documents the advantage of DSRS over total portal systemic shunt in the schistosomiasis population. This paper again emphasizes the importance of normal hepatocellular function in this population which is mentioned after DSRS. In contrast it shows how significant encephalopathy develops after total shunt, and advocates abandonment of such operations in this population.

## 7. Hemodynamic effects of DSRS

*The hemodynamic responses after DSRS differs by disease etiology. The paper discussed was presented at the American Surgical Association in 1983 and published in Annals of Surgery 1983 [60].*

Alterations in hepatic and systemic hemodynamics play a central role in the complications of portal hypertension. In considering the therapeutic options for variceal bleeding, one of the major considerations must be how the therapy will alter hemodynamics, either for better or worse. This has best been illustrated by the severely detrimental consequences of total portal systemic shunts depriving the liver of all prograde portal flow and thus accelerating liver failure [2 – 4].

This paper reports on the differing hemodynamic response between patients with alcoholic and non-alcoholic cirrhosis after DSRS [60]. The major difference by these disease etiologies was that portal venous perfusion was significantly ($P <$ 0.01) better maintained by non-alcoholic (seven of eight) than alcoholic patients (four of 16) at one year after standard DSRS. The alcoholic patients also showed an increase in the flow-dependent index of galactose clearance, which was paralleled by an increase in cardiac output. These hemodynamic changes were not associated with any change in functional hepatic reserve measured by galactose elimination capacity (GEC). Combining the function and flow-dependent measures of galactose removal from plasma, an index of the flow required to perform a specific function was derived. This index was significantly increased in the alcoholic patients.

The data thus showed that, 1 year after standard DSRS, alcoholic patients are at greater risk of loosing portal perfusion. Loss of portal perfusion is associated with an increase in cardiac output and an increase in liver blood flow. This combination of hemodynamic changes appears to indicate that when the liver depends solely on hepatic arterial inflow, a greater flow is required to perform the same function.

The further possible association to these changes discussed in this paper is the effect on survival. While posed as a question, it is certainly suggestive that the loss of portal flow seen in alcoholic patients after standard DSRS may be a factor in the significantly poorer long-term survival of this subset as presented in Section 3.

*Comment*
When considering the effect of DSRS on hepatic hemodynamics it is important to view it against the background of the natural history of hemodynamic changes in cirrhosis. Some patients with cirrhosis will spontaneously lose portal perfusion [61]. Patients with cirrhosis who have not undergone surgery may develop a hyperdynamic state with elevated cardiac output and low peripheral vascular resistance [62]. The best approximation to a 'control' group of patients with cirrhosis against whom to assess these hemodynamic changes after DSRS is the group of patients who have received endoscopic sclerosis.

In our prospective study of DSRS versus endoscopic sclerosis for variceal bleeding presented earlier [38] the two groups of cirrhotic patients entered were comparable. While the sclerosis group is not a 'control' group in the strictest sense, it is a group, matched by all parameters for the severity of cirrhosis, similar to those having DSRS. As in the above cited paper [60], the major difference between the two groups is in portal perfusion: seven of 15 (47%) of the DSRS patients, and only one of 19 (5%) of the sclerosis patients lost portal perfusion at one year. Loss of portal perfusion in this study was not the natural history, but a treatment effect of DSRS. Effective liver blood flow and cardiac output measures did not change in either group at one year (Table 4). It can be noted from the standard deviations that there is a fairly wide range, particularly in the DSRS group: some patients in this group became hyperdynamic although the group as a whole was not. Later follow-up at 2 years in this study shows a very similar pattern in these hemodynamic changes.

What factors lead to loss of portal perfusion after DSRS, and what makes the patients with alcoholic cirrhosis particularly susceptible? Loss of portal flow will occur if the sinusoidal pressure exceeds the portal pressure on the basis of (a) change in outflow resistance, (b) increased arterial inflow, (c) fall in portal pressure due to lower collateral resistance or (d) a combination of the above.

Increased outflow resistance may occur on a differing pathologic basis in alcoholic compared to post-hepatitic cirrhosis. The injury in alcoholic hepatitis is primarily perivenular, while that in viral hepatitis is mainly periportal. Does the cardiac output increase before or after loss of portal perfusion? Unpublished data shows that all patients become hyperdynamic to some degree in the first 2 days after DSRS, but precise day-by-day, week-by-week and month-by-month documentation of these changes is difficult to acquire.

The role of the shunt itself, and the development of collateral pathways from the high pressure portal vein to low pressure splenic vein after DSRS, have been extensively evaluated [63]. Review of pre- and 1year post-shunt angiograms in 50 patients (25 alcoholic and 25 non-alcoholic) showed the following. Ninety-eight percent of

TABLE 4  Effective liver blood flow and cardiac output changes at 1 year into sclerosis and DSRS

|  | Flow (ml/min) | Cardiac output (l/min) |
| --- | --- | --- |
| Normal | 1378 ± 218 | 5.0 |
| Sclerosis |  |  |
| Pre | 1125 ± 394 ($N = 21$) | 7.3 ± 2.3 ($N = 12$) |
| 1 year | 1229 ± 432 | 7.6 ± 2.8 |
| DSRS |  |  |
| Pre | 1059 ± 284 ($N = 17$) | 5.9 ± 1.8 ($N = 8$) |
| 1 year | 1063 ± 388 | 8.4 ± 5.2 |

There are no significant changes in these parameters.

patients had developed some collaterals at 1 year. This developed along three main pathways, transpancreatic 72%, transgastric 48% and colonic 46% (Fig. 5). Multiple pathways developed in 64% of patients. Grading the size of these collateral pathways showed that in 74% of patients these exceeded the size of the portal and/or superior mesenteric vein. The effect of these collaterals in this selected study population on portal flow showed that 32% lost portal perfusion at one year, with this being significantly ($P < 0.05$) more common in alcoholic (48%) than non-alcoholic (16%) patients. The size, site and number of pathways was not different by disease etiology. Finally, the pancreatic pathway was most commonly associated with loss of portal perfusion.

Other publications [64 – 66] have shown the development of similar collaterals, but no attempt has been made to quantitate their effects. Maillard's data [64] showed that 94% of his patients developed collaterals after DSRS but, as shown by his illustrations, some maintain portal flow, although the percentage is not given. In Belghiti's series all patients developed collaterals, but 80% maintained some portal flow [65].

However considered, these hemodynamic changes after DSRS amount to a varying portaprival syndrome in these patients. The definition of the changes as outlined above, has led to modifications in surgical technique as previously described – and new approaches to collateral interruption once they have developed.

DSRS with entire splenopancreatic disconnection (DSRS + SPD) has evolved as a method for better maintaining portal perfusion after DSRS [18]. As indicated from the above data the prime target population for this improvement are patients with alcoholic cirrhosis. But collateral pathways develop in *all* patients with cirrhosis managed by standard DSRS and, in theory at least, prevention of such portaprival pathways should be benefical in all such patients. Data at one year shows significantly ($P < 0.05$) better maintenance of portal perfusion following DSRS + SPD than after DSRS alone. Only one of 11 alcoholic and two of 17 non-alcoholic patients lost perfusion at one year after this modified procedure. The other measured hemodynamic parameters in this study, of galactose clearance and cardiac output, showed a course parallel to non-alcoholic patients after standard DSRS. Longer follow-up will show if these advantages translate to improved survival in alcoholic patients.

Further important data in this study [18] showed a significant reduction in the insulin levels in the shunts of patients after DSRS + SPD compared to standard DSRS. This data supports the concept of interruption of the pancreatic siphon seen after standard DSRS (Fig. 3) but, again, longer follow-up is required to show whether this translates to better delivery of hepatotrophic factors to the liver and improved maintenance of liver volume and function.

## 8. Metabolic changes with DSRS

*The metabolic responses following DSRS are superior to those after total portal systemic shunt. The paper discussed was presented at the American Surgical Association in 1974 and published in the Annals of Surgery 1974 [67].*

This paper presented and published in 1974 emphasizes Emory's early commitment to measure quantitatively the effects of shunt surgery in patients with cirrhosis [61]. This commitment to measure 'liver function', or how well the liver works rather than how much ungoing liver damage is present, has been an important factor which sets much of this work above that from other centers. Early in the history of the DSRS the questions were being asked as to whether the physiologically appealing selective variceal decompression really had a metabolic advantage to the liver. This paper epitomizes the investigative methods which have been a mark of the DSRS work.

Eighteen patients were studied prior to, and three to seven months after, shunt. Nine patients had DSRS and nine total shunts. Metabolic studies were done on the Clinical Research Unit during a 14 day stay under carefully controlled dietary conditions. Measurement of maximal rates of urea synthesis showed that patients with DSRS showed no change, while patients having total shunt showed a significant reduction in that index (Table 5). Likewise, ammonium chloride tolerance, defined as the smallest dose required to produce a 40 $\mu g/dl$ rise in plasma ammonia, was unchanged in the DSRS group, but was significantly worse in the total shunt group (Table 5). Concurrent with these metabolic changes of impaired nitrogen metabolism in the total shunt patients there was a significantly higher incidence of encephalopathy. Following DSRS, only one patient developed encephalopathy, while five of the nine patients having total shunts showed signs of encephalopathy.

This paper therefore, documented for the first time both the clinical advantage of low encephalopathy following DSRS and a metabolic basis on which this might occur.

## Comment

The majority (90%) of patients managed for variceal bleeding at Emory have portal hypertension secondary to cirrhosis. In considering overall patient management an equal weighting must be given to the stage of the cirrhosis, particularly as it affects metabolic function, as to the bleeding itself. Cirrhosis is a spectrum disease, ranging from virtually normal hepatic size, function and hemodynamics at one end, to the small liver with no portal perfusion and poor hepatocyte reserve at the other end. The above paper illustrates the way in which patients having DSRS have been

TABLE 5   Changes in maximal rate of urea synthesis and ammonium chloride tolerance in patients after DSRS and total shunts

| | MRUS | | Ammonia tolerance | |
| --- | --- | --- | --- | --- |
| | Pre | Post | Pre | Post |
| Normal | 55 – 70 mg urea N/h/kgBw 3/4 | | > 0.21 g NH$_4$Cl/kgBW 3/4 | |
| DSRS | 46.6 ± 4.1 | 43.0 ± 4.0 | 0.16 ± 0.02 | 0.14 ± 0.03 |
| Total shunt | 40.0 ± 4.2 | 24.6 ± 4.5[a] | 0.14 ± 0.02 | 0.06 ± 0.01[a] |

[a] $P < 0.05$.

studied from the initiation of this program at Emory. The emphasis in this paper was on nitrogen metabolism and the major associated clinical problem of hepatic encephalopathy. One of the primary reasons for the introduction of the DSRS was the hope of reducing this clinical problem, and the rationale behind that hope was improved maintainance of hepatic metabolic function. This study remains the best study in the literature which documents the advantage of DSRS over total shunts in terms of nitrogen metabolism and encephalopathy.

The three year follow-up report of the prospective randomized study comparing DSRS and total shunt [30] examined, more extensively, metabolic function in the two groups. Analysis by the groups as originally randomized showed no significant difference in MRUS, ammonia tolerance, GEC or antipyrine clearance. However, this paper did emphasize how metabolic changes depend on portal perfusion. When correlated to this parameter, patients with retained portal perfusion had significantly better maintenance of MRUS, GEC, fasting ammonia and ammonia tolerance.

Quantitative evaluation of hepatic function remains an evolving field for the Emory group. The ability to carefully stratify patients at initial evaluation, and then measure quantitatively how parameters change with therapy is a feature not found in most other studies. The current profile collected for all patients having elective management of variceal bleeding measures [62] was made up of the following.

(a) *Galactose elimination capacity.* At high plasma galactose levels this measures the functional hepatocyte mass.

(b) *Liver volume.* This is measured by serial computed tomography.

(c) *Galactose clearance.* At very low plasma concentrations this is limited by functional liver blood flow.

(d) *Systemic hemodynamics.* Radionuclide angiocardiography measures cardiac output and cardiac volume indices.

(e) *Portal venous perfusion* is semiquantitated on venous phase visceral angiography.

(f) *Liver biopsy* is done for assessment of the activity of the liver disease.

In addition, in selected subsets of patients, other quantitative measures such as amino acid and ammonia tolerance scores are measured following a standard protein meal [63].

Table 6 documents the changes in some of these parameters in subsets of patients undergoing DSRS, with their preoperative and 1 year postoperative data. These data emphasize the ability to maintain hepatic function after DSRS, but do document loss of liver volume and the variable hemodynamic changes previously discussed.

**Conclusions**

This review has attempted to bring together for the reader the evolution and results of a management method, the distal splenorenal shunt, for variceal bleeding. To those involved in this ongoing work these have been, and continue to be, exciting times. Some pre-conceived ideas have proved correct, while others were not. What sets this work apart is the willingness to formulate hypotheses and test them, design studies and complete them and collect and analyse data related to clinical manage-

TABLE 6 Quantitative liver function, mass and hemodynamic data prior to and one year after DSRS in patient subgroups (21 patients managed by chronic endoscopic sclerosis are included for comparison)

| | No. of patients | GEC (mg/min) | Liver volume (cc) | Liver blood flow (ml/min) | Portal perfusion | Cardiac output (l/min) |
|---|---|---|---|---|---|---|
| Normal | | 500 ± 50 | 1493 ± 230 | 1378 ± 218 | 1 | 5 |
| Cirrhosis, alcoholic | 16 | | | | | |
| Preoperative | | 337 ± 99 | 2113 ± 600 | 1133 ± 265 | 2.0 | 6.9 ± 1.7 |
| 1 Year | | 305 ± 69 | 1836 ± 637[a] | 1339 ± 406[b] | 3.5[a] | 10.0 ± 3.5[a] |
| Cirrhosis, non-alcoholic | 8 | | | | | |
| Preoperative | | 362 ± 98 | 1489 ± 433 | 1045 ± 269 | 2.0 | 6.9 ± 1.7 |
| 1 Year | | 324 ± 93 | 1311 ± 487[a] | 964 ± 169 | 2.0 | 7.3 ± 2.8 |
| Portal vein thrombosis | 6 | | | | | |
| Preoperative | | 378 ± 57 | 966 ± 253 | 979 ± 192 | 1 | – |
| 1 Year | | 353 ± 83 | 1028 ± 310 | 924 ± 169 | 1 | – |
| Endoscopic sclerosis | 21 | | | | | |
| Preoperative | | 306 ± 66 | 1712 ± 508 | 1079 ± 333 | 1.5 | 7.3 ± 2.3 |
| 1 Year | | 356 ± 82[a] | 1549 ± 422[a] | 1174 ± 396 | 1.4 | 7.6 ± 2.8 |

Significant preoperative to 1-year changes: [a] $P < 0.05$; [b] $P < 0.07$.

ment. The focus is on patients and their clinical problem of portal hypertension and variceal bleeding, who, through the endeavors outlined in this review, continue to receive improved management year-by-year.

### Acknowledgements

The authors thank Verna J. Stevens for her untiring patience and help in the preparation of this manuscript.

## References

1  Warren WD, Zeppa R, Foman JJ. Selective transsplenic decompression of gastroesophageal varices by distal splenorenal shunt. Ann Surg 1967; 166: 437 – 455.

2  Reynolds TB, Donovan AJ, Mikkelsen WP, et al. Results of a 12-year randomized trial of portacaval shunt in patients with alcoholic liver disease and bleeding varices. Gastroenterology 1981; 80: 1005 – 1011.

3  Jackson FC, Perrin EB, Felix RW, et al. A clinical investigation of the portacaval shunt. V. Survival analysis of the therapeutic operation. Ann Surg 1974; 174: 672 – 701.

4  Resnick RH, Iber FL, Ishihara AM, et al. A controlled study of the therapeutic portacaval shunt. Gastroenterology 1974; 67: 843 – 857.

5  Rueff B, Prandi D, Degos F, et al. A controlled study of the therapeutic portacaval shunt in alcoholic cirrhosis. Lancet 1976; i: 655 – 659.

6  Johnson G, Dart CH, Peters RM, MacFie JA. Hemodynamic changes with cirrhosis of the liver: control of arteriovenous shunts during operation for esophageal varices. Ann Surg 1977; 183: 369 – 376.

7  Mikkelsen WP, Edmondson HA, Peters RL, et al. Extra- and intrahepatic portal hypertension without cirrhosis (hepatoportal sclerosis). Ann Surg 1965; 162: 602 – 608.

8  Price JB, McCullough W, Peterson L, Britton RC, Voorhees AB. Increased intestinal absorption resulting from portal systemic shunting in the dog and man. Surg Forum 1966; 17: 367.

9  Warren WD, Millikan WJ. Selective transsplenic decompression procedure: changes in technique after 300 cases. Contemp Surg 1981; 18: 11 – 32.

10  Henderson JM, Millikan WJ, Warren WD. The distal splenorenal shunt: an update. World J Surg 1984; 8: 722 – 732.

11  Eckhauser FE, Pomerantz RA, Knol JA, Strodel WE, Williams DM, Turcotte JG. Early variceal rebleeding after successful distal splenorenal shunt. Arch Surg 1986; 121: 547 – 552.

12  Pera C, Visa J, Rodes J, et al. Preliminary trial of retroperitoneal approach for modified distal splenorenal shunt. World J Surg 1978; 2: 653 – 659.

13  Nagasue N, Ogawa Y, Yukaya H, Hirose S. Modified distal splenorenal shunt with expanded polytetrafluoroethylene interposition. Surgery 1985; 98: 870 – 878.

14  Rosenthal D, Barber WA, Lamis PA, et al. The jugular vein as an interposition graft in the distal splenorenal shunt. Surg Gynecol Obstet 1985; 161: 372 – 374.

15  Inockuchi K, Beppu K, Kayanagi N, et al. Exclusion of nonisolated splenic vein in distal splenorenal shunt for prevention of portal malcirculation. Ann Surg 1984; 200: 711 – 717.

16  Vang J, Simert G, Hansson JA, et al. Results of a modified distal splenorenal shunt for

portal hypertension. Ann Surg 1977; 185: 224 – 228.

17  Nabseth DC, Widrich WC, O'Hara ET, Johnson WC. Flow and pressure characteristics of the portal system before and after splenorenal shunt. Surgery 1975; 78: 739.

18  Warren WD, Millikan WJ, Henderson JM, et al. Splenopancreatic disconnection: Improved selectivity of distal splenorenal shunt. Ann Surg 1986; 204: 346 – 355.

19  Warren WD, Millikan WJ, Henderson JM, et al. Ten years portal hypertensive surgery at Emory: Results and new perspectives. Ann Surg 1982; 195: 530 – 542.

20  Warren WD, Henderson JM. Portal hypertension. In: Cameron JL, ed. Current Surgical Therapy, 2. St. Louis: C V Mosby Co, 1986; 176.

21  Zeppa R, Hensley GT, Levy JV, et al. The comparative survival of alcoholics versus nonalcoholics after distal splenorenal shunt. Ann Surg 1978; 187: 510 – 514.

22  Rikkers LF, Soper NJ, Cormier RA. Selective operative approach for variceal hemorrhage. Am J Surg 1984; 147: 89 – 96.

23  Brown SL, Busuttil RW. Survival of alcoholic v nonalcoholic patients after portasystemic shunts. Arch Surg 1984; 119: 1321 – 1324.

24  Adson MA, van Heerden JA, Ustrup DM. The distal splenorenal shunt. Arch Surg 1984; 119: 609 – 614.

25  Hutson DG, Livingstone A, Levi JV, et al. Early hepatic failure or upper gastrointestinal bleeding following a distal splenorenal shunt. Surg Gynecol Obstet 1982; 155: 46 – 48.

26  Hanna SS, Smith RB III, Henderson JM, Millikan WJ Jr, Warren WD, Reversal of hepatic encephalopathy after occlusion of total portasystemic shunts. Am J Surg 1981; 142: 285 – 289.

27  Potts JR III, Henderson JM, Millikan WJ Jr, Sones PJ, Warren WD. Restoration of portal venous perfusion and reversal of encephalopathy by balloon occlusion of portal systemic shunt. Gastroenterology 1984; 87(1) 208 – 212.

28  Millikan WJ Jr, Warren WD, Henderson JM, et al. The Emory prospective randomized trial: selective vs nonselective shunt to control variceal bleeding: Ten year follow-up. Ann Surg 1985; 201: 712 – 722.

29  Galambos JT, Warren WD, Rudman D, et al. Selective and total shunts in the treatment of bleeding varices. A randomized controlled trial. N Engl J Med 1976; 295: 1089 – 1095.

30  Rikkers LF, Rudman D, Galambos JT, et al. A randomized, controlled trial of the distal splenorenal shunt. Ann Surg 1978; 188: 271 – 282.

31  Smith RB, Warren WD, Salam AA, et al. Dacron interposition shunts for portal hypertension. An analysis of morbidity correlates. Ann Surg 1980; 192: 9 – 17.

32  Langer B, Taylor BR, Mackenzie DR, et al. Further report of a prospective randomized trial comparing distal splenorenal shunt with end-to-side portacaval shunt: an analysis of encephalopathy, survival, and quality of life. Gastroenterology 1985; 88: 424 – 429.

33  Reichle FA, Fahmy WF, Golsorkhi M. Prospective comparative clinical trial with distal splenorenal and mesocaval shunts. Am J Surg 1979; 137: 13 – 21.

34  Fischer JE, Bower RH, Atamian S, et al. Comparison of distal and proximal splenorenal shunts: a randomized prospective trial. Ann Surg 1981; 194: 531 – 544.

35  Conn HO, Resnick RH, Grace ND, et al. Distal splenorenal shunt vs portal-systemic shunt: current status of a controlled trial. Hepatology 1981; 1: 151 – 160.

36  Harley HAJ, Morgan T, Redeker AG, et al. Results of a randomized trial of end-to-side portacaval shunt and distal splenorenal shunt in alcoholic liver disease and variceal bleeding. Gastroenterology 1986; 91: 802 – 809.

37  Henderson JM. Variceal bleeding: which shunt? Gastroenterology (Editorial) 1986; 91: 1021 – 1023.

38 Warren WD, Henderson JM, Millikan WJ, et al. Distal splenorenal shunt versus endoscopic sclerotherapy for long-term management of variceal bleeding. Preliminary report of a prospective, randomized trial. Ann Surg 1986; 203(5): 454 – 462.

39 Crafoord C, Frenckner P. New surgical treatment of varicose veins of the oesophagus. Acta Otolaryngol 1939; 27: 422 – 429.

40 Whipple AO. The problem of portal hypertension in relation to hepatosplenopathies. Ann Surg 1945; 122: 449 – 475.

41 Conn HO, Grace ND. Portal hypertension and sclerotherapy of esophageal varices. Endoscopy Rev 1985: 39 – 53.

42 Paquet K-J, Feussner H. Endoscopic sclerosis and esophageal balloon tamponade in acute hemorrhage from esophagogastric varices: a prospective controlled randomized trial. Hepatology 1985; 5: 580 – 589.

43 Yassin YM, Sherif SM. Randomized controlled trial of injection sclerotherapy for bleeding oesophageal varices: an interim report. Br J Surg 1983; 70: 20 – 22.

44 Korula J, Balart LA, Radvan G, et al. A prospective, randomized controlled trial of chronic esophageal variceal sclerosis. Hepatology 1985; 5: 584 – 589.

45 Clark AW, Westaby D, Silk DBA, et al. Prospective controlled trial of injection sclerotherapy in patients with cirrhosis and recent variceal haemorrhage. Lancet 1980; ii: 552 – 554.

46 Westaby D, Macdougall BRD, Williams R. Improved survival following injection sclerotherapy for esophageal varices: final analysis of a controlled trial. Hepatology 1985; 5: 827 – 830.

47 Barsoum MS, Balous FI, El-Rooby AA, et al. Tamponade and injection sclerotherapy in the management of bleeding oesophageal varices. Br J Surg 1982; 69: 76 – 78.

48 Terblanche J, Bornman PC, Kahn D, et al. Failure of repeated injection sclerotherapy to improve long-term survival after oesophageal variceal bleeding: a five year prospective controlled trial. Lancet 1983; ii: 1328 – 1332.

49 Cello JP, Grendall JH, Cross RA, et al. Endoscopic sclerotherapy versus portacaval shunt in patients with severe cirrhosis and variceal hemorrhage. N Engl J Med 1984; 311: 1589 – 1594.

50 The Copenhagen Esophageal Varices Sclerotherapy Project. Sclerotherapy after first variceal hemorrhage in cirrhosis: a randomized multicenter trial. N Engl J Med 1984; 311: 1594 – 1600.

51 Warren WD, Millikan WJ, Smith RB, et al. Noncirrhotic portal vein thrombosis. Physiology before and after shunts. Ann Surg 1980; 192: 341 – 349.

52 Hahn M, Massen M, Nencki M, Pawlow J. Die Eck'sche Fistel zwischen der unteren Hohlvene und der Pfortader und ihre Folgen fur den Organismus. Arch Exp Pathol Pharmokol 1893; 32: 161 – 167.

53 Henderson JM, Millikan WJ Jr, Galambos JT, Warren WD. Selective variceal decompression in portal vein thrombosis. Br J Surg 1984; 71: 745 – 749.

54 El-Khishen MA, Henderson JM, Millikan WJ Jr, Kutner MH, Warren WD. Splenectomy is contraindicated for thrombocytopenia secondary to portal hypertension. Surg Gynecol Obstet 1985; 160: 233 – 238.

55 Fonkalsrud EW, Myers NA, Robinson MJ. Management of extrahepatic portal hypertension in children. Ann Surg 1974; 180: 487 – 490.

56 Voorhees AB, Chaitman E, Schneider S, et al. Portalsystemic encephalopathy in the noncirrhotic patient. Effect of portal systemic shunting. Arch Surg 1973; 107: 659.

57 Rodgers BM, Talbert JL. Distal spleno-renal shunt for portal decompression in childhood. J Pediatr Surg 1979; 14: 33 – 37.

58 Ezzat FA, Abu-Elmagd KM, Aly IY, et al. Distal splenorenal shunt for management of

variceal bleeding in patients with schistosomal hepatic fibrosis. Ann Surg 1986; 204: 566 – 573.

59 DaSilva LC, Macedo AL, Fermanian J, et al. A randomized trial for the study of the elective surgical treatment of portal hypertension in Mansonic Schistosomiasis. Ann Surg 1986; 204: 148 – 153.

60 Henderson JM, Millikan WJ Jr, Wright-Bacon L, Kutner MH, Warren WD. Hemodynamic differences between alcoholic and nonalcoholic cirrhotics following distal splenorenal shunt – effect on survival? Ann Surg 1983; 198: 325 – 334.

61 Warren WD, Muller WH. A clarification of some hemodynamic changes in cirrhosis and their surgical significance. Ann Surg 1959; 150: 413 – 420.

62 Kowlaski HJ, Abelman WH. The cardiac output at rest in Laemec's Cirrhosis. J Clin Invest 1953; 32: 1025.

63 Henderson JM, Gong-Liang J, Galloway J, Millikan WJ Jr, Sones PJ, Warren WD. Portaprival collaterals following distal splenorenal shunt: incidence, magnitude and associated portal perfusion changes. J Hepatol 1985; 1: 649 – 661.

64 Maillard JN, Flamant YM, Hay JM, et al. Selectivity of the distal splenorenal shunt. Surgery 1979; 86: 663 – 671.

65 Belghiti J, Grenier P, Nouel O, et al. Long-term loss of Warren's shunt selectivity. Angiographic demonstration. Arch Surg 1981; 116: 1121 – 1124.

66 Widrich WC, Robbins AH, Johnson WC, et al. Long-term followup of distal splenorenal shunts: evaluation by arteriography, shuntography, transhepatic portal venography and cinefluorography. Radiology 1980; 134: 341 – 345.

67 Warren WD, Rudman D, Millikan W, et al. The metabolic basis of portasystemic encephalopathy and the effect of selective vs nonselective shunts. Ann Surg 1974; 180(4): 573 – 579.

68 Henderson JM, Warren WD. A method of quantitating hepatic function and hemodynamics in cirrhosis: the changes following distal splenorenal shunt. Jpn J Surg 1986; 16: 157 – 168.

69 Ibrahim S, Millikan WJ Jr, Henderson JM, Wright-Bacon L, Warren WD, Noe B. Branched-chain amino acid tolerance following oral protein load in normal and cirrhotic subjects. American College of Surgeons 1983 Surgical Forum Volume XXXIV: 36 – 38.

© 1988 Elsevier Science Publishers B.V. (Biomedical Division)
Treatment of esophageal varices
Y. Idezuki, editor

239

Chapter 21

# The importance of hepatic functional reserve as a determinant of prognosis after portal decompression

FREDERIC E. ECKHAUSER, JEREMIAH G. TURCOTTE AND GEORGE D. ZUIDEMA

*Division of Gastrointestinal Surgery & Department of Surgery, University of Michigan Medical Center, Ann Arbor, MI, USA*

## Introduction

The clinical feasibility of decompressing the portal circulation in an effort to reduce the risk of recurrent variceal hemorrhage was first demonstrated in the mid 1940s and is now well-established. Although operative survival rates are acceptable, the operation may irreversibly alter the patient's quality of life. Despite extensive research efforts worldwide, there is to date no reliable method for predicting the severity of such changes. A variety of classification systems have been developed to equate differences between groups of patients that might influence the outcome. Of these, only the Child classification system which combined two laboratory and three clinical observations to estimate hepatic reserve, has withstood the test of time as an accurate predictor of patient survival.

### Natural history of cirrhosis and portal hypertension

The most inclusive study of survival among patients with cirrhosis was published in 1942 by Ratnoff and Patek [1]. They estimated that approximately one out of every four cirrhotics would die from variceal hemorrhage and predicted that one third would die after the initial bleed. A 25% one-year survival rate after the first episode of hematemesis was also projected. Thirteen years later Nachlas et al. published a retrospective study which associated outcome with identifiable risk factors such as jaundice and ascites [2]. They observed that 60% of cirrhotic patients died after the

Address Correspondence to: Frederic E. Eckhauser, M.D., Associate Professor of Surgery & Chief, Division of GI Surgery, 2920 K Taubman Center, 1500 E. Medical Center Drive, Ann Arbor, MI 48109, USA.

first bleed but noted that two-thirds of the survivors lived beyond one year. The wide variability in survival quoted by these and other authors is due to many factors, including the natural history of bleeding varices, associated risk factors and patient selection.

The natural history of variceal bleeding in patients with clinically demonstrated cirrhosis was studied comprehensively by Conn et al. and reported in 1972 [3]. Among patients included in the study they observed a 50% one-year risk of hemorrhage following identification of varices and a decreasing annualized risk thereafter. It is unclear why the risk of bleeding appeared to decrease over time after inclusion in the study. However, a plausible explanation may be that portal hemodynamics and liver function often improve after elimination of factors responsible for the underlying liver disease. Improvement in these parameters may be accompanied by decreased portal pressure and a reduced risk of variceal hemorrhage. It is interesting to note that, in some patients with cirrhosis, varices often lessen during periods of intensive medical management. Teleologically it would be tempting to assume that changes in intrahepatic vascular resistance and portal pressure correspond to fluctuations in clinical hepatic risk status but the literature addressing this question is ambiguous.

In a subsequent study, Graham and Smith analysed the clinical course of 85 consecutive patients with endoscopically documented variceal hemorrhage and reported a 6-week medical mortality rate of 42% [4]. They noted that nearly two-thirds of early deaths (within 6 weeks of the index bleed) resulted from bleeding while deaths occurring after 6 weeks were more likely related to hepatic failure or infectious complications. Attempts to correlate the risk of death from bleeding or other causes with factors such as the acuity and severity of bleeding and hepatic reserve status at the time of bleeding were unrewarding. While the study was mainly descriptive, the authors clearly demonstrated that death from bleeding affects primarily 'early' survival. The risk of late bleeding (32%) among survivors appears to be no greater than that observed in patients with a known history of varices who have never bled.

A variety of techniques have been utilized in an effort to identify patients with varices who are at risk of bleeding, including endoscopy, angiography, manometry and clinical assessment. Beppu and others recently evaluated the role of esophageal endoscopy in assessing the risk of variceal bleeding in 172 patients [5]. The criteria used were established by the Japanese Research Society for Portal Hypertension and included categories pertaining to the color, form and location of the varices. Of all the endoscopic features analysed, the red color sign, fundamental color (blue versus white) and esophagitis most closely correlated with the risk of bleeding. Form and location of varices were also important discriminants, but had less independent predictive value than the red color sign.

Some authors have suggested a relationship between portal pressure and the risk of variceal hemorrhage [6]. However, studies at the University of Michigan of portal pressure measured as the difference between the wedged hepatic vein and inferior vena cava pressure (corrected sinusoidal pressure) in 32 patients with histologically confirmed cirrhosis failed to show any association with either the size of the varices or the risk of bleeding [7]. Further, there was no apparent correlation between corrected sinusoidal pressure and variceal size, hepatic reserve status or survival after portasystemic shunting. The authors concluded that while measurement of portal pressure appears to have little prognostic importance, it may be useful for differentiating sinusoidal versus extrahepatic, presinusoidal etiologies of portal hypertension. This problem is compounded by the lack of precise or uniform methodology available for assessing preoperative portal hemodynamics.

## Patient selection criteria

The mortality and morbidity of portal decompression is dictated largely by whether the patient has sufficient hepatic reserve to tolerate a major operation. For many years surgeons have recognized that the presence of jaundice, ascites or encephalopathy adversely affects survival after portasystemic shunting. Child was the first to systematically utilize and recommend a multifactorial classification system which combined two laboratory and three clinical observations to estimate hepatic functional reserve [8]. Of these criteria the four most useful proved to be the patient's state of nutrition, the presence or absence of ascites and laboratory determination of serum bilirubin and albumin. Child showed retrospectivily, in 128 patients who underwent end-to-side portacaval shunt, that the capacity of the patient to tolerate the stress of portal decompression correlated closely with preoperative hepatic risk assessment. In this study Child demonstrated a 4.3% combined postoperative mortality rate among 80 patients with minimal or moderate impairment of hepatic reserve (Child risk classes A and B, respectively) compared to 53% among 48 patients with more severe impairment (Child risk class C). There was also a lower incidence of ammonia intoxication among good or moderate-risk patients compared to poor-risk patients.

Child also analysed late survival following portal decompression and reported strikingly disparate results for patients with different risk classifications. Among 102 cirrhotic patients undergoing either end-to-side or side-to-side portacaval shunts for variceal bleeding, the overall cumulative probability of 5-year survival was 30% [9]. Early mortality accounted for some of the observed differences in long-term survival. For example, if patients dying within 3 months of operation were deleted from the calculation, the cumulative probability of 5-year survival increased to 40%. However, long-term survival was most dependent upon hepatic risk at the time of operation. Among A and B risk patients the cumulative probability of surviving 5 years was 42 and 33%, respectively, whereas only 18% of C risk patients had a similar survival. Because of differences in patient selection and classification at the time, valid comparison of Child's results with those of other large series was difficult. However, Wantz and Payne used an identical risk classification system and reported similar differences in the rates of operative mortality and long-term survival [10]. In their series, 80% of group A and B patients survived for 2 or more years compared to 27% in group C patients.

Warren and colleagues advocated another form of patient selection based upon hemodynamic criteria [11]. This approach was based on the supposition that portal flow diversion adversely affects hepatic metabolism and hypothesized that patients with good preoperative portal blood flow would tolerate a portasystemic shunt procedure less well than patients with more severely compromised hepatopedal flow. Smith and associates assessed a variety of hemodynamic parameters in 67 patients undergoing shunt procedures and classified them into three hemodynamic stages [12]. The data included several static pressure and dynamic flow measurements but was weighted in favor of dynamic information. Stage I patients exhibited relatively normal prograde portal flow while Stage II or III patients showed evidence of progressively reduced or even reversed portal flow. In theory, Stage II patients should have the most favorable prognosis because of moderate portal flow reduction and 'presumed' compensation. While hemodynamic staging provided prognostic information regarding operative mortality and patient survival, it proved to be less predictive than Child's original hepatic risk classification based on clinical and laboratory assessment of hepatic functional reserve. For example, 3-year survival based on Child's approach was 64% for Class A patients, 20% for Class B patients and 8% for Class C patients. By comparison, 3-year survival based on hemodynamic staging was 33% for Stage I patients, 34% for Stage II patients and 29% for Stage III patients. The authors concluded that "despite the theoretical attractiveness of hemodynamic principles, it is more practical and more informative to base patient selection criteria upon clinical and biochemical information" [12].

Stratification of patients into risk categories according to hepatic pathology has received sporadic attention. Proponents of this approach argue that histologic evidence of acute alcoholic hepatitis is associated with prohibitive operative mortality, particularly in patients requiring emergency shunts [13, 14]. Mikkelsen demonstrated an association between the presence of Mallory bodies, increased operative mortality and decreased long-term patient survival [13]. In a more inclusive study, Eckhauser and associates at the University of Michigan examined patient survival in 124 shunted patients with liver biopsies obtained at the time of operation [14]. Survival was analysed according to several clinical and hepatic histologic criteria including Child risk classification, timing of operation, presence or absence of cirrhosis, etiology of cirrhosis and presence or absence of Mallory bodies. All of the criteria correlated with prognosis. However, only Child risk classification and the histologic presence of many Mallory bodies had independent predictive value. The prognostic value of the other criteria was largely dependent on differences in hepatic functional reserve.

Other authors have questioned the prognostic value of hepatic histology citing as detractors biases in patient selection and reporting inconsistencies [15]. It is true that Mallory bodies are found in a number of liver abnormalities including Wilson's disease, primary biliary cirrhosis and cholestasis, and are not peculiar to alcoholic cirrhosis. However, of the 24 patients with Mallory bodies reported in our study, 88% had alcoholic cirrhosis and only 12% had nonalcoholic etiologies. While the pathogenesis and clinical significance of these intracytoplasmic inclusions is unclear, our data suggests strongly that histologic evidence of many Mallory bodies is associated with a high operative mortality and poor long-term survival, irrespective of hepatic risk status.

## The timing of operation

Patients who experience variceal hemorrhage are at greatest risk of rebleeding or dying within a relatively short time of the bleeding episode. Smith and Graham analysed survival in 85 unselected variceal bleeders and showed that the life-table curve can be divided into two distinct periods of risk: an early phase of high risk and a long-term phase during which survival is dictated by the severity and progression of the underlying liver disease [16]. They suggested that the timing of intervention may be the single most important variable that influences early survival. In an earlier report, the authors followed the course of 13 patients in whom operation was delayed to allow improvement in liver function [4]. Only one patient improved significantly and four patients (31%) rebled and died before operation could be performed. Of the nine remaining patients in whom operation was delayed an average of 1.8 months (range 1 – 4 months), two (22%) died in the immediate postoperative period. One patient was lost to follow-up and the six surviving patients were followed for an average of 24 months with no intervening deaths. From this study they concluded that improvements in liver function or hepatic functional reserve should not be anticipated following an episode of acute variceal bleeding and that further management decisions should not be based on this expectation alone.

This observation is especially important because of ambiguities in the literature concerning the efficacy of immediate versus delayed portal decompression. In 1961 Orloff and associates undertook a study of emergency portal decompression based on data from their institution that all other therapies to control bleeding were associated with a mortality rate greater than 80% [17]. All patients entered into the study were stabilized rapidly and underwent portacaval shunt within 8 h of admission. Twenty-one of 40 patients survived operation and left the hospital for an early survival rate of 53%. Of the 19 deaths, nearly 80% resulted from liver failure. Follow-up was complete in all 21 early survivors for up to 50 months. Seventeen were alive for a long-term survival rate of 43% and all but one of the survivors lived for longer than one year.

Despite Orloff's evidence that improved early and late survival rates could be anticipated after immediate portal decompression in unselected patients with cirrhosis, many prominent surgeons including Dr. Child were reluctant to adopt this philosophy. Dr. Child advocated a more selective approach based on assessment of hepatic risk: "In general we do not apply the principle of emergent decompression to poor-risk (C) patients, for here the mortality of any operation appears to be equivalent or greater than that of medical therapy. If a patient in question becomes deeply jaundiced, if ascites collects, and if he cannot be aroused from coma, he is maintained upon continuing supportive therapy in the hope that bleeding will be controlled by prolonged tamponade. Some small proportion of patients will recover and become candidates for elective decompression. The remainder will die, but they would die just as surely as if a portacaval shunt were performed emergently" [8]. It remained for Smith and Graham to later suggest that the improved survival seen after delayed therapy resulted not from the subsequent intervention but from the delay itself [16]. In other words, patients who would have died regardless of the type of intervention were eliminated early resulting in a 'higher' early mortality rate but an improved long-term survival rate. These authors graphically demonstrated that survival curves for variceal bleeders could be altered dramatically by simply changing the time of the patient's entry into the study. One of the major conclusions of this study was that valid comparison of any therapeutic modalities used to manage patients with variceal bleeding must incorporate timing of randomization and intervention into the protocol design.

To further investigate the influence of operative timing on early and long-term patient survival, we performed a retrospective analysis of 77 patients undergoing selective distal splenorenal shunt at the University of Michigan. A numerical score for hepatic risk status (HRSS) was calculated at the time of the index bleed and again just prior to operation. This score was determined using the Campbell-Parker modification of the Child hepatic risk classification [18]. Additional variables were analysed including age, sex, number of previous bleeding episodes, time from index bleed to operation, transfusion requirements during operation and etiology of cirrhosis. Among 64 patients who underwent elective distal splenorenal shunt, there was a significant improvement in the HRSS from the time of the index bleed to operation. The most important predictor of the HRSS at the time of operation appeared to be the HRSS at the time of the index bleed. Simple survival analysis of elective cases demonstrated a mean survival time of 65 months and cumulative 3- and 5-year survival rates of 73 and 65%, respectively. Of elective cases that lived beyond 30 days of operation, the cumulative probability of surviving 5 years was 80%. We conclude that both HRSS measures are important predictors of survival. Early survival (operative mortality) is dependent upon the HRSS at the time of operation. By comparison, for patients who survive operation, the extent of underlying liver damage measured by HRSS at the index bleed is the only important variable. While the results of our study partly support Smith and Graham's contention that "the risk of dying is primarily dependent upon the severity of the underlying liver disease", we disagree with their observation that hepatic risk cannot be improved prior to operation. Adjunctive techniques such as endoscopic injection sclerotherapy and transhepatic variceal obliteration can be used to achieve temporary hemostasis. Each of these approaches is accompanied by unique complications but can be performed in specialized centers, by skilled individuals, with acceptable morbidity and low procedure-related mortality. We further suggest that delaying selective portal decompression can be justified by the expectation of improved operative mortality.

## References

1   Ratnoff OD, Patek AJ Jr. The natural history of Laennec's cirrhosis of the liver. An analysis of 386 cases. Medicine 1942; 21: 207 – 268.
2   Nachlas MM, O'Neil JE, Campbell AJA. The life history of patients with cirrhosis of the liver and bleeding esophageal varices. Ann Surg 1955; 141: 10 – 23.
3   Conn HO, Lindenmuth WW, May CJ, et al. Prophylactic portacaval anastomosis. A tale of two studies. Medicine 1972; 51: 27 – 40.
4   Graham DY, Smith JL. The course of patients after variceal hemorrhage. Gastroenterology 1981; 80: 300 – 309.

5   Beppu K, Inokuchi K, Koyanagi N, et al. Prediction of variceal hemorrhage by esophageal endoscopy. Gastroint Endosc 1981; 27: 213 – 218.

6   Adamson RJ, Butt K, Dennis CR. Prognostic significance of portal pressure in patients with bleeding esophageal varices. Surg Gynecol Obstet 1977; 145: 353 – 356.

7   McLeod MK, Eckhauser FE, Turcotte JG, Significance of corrected sinusoidal pressure in patients with cirrhosis and portal hypertension. Ann Surg 1981; 194: 562 – 567.

8   Child CG III and Turcotte JG. Surgery and Portal Hypertension. In: Child CG III, ed. The liver and Portal Hypertension. Philadelphia: W.B. Saunders Co. 1964; 1 – 85.

9   Turcotte JG, Wallin VW, Child CG III. End to side versus side to side portacaval shunts in patients with cirrhosis. Am J Surg 1969; 117: 108 – 116.

10  Wantz GE, Payne MA. Experience with portacaval shunt for portal hypertension. N Engl J Med 1961; 265: 721 – 728.

11  Warren WD, Restrepo JE, Respess JC, et al. The importance of hemodynamic studies in management of portal hypertension. Ann Surg 1963; 158: 387 – 404.

12  Smith GW, Maddrey WC, Zuidema GZ. Portal Hypertension As We See It. In: Child CG III, ed. Portal Hypertension As Seen By 17 Authorities. Philadelphia: W.B. Saunders Co. 1974; 1 – 35.

13  Mikkelsen WP. Therapeutic portacaval shunt: preliminary data on controlled trial and morbid effects of acute hyaline necrosis. Arch Surg 1974; 108: 302 – 305.

14  Eckhauser FE, Appelman HD, O'Leary TJ, et al. Hepatic pathology as a determinant of prognosis after portal decompression. Am J Surg 1980; 139: 105 – 112.

15  Chandler JC, Van Meter CH, Kaiser DL, et al. Factors affecting immediate and long-term survival after emergent and elective splanchnic-systemic shunts. Ann Surg 1985; 201: 476 – 487.

16  Smith JL, Graham DY. Variceal hemorrhage. A critical evaluation of survival analysis. Gastroenterology 1982; 82: 968 – 973.

17  Orloff MJ. Emergency portacaval shunt: a comparative study of shunt, varix ligation and nonsurgical treatment of bleeding esophageal varices in unselected patients with cirrhosis. Ann Surg 1967; 166: 456 – 478.

18  Campbell DP, Parker DE, Anagnostopolous CE. Survival prediction in portacaval shunts. A computerized statistical analysis. Am J Surg 1973; 126: 748 – 751.

© 1988 Elsevier Science Publishers B.V. (Biomedical Division)
Treatment of esophageal varices
Y. Idezuki, editor

Chapter 22

# Evaluation of shunting operation for the treatment of portal hypertension

YAN-TING HUANG

Department of Surgery, First Teaching Hospital, Beijing Medical University, China

## Current status of surgical treatment of portal hypertension in China

Portal hypertension is a common disease in China. Since the 1950s, surgical treatment of this condition has been widely adopted and approximately 7000 cases of different shunting and disconnective operations had been reported by the end of 1987, excluding those who received simple splenectomies only.

### Incidence and epidemiology [1]

As reported in the Chinese literature, 97.8% of portal hypertension is of the intrahepatic type and the remaining 2.2% are of the extrahepatic type. The number of liver cirrhosis cases are comprised of 49.1% post-necrotic, 41% schistosomal, 6.9% portal, 0.4% biliary and 2.6% pathologically unclear.

The pathogenesis of cirrhosis varies in different parts of this country: in north, northeast and northwest China, approximately 90% of the patients have post-necrotic cirrhosis caused by viral hepatitis, in east China and central China 77.9% and 54.7% suffer from schistosomal cirrhosis and in southwest China post-necrotic and schistosomal cirrhosis is about equally distributed. In recent years, however, the number of patients with post-necrotic cirrhosis has tended to increase in some regions, especially in northern and central China (Table 1).

### Operative procedures

Simple splenectomy may give better results in the treatment of portal hypertension caused by schistosomiasis, especially in patients without bleeding. 2145 cases of splenectomy were reviewed in 1979, the postoperative bleeding rate in patients without bleeding before operation was 3.8%, and that in patients with bleeding before operation was 7.5%. The ten-year survival rate was over 90%, and 58.6% of patients had various degrees of improved working capacity after operation [1].

From 1953 to 1982, 3215 patients treated with surgery other than splenectomy were analysed. Portosystemic shunting was performed in 1858 (88.9%) cases and porto-azygous disconnection was performed in 357 (11.1%) cases. But from 1983 to 1987, of 3851 cases reported, 2143 (55.6%) underwent portosystemic shunting operations and 1708 (44.4%) were treated with porto-azygous disconnection [1 – 3]. Although shunting has been the popular procedure for the treatment of portal hypertension, in the last 5 years its use has decreased, and porto-azygous disconnection has been more often used.

In 2143 cases of shunting operation performed in the last 5 years, there were 746 cases of splenorenal shunts, 269 cases of portocaval shunts, 429 cases of splenocaval shunts, 521 cases of mesocaval shunts, 121 cases of distal splenorenal shunts and 57 cases of coronary venous caval shunts. Before 1982, splenorenal and portocaval shunting were the predominant choices, while in recent years various other shunting procedures have been used.

TABLE 1  Geographic distribution of pathogenesis in 1526 cirrhotic patients

| Region | No. of patients | Number of patients (%) | | | | |
|---|---|---|---|---|---|---|
| | | Postnecrotic | Schistosomatic | Portal | Biliary | Not clear |
| Northeast, northern | 456 | 408 (89.5) | 0 | 22 (4.8) | 0 | 26 (5.7) |
| Eastern | 474 | 92 (19.4) | 369 (77.9) | 10 (2.1) | 1 (0.2) | 2 (0.4) |
| Central, south | 422 | 112 (26.5) | 231 (54.7) | 66 (15.6) | 1 (0.2) | 12 (2.8) |
| Southwest | 113 | 77 (68.1) | 26 (23.0) | 7 (6.2) | 3 (2.7) | 0 |
| Northwest | 61 | 60 (98.4) | 0 | 0 | 1 (1.6) | 0 |

TABLE 2  Results of different shunt operations

| Type of shunt | Operative mortality (%) | Rebleeding rate (%) | Incidence of encephalopathy (%) | Long-term[a] survival, (%) |
|---|---|---|---|---|
| SRS | 0 – 7.7 | 4.8 – 24.1 | 5.9 – 12.2 | 72.5 – 83 |
| PCS | 2.9 – 3.3 | 4.0 – 8.6 | 7.7 – 11.0 | 63.8 – 70.3 |
| MCS-H | 1.5 – 8.9 | 6.1 – 7.4 | 0 – 7.7 | 72.7 – 82.0 |
| MCS-SS | 0 – 8.0 | 4.3 – 25.0 | 0 – 15.1 | 83.3 |

SRS, splenorenal; PCS, portocaval; MCS-SS, mesocaval, side-to-side.
[a] Survival for at least 5 years.

Of the cases treated with porto-azygous disconnection, 93.9% cases had lower esophageal and proximal perigastric devascularization and removal of the spleen. Gastric fundal transection, fundal extramucosal disconnection and the use of EEA staple instruments to transversely sever the lower esophagus were also reported. Recently, the combined lower esophageal transection and fundal perigastric devascularization (Sugiura's operation), which is widely used in Japan, has also been carried out in China, but only on a small scale [1 – 3].

*Results of surgical treatment*

Because the conditions of the cirrhotic patients varied, it is difficult to analyse the results reported in any depth and the following data presented in Table 2 can only serve as reference data.

Of 1369 cases of porto-azygous disconnection, the mortality rate for elective operation was 1.1 – 9% and the rebleeding rate was 4.1 – 17.3%; the incidence of encephalopathy was 0 – 1.7%; 5-year survival rate was 75 – 92.4%.

## Clinical data on shunting operations in the First Teaching Hospital, Beijing Medical University

Various shunting operations were adopted in 443 patients from 1961 to the end of 1986. Excluding six cases of the extrahepatic type, 437 cases of intrahepatic portal hypertension are summarized as follows.

*General material*

Of the 437 cases 322 were male and 115 female; their age varied from 12 to 68 years, with 28 cases above the age of 55.

Therapeutic shuntings were performed in 298 cases with a history of variceal bleeding, these shuntings included 45 emergency cases. Prophylactic shuntings were performed in 139 cases with proved esophageal varices. Child's classification was used according to the results of the latest liver function test before surgery. 87 cases were classified as A (19.9%), 212 cases as B (48.5%) and 138 cases as C (31.6%).

TABLE 3   Shunting procedures and operative mortality

| Type of shunt | No. of cases | Elective shunting | | | Emergency shunting | | |
|---|---|---|---|---|---|---|---|
| | | No. of cases | No. of deaths | Mortality (%) | No. of cases | No. of deaths | Mortality (%) |
| SRS | 246 | 230 | 9 | 3.9 | 16 | 3 | 18.8 |
| PCS | 146 | 122 | 4 | 3.3 | 24 | 5 | 20.8 |
| MCS | 30 | 25 | 2 | 8.0 | 5 | 3 | 60.0 |
| SCS | 5 | 5 | 0 | 0 | 0 | 0 | 0 |

*Shunting procedures and operative mortality*

Four kinds of shunting operation were performed (Table 3).

Of 30 cases of mesocaval shunting, there were end-to-side shunts in eight, side-to-sides shunts in 17 and H-graft shunts in five cases. In addition, ten cases of distal splenorenal shuntings were performed as elective operation without death.

Twenty-six cases died after operation: nine cases (34.6%) from liver failure; nine from upper digestive tract bleeding, including two cases of stress ulcer proved by endoscopy; seven (26.9%) from variceal bleeding. Eleven cases died after emergency surgery (mortality rate of 24.4%), three from persistent bleeding.

*Liver function and operative mortality*

The relationship between liver function and operative mortality is shown in Table 4.

Three cases (27.3% of 11 deaths) from Child's class B died of liver failure, six cases (42.9% of 14 deaths) of class C died of liver failure and the only one class A patient died from respiratory complications.

*Results of shunting operation*

Forty of the 45 patients who underwent emergency shuntings had their bleeding stopped (88.9%). The remaining five patients had persistent bleeding, three died (two received mesocaval shunting and one received splenorenal shunting) and in two the bleeding stopped spontaneously after 2 – 3 days.

Of 411 cases who were discharged from hospital after operation, 376 (91.5%) were followed-up, the longest period being 20 years, with an average of 8 years and 6 months.

Bleeding occurred in 53 patients (14.4%) after shunting operation (Table 5).

Postshunting encephalopathy developed in 76 patients with an incidence of 20.7%.

The relationship between the incidence of encephalopathy and different shuntings is shown in Table 6.

The number of patients who received mesocaval, splenocaval and distal splenorenal shunting may be too small to give meaningful results regarding the incidence of rebleeding and encephalopathy.

The long-term survival of 422 patients after shuntings is shown in Table 7.

TABLE 4   Liver function and operative mortality

| Classification of liver function | No. of cases | No. of deaths | Mortality (%) |
|---|---|---|---|
| A | 87 | 1 | 1.2 |
| B | 212 | 11 | 5.2 |
| C | 138 | 14 | 10.2 |

TABLE 5  Bleeding rate in various shuntings

| Type of shunt | No. of cases | No. of bleeding episodes | Bleeding[a] rate (%) |
| --- | --- | --- | --- |
| SRS | 216 | 35 | 16.2 |
| PCS | 122 | 14 | 11.5 |
| MCS | 23 | 2 | 13.1 |
| SCS | 5 | 0 | 0 |
| DSRS | 10 | 2 | 20.0 |

[a] $P > 0.25$, difference is not significant.

TABLE 6  Type of shunt and encephalopathy

| Type of shunt | No. of cases | No. of encephalopathies | Incidence (%) |
| --- | --- | --- | --- |
| SRS | 216 | 40 | 18.5 |
| PCS | 122 | 31 | 25.4 |
| MCS | 23 | 4 | 17.4 |
| SVS | 5 | 1 | 20.0 |
| DSRS | 10 | 1 | 10.0 |

TABLE 7  The long-term results of shunting operations[a]

| | 1 year | | | | 5 year | | | |
| --- | --- | --- | --- | --- | --- | --- | --- | --- |
| Type of shunt | No. of cases | No. of survivors | Survival rate (%) | Corrective survival rate (%)[b] | No. of cases | No. of survivors | Survival rate (%) | Corrective survival rate (%)[b] |
| SRS | 246 | 217 | 88.2 | 89.1 | 169 | 129 | 67.3 | 72.4 |
| PCS | 146 | 126 | 86.3 | 87.5 | 109 | 82 | 64.9 | 72.8 |
| MCS | 30 | 21 | 70.0 | 70.9 | 17 | 14 | 57.7 | 57.2 |

| | 10 year | | | | 20 year | | | |
| --- | --- | --- | --- | --- | --- | --- | --- | --- |
| Type of shunt | No. of cases | No. of survivors | Survival rate (%) | Corrective survival rate (%)[b] | No. of cases | No. of survivors | Survival rate (%) | Corrective survival rate (%)[b] |
| SRS | 102 | 68 | 44.9 | 52.2 | 40 | 6 | 6.7 | 16.3 |
| PCS | 65 | 39 | 38.9 | 51.3 | 22 | 4 | 7.1 | 21.5 |
| MCS | 11 | 7 | 36.7 | 43.7 | 4 | 1 | 9.2 | 26.2 |

[a] Death in the first year includes operative death. The survival rate is calculated according to the life table. Patients who died of causes other than portal hypertension and those who were lost to follow-up were classified as 'dead' cases.
[b] The survival rates between different periods for various types of shunt were not significantly different ($P > 0.1$).

## Evaluation and prospect of total portosystemic shunting operation for the treatment of portal hypertension

The main aim of surgical treatment of portal hypertension is to eliminate the risk of bleeding from gastroesophageal varices. Once massive bleeding occurs, it may cause death directly or cause deterioration of the liver function. Although the bleeding may cease after conservative treatment, rebleeding often occurs leading, in most patients, to a poor prognosis. A dozen different portosystemic shunts have been developed since Whipple's end-to-side portocaval shunt and Blalock's end-to-side splenorenal shunt reported in 1945 [4]. In 1967, Warren advanced a procedure of selective gastro-esophageal varices decompression by distal splenorenal shunt [5], thus the traditional shunt may be called total portosystemic shunt (TPSS) [6]. Generally speaking, if there are many different approaches suggested to treat a given disease, it means that none of them are totally satisfactory, and this is the case with portal hypertension.

It is generally recognized that TPSS can effectively decrease the portal pressure and keep it stable after shunting [7]. In most patients, TPSS is able to prevent and control the bleeding from the ruptured esophageal varices. According to the literature, 95% of acute variceal bleedings stopped after emergency shunting [8].

In our patients, only three bleedings failed to stop in 45 emergency shuntings, a rate of bleeding stoppage of 93,3%. Other Chinese surgeons have reported the rebleeding rate to be 3.8 – 20%, which is similar to that reported in other countries [9]. In our series the rebleeding rate was 11.5 – 16.2%. By reviewing some randomized and prospective controlled records, Conn found that the rebleeding rate in patients with esophageal variceal hemorrhage who received portosystemic shunting was much lower than in those treated with conservative measures [10]. We have analysed, retrospectively, 407 patients with esophageal varices proved by barium study but with no history of bleeding. 139 patients received prophylactic shuntings and three died from the operation (mortality rate, 2.2%). 136 postoperative survivors were followed-up for an average of 6 years and 4 months; bleeding occurred in 21 patients (15.4%). The remaining 268 patients treated medically were followed-up for an average of 5 years and 3 months; 97 patients had bleeding episodes (36.2%) ($P < 0.005$) [11]. The above results show that the shunting operation is effective for prevention of esophageal variceal bleeding, so prophylactic shunting has its place despite the controversy [12]. Because of the possibility of developing postshunting encephalopathy, we recently limited our indications for prophylactic shuntings as follows (although the prediction of bleeding is difficult): (1) progressively severe esophageal varices proved by repeated barium study in an interval of 3 months; (2) definite RC signs shown by endoscopy; (3) the patient being highly nervous about variceal bleeding; (4) fair liver function.

In recent years, the mortality of shunting operations has been successfully lowered to an acceptable level, below 4% for elective shuntings [9]. The operative mortality in our series was 5.9%, it was 3.8% for elective shunting and only 1.2% in class A patients. Emergency shunting still has a high operative mortality, in our patients it was up to 24.4%, therefore it is better to use all kinds of nonoperative managements, including esophageal tamponade, intravenous vasopressin and injection sclerotherapy via endoscopy, etc., to stop the bleeding and perform an elective shunting within 2 to 3 weeks. If the conservative treatment fails to control bleeding, since 1975 we have elected to perform emergency porto-azygous disconnection.

The main disadvantage of TPSS is that hepatopetal blood flow is reduced to a half of the original total liver blood flow [13]. Thus, the metabolism and regeneration of the liver cells are definitely impaired. TPSS also makes the intestine-absorbed toxic substances bypass the liver, contributing to the development of postshunting encephalopathy [14]. The incidence of encephalopathy in our patients was 20.8% and was as high as 25.4% after portocaval shunting. Fifty of 76 patients had moderate and severe postshunting encephalopathy. The patients lost the ability to work and had difficulty in taking care of themselves. Selective angiography for 20 moderate encephalopathic patients (nine PCS, seven SRS and four MCS) showed patent anastomotic stoma. To identify the correlation between encephalopathy and liver function before shunting, 118 PCS (30 with encephalopathy) were analysed (Table 8).

The material mentioned above shows that there was no definite correlation between liver function and encephalopathy [15]. Unshunted patients also may develop encephalopathy due to spontaneous collateral shunts and impaired liver function. 268 unshunted patients with proved esophageal varices and without bleeding, with their liver function classified as A (36.2%), B (44.8%), and C (19%) were followed-up for an average of 5 years and 3 months; ten patients developed encephalopathy (3.7%) [11].

It is generally believed that the larger the anastomotic stoma the more the blood volume bypassing the liver, and the more likely the development of encephalopathy. Bismuth had challenged the general viewpoint by showing both almost identical incidences [25%] in his small controlled study, in which 13 patients had anastomotic stomas larger than 2 cm in diameter and 23 less than 1.5 cm [16]. Chinese surgeons usually prefer to make a smaller anastomotic stoma of 1.2 cm in diameter or less. Most of our anastomotic stomas were between 1.0 and 1.2 cm in diameter. Seven of 23 patients with the portocaval anastomotic stomas larger than 1.3 cm developed postoperative encephalopathy (an incidence of 30.4%), which was not significantly different from that of the total group of portocaval shunting (25.4%). In addition, smaller anastomic stoma more easily produce thrombosis after operation.

A correlation between the incidence of encephalopathy and the magnitude of decrease of portal pressure after portocaval shunting has been observed in our patients. The portal pressure of 88 patients without encephalopathy was lowered by an average of 76 mmH$_2$O after shunting and that of 30 patients with

TABLE 8   Liver function and encephalopathy (EP)

| Liver function grading | No. of patients with EP (%) | No. of patients without EP (%) |
|---|---|---|
| A | 7 (23.3) | 20 (22.7) |
| B | 15 (50.0) | 45 (51.1) |
| C | 8 (22.7) | 23 (16.2) |

encephalopathy by an average of 406 mmH$_2$O. The difference between the two groups was statistically significant ($P < 0.05$). Similar condition was noticed in the mesocaval shunting patients. In four patients with encephalopathy, portal pressure decreased after shunting by an average 527 mmH$_2$O, and only 104 mmH$_2$O in 21 patients without encephalopathy. In contrast with the shunting operation, 75 patients who received porto-azygous disconnection were followed-up for an average of 5 years and 6 months; only two patients had encephalopathy and 14 (18.7%) rebled during this period. The changes in portal pressure of these patients were studied. It increased to a certain extent in 69 of 76 patients, to an average of 39 mmH$_2$O higher than the original level before the disconnection procedure. Hence, it seemed that the development of postoperative encephalopathy is parallel to the extent of decreased portal perfusion or the magnitude of decreased portal pressure. The reduction of portal perfusion is also related to the prognosis and even to the survival of the cirrhotic patients [17].

Because of the high incidence of postshunting encephalopathy, reduction of liver perfusion and harmful effects on the recovery of the cirrhotic liver, the frequency of selection of total portosystemic shunting seems to have the tendency to decrease over the last 5 years in China. The percentage of patients receiving TPSS has decreased from 88.9 to 55.6%.

Distal splenorenal shunt is recognized as a rational design for selectively reducing the pressure of the varices in the gastro-esophageal region, a highly risky area from which to bleed, while keeping the hepatic portal perfusion at its original high pressure. This type of regional decompression operation was started in 1975 in China, and since then a total of 121 cases have been reported with no development of postoperative encephalopathy, but with a higher rebleeding rate of 4.7 – 17.5%. It seems that the procedure for completing a distal splenorenal shunt is rather difficult, we had two failures in 12 such procedures, and another two suffered unsatisfactory anastomosis. Recently, research into the long-term effects of distal splenorenal shunt on hepatopetal blood flow has been under way in some centers [19].

In order to maintain the portal blood flow and simultaneously eliminate the risk of rebleeding, in 1987 we began a new approach to treat portal hypertension with splenectomy and coronary vein embolization. The embolization agent is $n$-octyl alpha-cyanoacrylate mixed with radiopaque material which is able to polymerilyze in 10 – 15 s. This agent was injected through coronary venocatherization after ligation of the proximal end of the coronary vein. Embolization can not only reach the coronary venous trunk but also its gastric and esophageal branches supplying the gastro-esophageal varices, thus the plexus of veins at the gastric fundus and lower portion of the esophageal varices were occluded. The Second Affiliated Hospital of Si-An Medical University have reported their experience in 84 cases receiving this operation. There was one operative death, and no rebleeding or encephalopathy was found during the period of 2-year follow-up [20]. We have performed 17 such operations with no operative mortality, rebleeding or encephalopathy within one year after surgery. The portal pressure dropped 15 mmH$_2$O after splenectomy, and went up to well above the original level (an average of 17 mmH$_2$O) after the embolization of the coronary venous system. According to these findings, we suggest that the rise in portal pressure created by porto-azygous disconnection would contribute to the reopening of the occluded collaterals between the area drained by portal vein and that by the coronary vein. In the last six months, we have added the traditional splenorenal shunt to coronary venous embolization in ten cases. The portal pressure elevated (an average of 19 mmH$_2$O) after splenectomy and coronary venous embolization while, when the shunting was completed, it fell by an average of 75 mmH$_2$O, with an actual fall of 56 mmH$_2$O from the original level. Our argument for this combined procedure is: **(1)** coronary venous embolization is effective in preventing variceal bleeding; **(2)** shunting can lower the elevated portal pressure, consequently the reopening of the occluded collaterals will be delayed or avoided; **(3)** the drastic fall of portal pressure after total portosystemic shunt can be corrected, thereby the possibility of developing postshunting encephalopathy may be reduced; **(4)** technically, splenorenal shunting is easy to complete. Warren and co-workers have reported a similar observation in which they found a higher 2-year survival rate and much more improved liver function in a group of patients who received a further distal splenorenal shunt after an ineffective injection sclerotherapy by endoscopy than those who received selective shunting only. It is recognized that liver blood flow is not impaired after the occlusion of lower esophageal varices by sclerotherapy, whereas distal splenorenal shunt was shown to decrease the portal blood flow by 47% after a long-term observation [19]. Our new approach has only been adopted in a very small group of patients with a very short period of observation, so we need longer follow-up and further analysis.

As mentioned in the beginning, cirrhosis in China is mainly postnecrotic or schistosomal not alcoholic, so there was no problem of giving up drinking alcohol after surgery. The pathological course of alcoholic cirrhosis is different from that of non-alcoholic [18]. Many problems concerning portal hypertension remain to be solved.

## References

1   Huang Yan-Ting. Operations for portal hypertension in China. Arch Surg 1985; 120: 1197 – 1199.
2   Huang Yan-Ting. The present status of surgical treatment for portal hypertension in China. Chin Med J 1983; 63: 175 – 178.
3   Résumé of Second National Symposium of portal hypertension. Chung Hua Wai Ko Tsa Chih (Chin J Surg) 1986; 24: 659 – 661.
4   Donovan AJ. Surgical treatment of portal hypertension. A historical perspective. World J Surg 1984; 8: 626 – 645.
5   Warren WD, et al. Selective trans-splenic decompression of gastroesophageal varices by distal splenorenal shunt. Ann Surg 1967; 166: 437 – 455.
6   Galambos JT, et al. Surgery for hypertension. Clin Gastroenterol 1979; 8: 525 – 534.
7   Huang Yan-Ting, et al. Short-term observation of portal pressure after portosystemic shunt. Chung Hua Wai Ko Tsa Chih (Chin J Surg) 1986; 24: 711 – 712.
8   Orloff MJ, et al. Long-term results of ermergency portocaval shunt for bleeding esophageal varices in unselected patients with alcoholic cirrhosis. Ann Surg 1980; 192: 325 – 337.

9 Levine BA, et al. Portasystemic shunting remains the procedure of choice for control of variceal hemorrhage. Arch Surg 1985; 120: 296 – 300.

10 Conn H. Ideal treatment of portal hypertension in 1985. Clin Gastroenterol 1985; 14: 259 – 264.

11 Bai Chun-Nian, et al. A further evaluation on prophylactic portosystemic shunt. Chung Hua Wai Ko Tsa Chih (Chin J Surg) 1986; 24: 719 – 721.

12 Leading articles (Editorial). Current thought on surgery for portal hypertension. Br Med J 1977; 2: 978 – 979.

13 Reynolds TB. Hepatic circulatory changes after shunt surgery. Ann NY Acad Sci 1970; 170: 379 – 391.

14 Fraser CL, Arieff AI. Hepatic encephalopathy. New Engl J Med 1985; 313: 865 – 873.

15 Huang Yan-Ting. Encephalopathy after porto-systemic shunt. Shyr Yung Wai Ko Tsa Chih (J Prac Surg) 1987; 7: 367 – 368.

16 Bismuth H, et al. Portal-systemic shunt in hepatic cirrhosis. Does the type of shunt decisively influence the clinical result? Ann Surg 1974; 179: 205 – 218.

17 Hendersen JM, et al. Hemodynamic differences between alcoholic and nonalcoholic cirrhosis following distal splenorenal shunt effect on survival? Ann Surg 1983; 198: 325 – 334.

18 Warren WD, et al. Distal splenorenal shunt versus endoscopic sclerotherapy for long-term management of variceal bleeding. Ann Surg 1986; 203: 454 – 462.

19 Rikkers LF, et al. Effects of altered portal hemodynamics after distal splenorenal shunts. Am J Surg 1987; 153: 80 – 83.

20 Liu Xiao-Gong, et al. Embolization of gastric coronary vein in the treatment of portal hypertension. Chung Hua Wai Ko Tsa Chih (Chin J Surg) 1986; 24: 648 – 651.

© 1988 Elsevier Science Publishers B.V. (Biomedical Division)
*Treatment of esophageal varices*
*Y. Idezuki, editor*

Chapter 23

# Mesocaval shunts

KENNETH G. SWAN, JOHN J. FLANAGAN AND JOYCE M. ROCKO

*Department of Surgery, UMDNJ – NJMS, Newark, NJ 07103-2757, USA*

The mesocaval shunt was introduced almost simultaneously by Marion [1] in France and Clatworthy [2] in the United States in 1951. It was initially used to control bleeding from the esophageal varices associated with congenital abnormalities of the hepatobiliary system in children. The procedure consisted of transposition of the divided inferior vena cava and the divided superior mesenteric vein, hence its name, mesocaval shunt. Up until his death in 1975 the procedure was also called the Drapanas shunt in attribution of that surgeon's modification with a Dacron® prosthesis to an 'H' configuration of a side-to-side shunt between superior mesenteric vein and inferior vena cava. The mesocaval shunt is currently configured with polytetrafluoro-ethylene (Goretex®) or autologous tissue (internal jugular vein) in addition to woven or knitted Dacron®. The mesocaval shunt is today one of the most popular techniques for elective or emergency control of variceal hemorrhage [3]. It will probably continue to be a mainstay in the surgical management of variceal hemorrhage.

In the United States, hemorrhage from esophageal varices is the most common cause of death from cirrhosis of the liver [4]; and cirrhosis of the liver is now the fifth leading cause of death in the United States [5]. A report of a recent survey [6] indicates that while young adults in the United States exhibit a continued downward trend in the use of most illicit drugs, their alcohol consumption has continued with little decline in the past three years.

The most common form of cirrhosis in the United States is that attributed to alcohol consumption. These and other observations indicate a probable sustained requirement for surgery in the foreseeable future in the United States. This is especially so when one considers the disappointing long-term results with sclerotherapy. The rebleed rate is lowest (18 – 65%) among non-alcoholic cirrhotics in Japan [7]. Amongst alcoholic cirrhotics the figures are higher. The rebleed incidence in Cello's series was 75%. This figure was in sharp contrast to the 0%

rebleed incidence in his patients who underwent portacaval shunt [8]. In Rikkers' recent report the rebleed rate was 57% following sclerotherapy versus 26% for shunt surgery [9]. The list of complications associated with sclerotherapy is long [10] and ranges from 'sclerotherapist's eye' to pericardial tamponade [11].

In the seventies, Orloff called attention to the fact that only a small percentage (10 – 20%) of the bleeding cirrhotic patient population ever came to elective surgery [12]. The explanation related to the fact that the mortality of the first bleed was high or, if controlled, was followed too soon by additional bleeding, which prevented elective surgery from becoming a realistic possibility. Terblanche pointed out that bleeding from esophageal varices was a probability in 30% of patients whose varices had not yet bled but that the figure increased to 70% once bleeding occurred [13]. Orloff thus advocated prompt (within eight hours) surgical intervention (emergency portocaval shunt) once the diagnosis of bleeding esophageal varices had been made [14]. Unfortunately, a high operative mortality of almost 50% gained little support for his protocol. This was especially so when he subsequently indicated that Child's 'C' patients were not candidates for surgery [15]. Some believe Child's 'C' classification to be a contraindication to any surgery [16]. Orloff subsequently reported a significant improvement in this percentage (17% operative mortality among 84 emergency shunts performed between 1978 and 1983) [17] but even surgeons remain unconvinced. Fischer described a 38 – 48% operative mortality for emergency mesocaval and portacaval shunts, respectively [18]. Welch and Malt described the operative mortality rate associated with emergency shunt surgery as 'unacceptably high' [19].

Among the generally accepted contraindications to portasystemic shunt surgery for bleeding esophageal varices are: (1) Child's classification 'C'; (2) uncontrollable ascites; (3) encephalopathy; and (4) alcoholic hepatitis. Unfortunately, the diagnosis of alcoholic hepatitis is possible only with liver biopsy and this is often not available for decision-making, especially when an emergency shunt is contemplated. Likewise, definitions of encephalopathy and the 'uncontrollability' of ascites are also elusive. And the determination as to when a Child's classification 'B' becomes a 'C' or vice versa is imprecise. We believe that the only real contraindication to emergency surgery is encephalopathy and have facetiously stated that '. . . if you don't need anesthesia to perform the operation you probably shouldn't operate!' The survival of Child's 'C' patients undergoing emergency surgery to prevent exsanguination has been sufficient for us to continue to recommend surgery under such circumstances. If bleeding can be controlled, we prefer to wait as long as possible before elective surgery in an effort to improve Child's classification. We keep the patient hospitalized, however. Thus such patients fall into the 'urgent' category.

Our interest in the mesocaval shunt was prompted by reports in the literature regarding the four conventional shunting procedures currently most popular. These are the portacaval (Eck fistula) shunt, the mesocaval (Drapanas) shunt, the distal splenorenal (Warren) shunt and the (Linton) proximal splenorenal shunts. Of these four, the portacaval shunt, whether side-to-side or end-to-side, has been, by far, the most commonly performed [20]. In Mehigan's analysis of 255 articles in the medical literature, dealing with shunting procedures during the decade ending in 1978, the next most commonly performed procedures were the mesocaval shunt (572), the

Linton shunt (550) and the Warren shunt (319). These numbers contrasted with 1894 portacaval shunts, most of which (1586) were end-to-side. Undoubtedly, more current data would probably show an increase in mesocaval shunts and Warren shunts as these two are the most recently introduced of the four.

Relative risks to the patient of either of these four procedures regarding operative mortality, incidence of encephalopathy and five-year survival are largely dependent upon observer selectivity. Conn's review of four separate randomized controlled trials of elective portacaval shunts (208 patients) compared with 195 medically treated variceal bleeders revealed an operative mortality of 11% which resulted in an encephalopathy rate of 32% but a rebleed rate of only 8%. These figures contrast with a rebleed rate of 58% but an encephalopathy rate of only 6% in the nonoperative group. Five-year survival rates (59% medical, 49% surgical) were comparable [21]. Langer [22] compared elective distal splenorenal shunt with elective end-to-side portacaval shunt and reported a slightly higher operative mortality (13% vs. 0%) and rebleeding incidence (15% vs. 10%) with the Warren shunt. The encephalopathy incidence was slightly lower with the latter procedure (23% vs. 40%) and five-year survival was comparable (51%, 56%). In Smith's cooperative Veterans Administration study [23] there were 162 Warren shunts performed and 376 'total shunts' (i.e., mesocaval, portacaval or Linton shunts) from 37 university affiliated hospitals. Operative mortality for elective procedures was 15% and for emergency procedures 43%, results which ". . . compare favorably with those from many private institutions." Of interest was their observation (reminiscent of Orloff's earlier one) that only 20 – 25% of patients with bleeding esophageal varices undergo surgery. Cameron's experience with the mesocaval shunt [24] indicated that long-term patency (100%, up to six years) was possible but operative mortality was high for nonelective procedures (urgent 33%, emergency 50%). Rypins [25] advocates a small-diameter (8 mm) mesocaval shunt which has a long-term patency if the early perioperative thrombosis, if it occurs, is eliminated with balloon angioplasty. Thus, patency of mesocaval shunts, regardless of configuration, does not appear to be as problematic as had earlier been predicted by Orloff.

Conversely, the distal splenorenal shunt, which had appeared to offer the highest probability of long-term success, was recently called into question by Warren himself. In a report to the American Surgical Association he pointed out that the distal splenorenal shunt was applicable only to nonalcoholic cirrhotics and that unless splenopancreatic disconnection (i.e., division of all pancreatic branches of the splenic vein) was carried out the likelihood of the 'selective' shunt remaining so was not high [26]. When this modification of the Warren shunt is not possible for technical reasons, the Linton shunt is an alternative. The incision for surgical exposure (i.e. long left subcostal) of each is the same.

Ottinger reported the largest series of Linton, or proximal splenorenal, shunts [27]. Among his 140 elective cases the operative time was seven hours and operative mortality was 12%; the five-year survival was 41%; the rebleed rate was 10% and encephalopathy occurred in 19% of those who survived surgery. Average blood loss was 4.3 units per operation. We admire those who have, but we have not, had personal experience with the Sugiura procedure [28] or splenopneumopexy [29] in the non-shunting operative approach to bleeding esophageal varices. With these obser-

from the recent literature in mind, we elected to compare in a prospective
ized fashion the distal splenorenal (Warren) shunt with the mesocaval shunt
in patients who were candidates for elective surgical intervention of bleeding
esophageal varices. We were interested in operative technique, mortality, patency,
encephalopathy and long-term survival. We performed mesocaval shunts, almost
exclusively, for emergency control of bleeding. We placed 'urgent' patients in the
elective category. We reserved the Linton shunt for patients with hypersplenism
(WBC $<4000$ mm$^{-3}$, platelets$<100$ 000 mm$^{-3}$). Since we performed more
mesocaval shunts we attempted to make conclusions regarding what we determined
was the optimal shunt.

TABLE 1   UMDNJ patient population ($n = 93$)

| | |
|---|---|
| Males | 86% |
| Caucasians | 89% |
| Age in years | |
| Mean | 45.3 ± 1.9 |
| Range | 22 – 69 |
| Laennec's cirrhosis | 96% |
| Childs classification | |
| A | 21% |
| B | 45% |
| C | 34% |

TABLE 2   Technical points for consideration in mesocaval shunting

1. Midline incision
2. Meticulous dissection
3. Mobilize SMV  –  2 fingers
4. Mobilize IVC  –  3 fingers
5. Protect right ureter
6. Large prosthesis, 22 – 24 mm
7. Short prosthesis, 2 – 4 cm
8. Prolene 5-0, C-1 needle
9. No pressure gradient

TABLE 3   Operative manometrics (cmH$_2$O) among patients undergoing mesocaval shunts

| | Portal | Shunt | Inferior vena caval | Central venous |
|---|---|---|---|---|
| $\bar{x}$ | 40.5 | 13.4[a, b] | 12.7[a] | 12.3[a] |
| S.E. | 2.1 | 0.8 | 0.9 | 0.7 |

[a] Values not significantly different ($P > 0.10$), but each significantly different ($P < 10^{-8}$) from portal pressure.
[b] Reduction in portal pressure 67%.

Our patient population is summarized in Table 1. The patients were mostly middle-aged white males whose varices were the result of alcoholic cirrhosis of the liver. Child's classification 'B' was most common. All patients had liver biopsies as the first step in the operative procedure following intra-abdominal exploration. All patients had angiography preoperatively to determine the patency of the portal venous system. The latter was shown to have a 17% chance of thrombosis in a recent large series by Belli [30]. In addition, we need to know the status of the splenic and left renal veins (Fig. 1), since their patency and proximity determine the feasibility

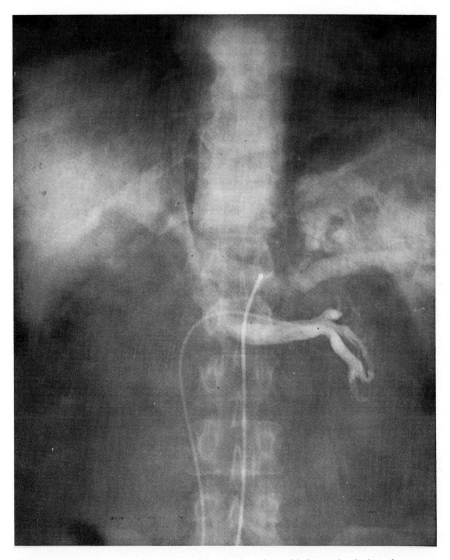

FIG. 1   Preoperative angiography with splenic vein and left renal vein less than one vertebral body apart.

of a Warren shunt (e.g., no more than one vertebral body apart) [31]. The only shortcoming of angiography is the inability to predict the relationship of the splenic vein to the pancreas. Ideally, the splenic vein is just inferior and slightly deep to the inferior border of the pancreas with the left renal vein deep to the splenic vein. Ideally, both are 10 – 15 mm in diameter. Unfortunately, the splenic vein can be directly behind, even superior to the pancreas; worse yet, it may run within the substance of the gland. This relationship precludes the Warren, but not necessarily the Linton, shunt in our experience.

Following randomization, we performed the mesocaval shunt (Fig. 2) through a midline abdominal surgical incision or the Warren shunt (Fig. 3) through a left subcostal incision. We never had to abandon a planned mesocaval shunt but did fail, in two patients, to perform a Warren shunt because of unsuitability of the splenic vein not appreciated angiographically preoperatively. The details of our technique for mesocaval shunt are summarized in an earlier report [32].

Certain technical points regarding the procedure deserve emphasis (Table 2). A midline abdominal surgical incision provides excellent exposure. Meticulous dissection reduces operative blood loss. We mobilize the superior mesenteric vein so as to permit its encirclement with two fingers. This requires dissection proximally to the level of the middle colic artery and requires division of the right colic artery and vein. We have never seen ischemic injury of the ascending colon as a result of this latter procedure. We use the right colic vein as part of the mesenteric venous

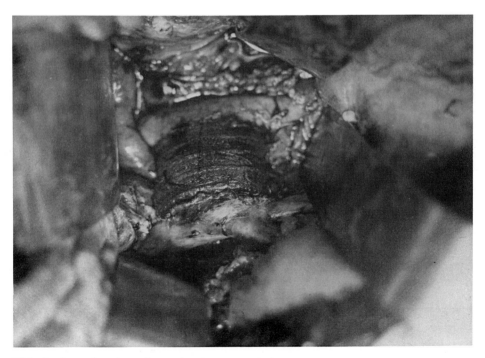

FIG. 2 Operative view of completed mesocaval shunt.

anastomatic suture line. The inferior vena cava is dissected up to permit its encircle-ment with three fingers. This procedure requires division and ligation of all lumbar veins and is time-consuming; however, this step is critical to shortening of the pro-sthetic length and even more importantly short-cutting the problematic duodenal loop which invariably vexes the shunt. The right ureter is variable in location (Fig. 4) and can be damaged easily during the course of the vena caval dissection. Thus we routinely look for, identify and encircle the right ureter with an umbilical tape in order to retract it out of the operative field.

We advocate a large in diameter (22 – 24 mm) cloth (Dacron®) prosthesis for the shunt (Fig. 2). Whether it is of knitted or woven construction is not important, since bleeding from graft or its suture lines is rarely a problem in our experience. Addi-tionally, we advocate as short a length as possible (2 – 4 cm) to the shunt. We believe patency of the shunt will be enhanced by its large size and short length. We have not had experience with polytetrafluoro-ethylene (Goretex®) in mesocaval shunting but do not recommend against its use. We have used polypropylene (Prolene®) suture material for anastomoses and favor 5 – 0 on a BB needle (Ethicon®). The vena caval anastomosis is made difficult because the depth of the operative field hinders rotation of the needle holder. Thus needle size assumes greater importance than does size of suture material. The inferior vena cava is a relatively thick-walled vein and is very forgiving to the surgeon. The same is not true of the superior mesenteric vein, which is often tissue-paper thin, tears easily and frustrates the most

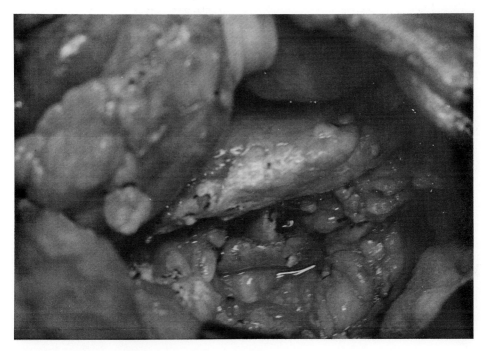

FIG. 3   Operative view of completed Warren shunt.

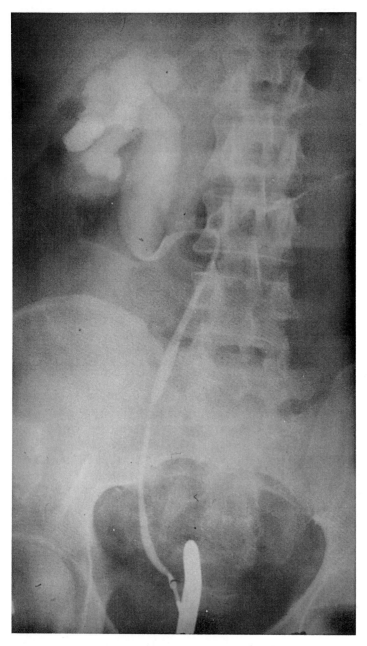

FIG. 4   Right ureter seen retrograde pyelographically to identify retrocaval ureter as congenital anomaly.

patient surgeon. Extensive mobilization of inferior vena cava and superior mesenteric vein, as previously described, facilitates these technically difficult anastomoses.

Following completion of the mesocaval shunt we routinely assess shunt effectiveness hemodynamically by measuring pressures across each suture line with a manometer connected to a 21 gauge needle inserted into the prosthesis. We compare these measurements with central venous pressure recorded by the anesthesiologist. We believe there should be no pressure gradient across either suture line other than that attributed to altitude. These values are summarized in Table 3. Mean portal pressure (shunt occluded) was $40.5 \pm 2.1$ (S.E.) $cmH_2O$. Shunt pressure (shunt open) was $13.4 \pm 0.8$ $cmH_2O$, which was a highly significant ($P < 10^{-8}$) decrease [33]. Inferior vena caval pressure, $12.7 \pm 0.9$ $cmH_2O$, and central venous pressure, $12.3 \pm 0.7$ $cmH_2O$, were not significantly ($P > 0.10$) different from shunt pressure. This reduction (67%) in portal pressure is the largest in the literature to our knowledge. Whether or not this physiological effect on portal pressure is beneficial or harmful to the patient, his liver or his central nervous system is unknown. What is known is that portal hypertension causes esophageal varices and that the most effective cure for bleeding from esophageal varices is reduction in blood pressure within the varices. The mesocaval shunt, constructed as described above, will effectively achieve this result. The effect is of course immediate and persistent as long as the shunt remains patent.

Table 4 summarizes our observations regarding performance of the procedure. Mean shunt diameter was $22.1 \pm 0.5$ (range $16.0 - 26.0$) mm; mean length was $3.26 \pm 0.10$ (range $7.5 - 2.2$) cm. Length of procedure ranged from 3.5 to 10 (mean $5.91 \pm 0.16$) hours. This parameter was offset in our opinion by the small value for operative blood loss/replacement, $0.44 \pm 0.15$ (range $0-4$) units per patient, including emergencies. What have been our results with these procedures? Table 5 summarizes our experience.

There were 93 patients in our series. This was comprised of 61 elective and 32 emergency operations. We considered electively scheduled procedures to be in the 'elective' category, thus 'urgent' cases are tabulated as elective, not 'emergency,' procedures. There were two operative mortalities associated with the elective procedures. One patient died following a mesocaval shunt and one died following a Warren shunt. Operative mortality for elective procedures was thus 3%. Thirty-two emergency procedures, almost all mesocaval shunts, were performed and four

TABLE 4   Operative observations among patients undergoing mesocaval shunts

|  | Shunt | | Time (hours) | Blood replacement (units) |
|---|---|---|---|---|
|  | Diameter (mm) | Length (cm) | | |
| Mean | 22.1 | 3.26 | 5.91 | 0.44 |
| SE | 0.05 | 0.10 | 0.16 | 0.15 |
| Range | 16.0 – 26.0 | 2.2 – 7.0 | 3.5 – 10.0 | 0 – 4 |

deaths occurred within 30 days. Operative mortality for emergency surgery was thus 13%. Overall operative mortality for the entire series was 6%. These data compare favorably with results from nonoperative management of bleeding esophageal varices in the medical service of our institution.

During the years 1980 – 1984 we identified and reviewed the records of 50 patients admitted to our Gastrointestinal Service with a diagnosis of bleeding from esophageal varices secondary to alcoholic cirrhosis of the liver (Table 6). Seventeen died within 30 days of admission, a hospital mortality of 33%. This figure is modest when compared to comparable studies within Veterans Administration Centers across the United States [23].

It is our policy to perform angiography to assist shunt patency postoperatively before discharge from the hospital (Figs. 5 and 6). We have been satisfied that *all* of our shunts have been patent at least during the early postoperative period. Upper gastrointestinal bleeding, even hemorrhage, is not uncommon in our experience during the early (first week) postoperative period;. Eckhauser made similar observations following distal splenorenal shunt [34]. This is particularly true following

TABLE 5   Operative mortality among shunted patients

|  | Patients | Mortality | |
|---|---|---|---|
|  |  | Number | Percent |
| **Elective** |  |  |  |
| Distal splenorenal (Warren) | 26 | 1 | 4 |
| Mesocaval (Drapanas) | 30 | 1 | 3 |
| Proximal splenorenal (Linton) | 5 | 0 | 0 |
| **Emergency** |  |  |  |
| Distal splenorenal | 1 | 0 | 0 |
| Mesocaval | 31 | 4 | 13 |
| Total | 93 | 6 | 6[a] |

[a] Operative mortality for elective procedures 3%.

TABLE 6   Non-operative mortality among patients hospitalized with bleeding esophageal varices

| Number | Etiology | Hospital mortality | |
|---|---|---|---|
|  |  | Number | Percent |
| 50 | Alcoholic cirrhosis | 17 | 33 |

Medical Service, UMDNJ, 1980 – 1984.

emergency procedures. Regarding this complication several observations are pertinent. Initially we returned to the operating room with these patients, assuming that
the shunt was clotted. We found patient shunts in all cases and no explanation for
the bleeding. Endoscopy usually revealed no specific source of the bleeding;
however, gastritis was seen with greater frequency than variceal hemorrhage under

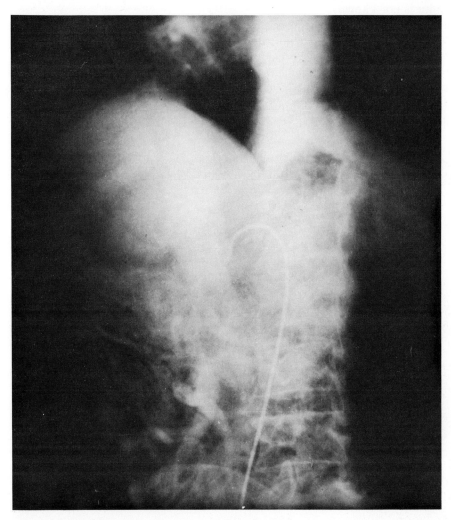

FIG. 5   Angiographically patent mesocaval shunt. Inferior vena cava is visualized in venous
phase of a superior mesenteric arterial injection.

these circumstances. Finally, varices often remain enlarged despite patent shunts. We treat such patients supportively and have been satisfied to observe spontaneous cessation of bleeding over a few days time. More recently we have routinely devascularized the stomach as a first step in emergency surgery and we seen less early postoperative hemorrhage today. Whether there is a causal relationship with this procedure is not known.

Our long-term follow-up studies are incomplete at this writing. If our patients stop alcohol ingestion they generally do well and we have 11-year survivors among both mesocaval and distal splenorenal shunt series. Those who continue alcohol ingestion progressively deteriorate with endstage liver disease, are lost to follow-up and presumably have died. We have not observed a difference in encephalopathy postoperatively when operative procedure was the variable. We have seen little encephalopathy among the abstinent patients in either group.

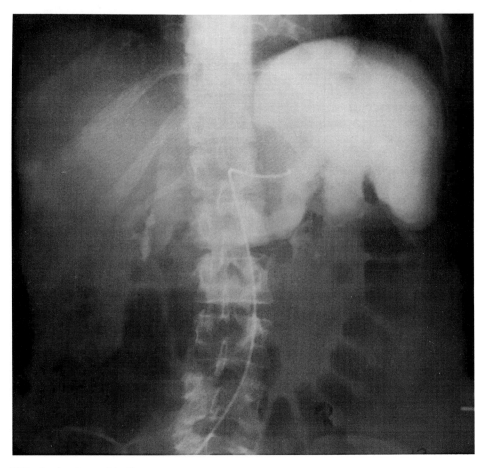

FIG. 6  Angiographically patent Warren shunt. Inferior vena cava is visualized in venous phase of a splenic arterial injection.

## Summary

The mesocaval shunt remains a good operation for control of variceal hemorrhage. The procedure is useful for elective as well as urgent or emergency control of bleeding esophageal varices. Concern for long-term patency appears to be unjustified if the procedure is properly performed. We advocate a large in diameter (22 – 24 mm) prosthesis which is made as short as possible (2 – 4 cm) by extensive mobilization of the inferior vena cava and the superior mesenteric vein. There should be no pressure gradient across either suture line; operative manometrics should so verify. Mortality rates for either elective or emergency surgery should be acceptably low, < 5% and < 15% respectively. The only contraindication to surgery is encephalopathy. The generally accepted high encephalopathy rate following classical portocaval shunt, along with increasing concern for the 'selectivity' of the distal splenorenal shunt, supports an increasing role for the mesocaval shunt. Encephalopathy following the operation is not high and certainly not higher than that following the Warren shunt in our experience.

## References

1 Marion P. Les Obstructions portales. Sem Hop Paris 1953; 29: 2781 – 6.
2 Clatworthy WH, Wall T, Watman RW. A new type of portal-to-systemic venous shunt for portal hypertension. Arch Surg 1955; 134: 146 – 52.
3 Mehigan DG, Zuidema GD, Cameron JL. The incidence of shunt occlusion following portosystemic decompression. Surg Gynecol Obstet 1980; 150: 661 – 663.
4 Burroughs AK, D'Heygere F, McIntyre N, Pitfalls in studies of prophylactic therapy for variceal bleeding in cirrhotics. Hepatology 1986; 6: 1407 – 1413.
5 Report of the National Center for Health Statistics, Bethesda, MD, 1987.
6 Johnston LD. University of Michigan's Institute for Social Research, Research Center, 13 Jan., 1987.
7 Terabayashi H, Ohnishi K, Tsunoda T, et al. Prospective controlled trial of elective sclerotherapy in comparison with percutaneous transhepatic obliteration of esophageal varices in patients with nonalcoholic cirrhosis. Gastroenterology 1987; 93: 1205 – 9.
8 Cello JP, Grendell JH, Crass RA, et al. Endoscopic sclerotherapy versus portacaval shunt in patients with severe cirrhosis and acute variceal hemorrhage. N Engl J Med 1987; 316: 11 – 15.
9 Rikkers LF, Burnett DA, Volentine GD, et al. Shunt surgery versus endoscopic sclerotherapy for long-term treatment of variceal bleeding. Ann Surg. 1987; 206: 261 – 271.
10 Conn HO, Grace NA. Portal hypertension and sclerotherapy of esophageal varices: A point of view. *Endosc Rev* 1985; 39 – 53.
11 Tabibian N, Schwartz JT, Smith L, et al. Cardiac tamponade as a result of endoscopic sclerotherapy: Report of a case. Surgery 1987; 102: 546 – 547.
12 Orloff MJ, Charters AC, Chandler JG, et al. Portacaval shunt as emergency procedure in unselected patients with alcoholic cirrhosis. Surg Gynecol Obstet 1975; 141: 59 – 68.
13 Terblanche J. Injection sclerotherapy for esophageal varices. Surgical Rounds 1979; 48 – 57.
14 Orloff MJ, Charters AC, Chandler JG, et al. Portacaval shunt as emergency procedure

in unselected patients with alcoholic cirrhosis. Surg Gynecol Obstet 1975; 141: 59 – 68.

15    Orloff MJ, Duguay LR, Kosta LD. Criteria for selection of patients for emergency portacaval shunt. Am J Surg 1977; 134: 146 – 152.

16    Wright PD, Loose HW, Carter RF, et al. Two-year experience of management of bleeding esophageal varices with a coordinated treatment program based on injection sclerotherapy. Surgery 1986; 99: 604 – 609.

17    Orloff MJ, Bell RH. Long-term survival after emergency portacaval shunting for bleeding varices in patients with alcoholic cirrhosis. Am J Surg 1986; 151: 176 – 183.

18    Fischer JE. Current concept of surgery in portal hypertension. Seminars in Liver Disease 1983; 3: 225 – 234.

19    Welch CE, Malt RA. Abdominal surgery. N Engl J Med 1983; 308: 685 – 695.

20    Mehigan DG, Zuidema GD, Cameron JL. The incidence of shunt occlusion following portosystemic decompression. Surg Gynecol Obstet 1980; 150: 661 – 663.

21    Conn HO. Ideal treatment of portal hypertension in 1985. Clin Gastroenterol 1985; 14: 259 – 288.

22    Langer B, Taylor DR, Mackenzie TG, et al. Further report of a prospective randomized trail comparing distal splenorenal shunt with end-to-side portacaval shunt. Gastroenterology 1985; 88: 424 – 9.

23    Fulenwider JT, Smith RB, Millikan WJ, et al. Variceal hemorrhage in the veteran population. Am Surg 1984; 50: 264 – 269.

24    Sarr MG, Herlong HF, Cameron JL. Long-term patency of the mesocaval C shunt. Am J Surg 1986; 151: 98 – 103.

25    Rypins EG, Milne N, Sarefeh IJ, et al. Quantitation and fractionation of nutrient hepatic blood flow in normals, portal hypertensive cirrhosis and after small diameter portacaval shunts. Ann Surg in press, 1988.

26    Warren WD, Millikan WJ, Henderson JM, et al. Splenopancreatic disconnection. Ann Surg 1986; 204: 346 – 355.

27    Ottinger LW. The Linton splenorenal shunt in the management of the bleeding complications of portal hypertension. Ann Surg 1982; 196: 664 – 668.

28    Abona GM, Baissony H, Al-Nakib BM, et al. The place of Sugiura operation for portal hypertension and bleeding esophageal varices. Surgery 1987; 101: 91 – 98.

29    Ono J, Taketo K, Kodama Y. Combined therapy for esophageal varices: Sclerotherapy, embolization and splenopneumopexy. Surgery 1987; 101: 535 – 543.

30    Belli L, Romani F, Sanalone CV, et al. Portal thrombosis in cirrhotics. Ann Surg 1986; 203: 286 – 291.

31    Warren WD, Salam AA, Hutson D, et al. Selective distal splenorenal shunt. Arch Surg 1974; 108: 306 – 314.

32    Rocko JM, Swan KG, Howard MM. Surgical management of bleeding esophageal varices: Results of 80 cases. Am Surg 1986; 52: 81 – 86.

33    Snedecor GW, Cochran WG. Statistical Methods. Sixth Edn. Ames, IA: Iowa State University Press, 1967.

34    Echauser FE, Pomerantz RA, Knol JA, et al. Early variceal rebleeding after successful distal splenorenal shunt. Arch Surg 1986; 121: 547 – 552.

© 1988 Elsevier Science Publishers B.V. (Biomedical Division)
*Treatment of esophageal varices*
*Y. Idezuki, editor*

Chapter 24

# Indication, results and prognosis of distal splenorenal shunt

K.-J. Paquet

*Department of Surgery, Heinz-Kalk Hospital, Am Gradierbau, D-8730 Bad Kissingen, FRG*

Selective variceal decompression by the distal splenorenal shunt (DSRS) is 20 years old. In that time it has been clearly shown that this procedure controls bleeding, but controversy exists as to how far the physiological goals of maintaining portal perfusion and hepatocyte function are achieved, and whether survival is improved. It is important [1 – 11] to emphasize that this not a portal systemic shunt: the varices are selectively decompressed, and portal hypertension must be maintained in the splanchnic-hepatic axis to retain portal perfusion. Thus the development of a portal systemic encephalopathy is prevented.

## Materials and methods

### Selection of the patients
Initial management of hemorrhage from esophageal varices consisted of the insertion of a Linton-Nachlas tube, restoration of blood volume, correction of metabolic imbalance, reduction of ascites and maximal nutritional improvement of liver function. When bleeding was not arrested by balloon tamponade, emergency endoscopic paravariceal sclerotherapy was undertaken.

The selection criteria for distal splenorenal shunt were Child-Pugh classification A or B [12, 13] and also the following criteria (Table 1): the sonographic volume of the liver should be 1000 – 2500 ml and the portal perfusion at sequential scintigraphy more than 30% [14 – 17]. Further visceral angiography should rule out stenosis of the hepatic artery supply and 'portal pseudoperfusion' [18] and demonstrate adequate length and caliber of the splenic vein, and liver biopsy at laparoscopy should not show activity or progression of cirrhosis.

From the 1st of April, 1982, to the 1st of July, 1987, 299 patients were admitted to our hospital with bleeding esophageal varices. The 161 in Child-Pugh class C were not considered for splenorenal shunt, nor were 17 with encephalopathy diagnosed from extensive neurological investigations (Table 2). The remaining 121 patients were selected using the above-mentioned criteria. They included 32 with portal perfusion; over 30% elected for a Warren shunt. Twenty-four fulfilled the criteria for a mesocaval interposition shunt [19]; in the remaining 65 an elective and chronic endoscopic paravariceal sclerotherapy was performed. In all 32 patients the distal splenorenal shunt was performed as an elective procedure. The underlying disease was liver cirrhosis, mainly of alcoholic origin (62.5%) in almost 90% of the series (Table 3); prehepatic block (2 cases), schistosomiasis and a cystic liver fibrosis were the other causes of portal hypertension and recurrent variceal bleeding. The male/female ratio was 20 to 12 and the mean age 48 (16 – 65) years. There were 11 cases of Child-Pugh A and 19 of Child-Pugh B.

*Surgical technique*
After measurement of the portal pressure via the superior mesenteric vein, the great omentum and transverse colon were lifted and the identification of the splenic vein was performed through the mesenterium and retroperitoneum along the inferior mesenteric vein. The splenic vein was dissected from confluence to the portal vein up to the hilus of the spleen. After the preparation of the left renal vein the splenic vein was disconnected from the portal vein and an end-to-side anastomosis with the renal vein was performed. Thereafter all varices along the distal greater curvature of the stomach were devascularized and the left gastric vein was ligated. In 7 cases the construction of a distal splenorenal shunt was technically impossible or too risky because of a severe chronic pancreatitis; in all cases a mesocaval interposition shunt with a 14 or 16 mm Dacron prothesis was performed.

TABLE 1   Selection criteria for elective distal splenorenal shunt in portal hypertension

1. Liver volume, sonographically determined as 1000 – 2500 ml [7, 10]
2. Portal perfusion $\geq$ 30% at sequential scintigraphy [1, 20]
3. No activity or progression of cirrhosis seen at laparoscopy and biopsy
4. No stenosis of the hepatic arterial circulation, and suitable lumen and length of the splenic vein, found at angiographic studies

TABLE 2   Methods in assessment of portal-systemic encephalopathy

1. Writing test
2. Number-connection test, trail test
3. Neurologic – psychiatric examination
4. EEG
5. Psychometric tests

TABLE 3   Etiology of the portal venous block

| Primary disorder | Causal factor | No. of cases |
|---|---|---|
| Intrahepatic | | |
| Cirrhosis | Alcoholism | 20 |
| Cirrhosis | Hepatitis | 5 |
| Cirrhosis | Unknown | 2 |
| Cirrhosis | Primary biliary | 1 |
| Cystic liver fibrosis | Congenital | 1 |
| Schistosomiasis | Infection | 1 |
| Total | | 30 (94%) |
| Extrahepatic | | |
| Portal vein thrombosis | Idiopathic or congenital | 2 (6%) |

TABLE 4   Prognosis of distal splenorenal shunt ($n$ = 26%): 0.1.01.1982 – 01.07.1987 (01.01.1988)

| | | |
|---|---|---|
| Early death | 2 | (7.7%) |
| Late death | 2 | (7.7%) |
| Shunt thrombosis | 0 | |
| Portal thrombosis | 0 | |
| Recurrence of hemorrhage | 0 | |
| Encephalopathy | 0 | |
| Five-year life expectancy | 82% | |

## Early and long-term results

There were 2 postoperative deaths (6.2%); the causes were liver and renal failure. At autopsy all the shunts were patent. Both patients were in class Child-Pugh B. Thus the hospital mortality of the splenorenal shunt was 7.7%. In no case was a recurrent variceal hemorrhage observed. Postoperative evaluation of the portal system was performed by selective visceral angiography in all patients. These investigations demonstrated the patency of all shunts performed 14 days and one year after the shunt and ruled out a portal thrombosis (Table 4).

The incidence of portal systemic encephalopathy was carefully investigated (see Table 2). No encephalopathy developed in any patient. The liver function remained stable. All patients could be followed up to the 1st of January 1988. There were two further deaths, one because of liver failure and one because of hepatocellular carcinoma. The five-year survival time according to Kaplan-Meier is over 80% (Fig. 1).

Thus elective distal splenorenal shunt after a strict selection of the patients offers the current best decompressive management method for bleeding esophageal

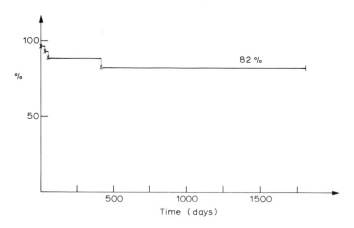

FIG. 1    Five-year life expectancy according to Kaplan-Meier (n = 26).

varices. The concept has proven valid, the technique has continued to evolve, and objective data have supported its ability to control bleeding, maintain portal flow and hepatic function and prevent portosystemic encephalopathy. If our series is compared to a series of patients with chronic elective sclerotherapy with the same selection criteria after refusal of a selecive shunt operation the results with distal splenorenal shunt seem to be superior to those with chronic elective sclerotherapy. It guarantees the longest survival without any fear of another recurrence of life-threating variceal hemorrhage.

## References

1    Conn HO, Resnick RH, Grace ND, et al. Distal spleno-renal shunt vs. portal-systemic shunt: current status of a controlled trial. Hepatology 1983; 1: 151–160.
2    Fischer JE, Bower RH, Atamian S, et al. Comparison of distal and proximal spleno-renal shunt: a randomized prospective trial. Ann Surg 1981; 194: 531–544.
3    Harley HAJ, Morgan T, Redeker AG, et al. Results of a randomized trial of end to side portacaval shunt and distal spleno-renal shunt in alcoholic liver disease and variceal bleeding. Gastroenterology 1987; 92: 1301–1310.
4    Langer B, Taylor BR, McKnee GR, et al. Further report of a prospective randomized trial comparing distal spleno-renal shunt with end to side portacaval shunt: an analysis of encephalopathy, survival and quality of life. Gastroenterology 1985; 88: 424–429.
5    Millikan WJ Jr, Warren BW, Henderson JM, et al. The Emory prospective randomized trial: selective vs. nonselective shunt to control variceal bleeding. Ann Surg 1985; 201: 712–722.
6    Reichle FA, Fahmy WF, Golsorskhi M. Comparative clinical trial with distal splenorenal and mesocaval shunt. Am J Surg 1981; 194: 531–544.
7    Rikkers LF, Rudan D, Galambos JT, et al. A randomized, controlled trial of the distal splenorenal shunt. Ann Surg 1978; 188: 271–282.
8    Warren WD, Zeppa R, Foman JJ. Selective transsplenic decompression of gastroesophageal varices by distal splenorenal shunt. Ann Surg 1967; 166: 437–455.

9   Warren WD, Millikan WJ. Selective transsplenic decompression procedure: changes in technique after 300 cases. Contemp Surg 1981; 18: 11 – 32.

10  Warren WD, Henderson JM. Distaler splenorenaler Shunt: seine gegenwärtige Bedeutung in der Therapie der Varizenblutung. Chir Gastroenterol 1987; 3: 63 – 72.

11  Zeppa R, Hensley GT, Levy JV, et al. The comparative survival of alcholics vs non-alcoholics after distal splenorenal shunt. Ann Surg 1978; 187: 510 – 514.

12  Child CG. Surgery and portal hypertension. In: Engelbert J, Dunfield H, eds. Major problems in clinical surgery, Vol. I. Philadelphia: WB Saunders, 1964.

13  Pugh PNH, Murray-Lyon IM, Dawson JM, Pietroni MC, Williams R. Transection of esophagus for bleeding esophageal varices. Br J Surg 1973; 60: 46 – 52.

14  Biersack H-J, Thelen M, Paquet K-J, Knopp R, Schmitt R, Winkler C. Die sequentielle Hepato-spleno-Szintigraphie zur quantitativen Beurteilung der Leberdurchblutung. Fortschr Röntgenstr 1977; 126: 47 – 58.

15  Koischwitz D. Sonographische Lebervolumenbestimmung: Problematik, Methodik und praktische Bedeutung der Quantifizierung des Lebervolumens. Fortschr Röntgenstr 1979; 131: 243 – 254.

16  Paquet K-J, Tholen M, Koischwitz G, Biersack H-J. Ein neues therapeutisches Konzept für die Auswahl von Leberzirrhotikern mit rezidivierender Ösophagusvarizenblutung für den elektiven Shunt. Chirurg 1979; 50: 313 – 318.

17  Paquet K-J, Zöckler CE, Draese K. Indikation und Auswahl von Leberzirrhotikern mit rezidivierender Ösophagusvarizenblutung zur elektiven Shuntoperation. Chir Gastroenterol 1987; 3: 15 – 22.

18  Fulenwider JT, Nordlinger BM, Millikan WJ, Sones PJ, Warren WD. Portal perfusion an angiographic illusion? Ann Surg 1979; 189: 257 – 262.

19  Paquet K-J, Kalk J-Fr, Koussouris P. Prospective evaluation and long-term results of mesocaval interposition shunts. Acta Chir Scand 1987; 153: 423 – 429.

© 1988 Elsevier Science Publishers B.V. (Biomedical Division)
*Treatment of esophageal varices*
*Y. Idezuki, editor*

Chapter 25

# Selective shunts for esophageal varices via trans-left gastric venous and trans-splenic routes – their rationale and clinical results

MICHIO KOBAYASHI[1], KIYOSHI INOKUCHI[2] AND KEIZO SUGIMACHI[3]

[1] *Department of Surgery I, Medical College of Oita, Oita,* [2] *Saga Prefectural Hospital, Koseikan Saga, Saga, and* [3] *Department of Surgery II, Faculty of Medicine, Kyushu University, Fukuoka, Japan*

## Introduction

There are two approaches to the selective decompression of esophageal varices: (1) a trans-left gastric venous route which was originated by Inokuchi as left gastric vena caval shunt (LGCS) [1], (2) a trans-splenic route proposed by Warren et al. as distal splenorenal shunt (DSRS) [2]. Because the serious drawback of the Warren shunt, namely 'loss of the selectivity', has been recently claimed at a remote follow up [3 – 7], we have devised an alternative way in which we tried to disconnect splenopancreatic communications after the distal splenorenal shunt (DSRS with splenopancreatic disconnection), in order to ensure a satisfactory selective shunting [8]. We herewith present the rationale and clinical results of our procedures, LGCS on the one hand and DSRS with splenopancreatic disconnection on the other, for the selective decompression of esophageal varices.

## Clinical results

*Left gastric vena caval shunt (LGCS)*
Left gastric vena caval shunt has been carried out on 250 cases since 1967. The patients include 189 cirrhotics and 56 patients with idiopathic portal hypertension. The follow-up period averaged 9 years and 7 months, ranging from 6 months to 19 years and 2 months.

Requests for reprints should be addressed to M. Kobayashi, M.D., Department of Surgery I, Medical College of Oita, Oita, Japan.

*Operative results (Table 1)* The operative mortality rate was satisfactorily low; 2.8% overall, and 3.7% in the cirrhotic cases. The bleeding after surgery was found only in 8.0% of all patients, and 7.9% in the cases with liver cirrhosis.

*Portal hemodynamics (Table 2)* The portal hemodynamics were assessed by angiography or ultrasonic examination. The diameter of the portal vein was marginally changed from the preoperative mean of 15.9 mm to 13.2 mm at the follow-up period. There was no case of thrombosis, stenosis or retrograde flow of the portal vein. The portal flow was well maintained at the mean of 680 ml/min at a remote follow-up. The shunt proved to be patent in 87.8%. Fig. 1 shows the representative angiograms of a patient who received this operation 12 years ago. Top left panel is an original angiogram from 12 years ago. Bottom right is the present film showing shunt open, and bottom left shows a forward flow of portal blood similarly to the preoperative status. Therefore, the purpose of selective decompression has been realized by our left gastric vena caval shunt.

### Distal splenorenal shunt (DSRS)

*Operative results* On the other hand, we have performed the Warren shunt on 39 patients. Table 3 shows its clinical results. Although 5.1% of operative mortality was acceptable, there was a high incidence of Eck's syndrome, more or less 20%, with concomitant low survival.

TABLE 1   Results of left gastric vena-caval shunt (250 cases)

|                   | Overall (250 cases) | Cirrhosis (187 cases) |
| ----------------- | ------------------- | --------------------- |
| Early death       | 7 ( 2.8%)           | 7 ( 3.7%)             |
| Late death        | 77 (30.8%)          | 70 (37.0%)            |
| Survivors         | 165 (66.4%)         | 112 (59.3%)           |
| Postop. bleeding  | 20 ( 8.0%)          | 15 ( 7.9%)            |

TABLE 2   Portal hemodynamics after LGCS

|                                  | Preop.      | Discharge   | Follow-up   |
| -------------------------------- | ----------- | ----------- | ----------- |
| Angiography (37 cases)           |             |             |             |
| Diameter PV (mm)                 | 15.9 ± 21   | 15.3 ± 2.4  | 13.2 ± 2.5  |
| Hepatofugal collat.              | 100%        | 0%          | 5.8%        |
| Portal thrombosis or stenosis    | 0           | 0           | 0           |
| Echo-Doppler (31 cases)          |             |             |             |
| PV Flow (ml/min)                 | 721 ± 186   | 743 ± 136   | 680 ± 231   |
| Retrograde flow                  | 0           | 0           | 0           |
| Shunt patency rate (147 cases)   |             |             | 87.8%       |

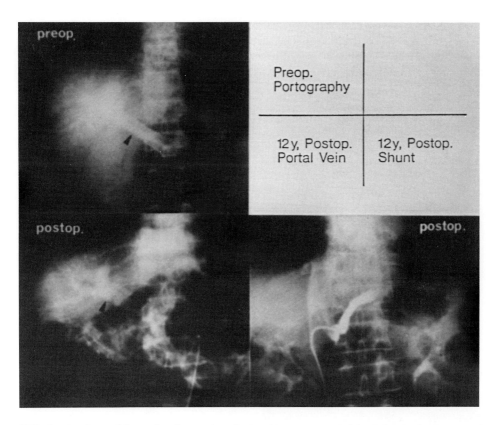

Preop.
Portography

12 y, Postop.
Portal Vein

12 y, Postop.
Shunt

preop.

postop.

postop.

FIG. 1  Angiographic study of portal perfusion in a case treated by left gastric vena caval shunt 12 years ago.

TABLE 3  Results of distal splenorenal shunt (39 conventional cases)

|  | Overall (39 cases) | Cirrhosis (30 cases) |
|---|---|---|
| Early death | 2 ( 5.1%) | 0 ( 0%) |
| Late death | 19 (48.7%) | 16 (53.3%) |
| Survivors | 18 (46.5%) | 14 (36.6%) |
| Postop. bleeding | 5 (12.8%) | 2 ( 6.6%) |
| Eck syndrome | 8 (20.5%) | 6 (20.0%) |

280

*Portal hemodynamics* Fig. 2 shows the venograms and the pulsed Doppler flowmetry at a remote follow-up after distal splenorenal shunt. As shown in the top panel, there was a leaking of portal blood flow from the proximal splenic vein via abundant intrapancreatic collaterals to the established shunt. The reversal portal flow ensued as shown at the bottom. Fig. 3 indicates the ways in which the porto-

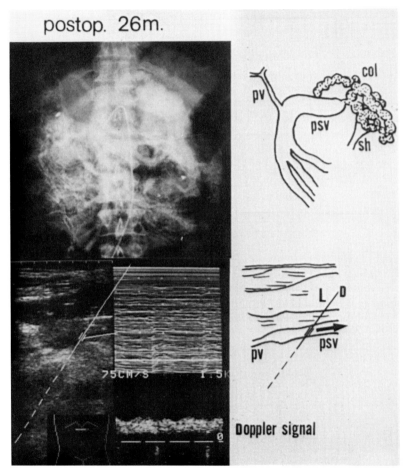

FIG. 2  Venous phase of the superior mesenteric arteriography in a cirrhotic patient 26 months after distal splenorenal shunt and measurement of blood flow volume and direction through the proximal splenic vein by pulsed Doppler flow meter. A marked narrowing of the portal vein was noted. The mesentric blood flow was hepatofugal through the proximal splenic vein and prominently developed collaterals which led to the shunt (upper). The proximal splenic vein was visualized on the B-mode scanning of the epigastrium. Doppler signals obtained from that vein indicated a hepatofugal flow in the leftward direction, estimated as 825 ml/min (below). pv = portal vein; psv = proximal splenic vein; col = collateral veins; sh = shunt; L = liver; and D = Doppler beam with sampling site represented by double bars.

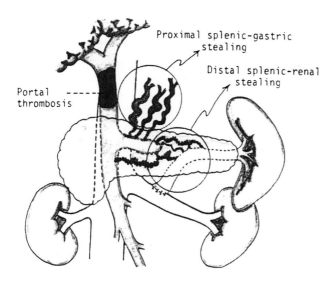

FIG. 3   Assumed mode of malcirculation in portal system after distal splenorenal shunt (DSRS).

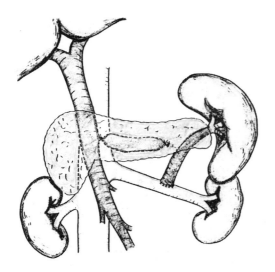

FIG. 4   Distal splenorenal shunt with splenopancreatic disconnection.

deprived malcirculation can occur in patients after DSRS. Two types of leakage in portal blood flow are possible, such as proximal splenic-gastric leakage and distal splenic-renal leakage. These were thought to cause the reduction of the portal vein, thus inducing stenosis or thrombosis of the portal vein.

*DSRS with splenopancreatic disconnection*
Hence, we have devised an alternative procedure (DSRS with splenopancreatic disconnection) in order to prevent such portal malcirculation. Fig. 4 shows the scheme of our procedure, namely splenic hilar renal shunt with proximal flush ligation of splenic vein. The point is that in addition to the ligation of the splenic vein adjacent to the portal vein, the shunt passageway was isolated as much as possible from the embedded pancreas. This method is principally the same as Dr. Warren's proposal in which he emphasized entire splenopancreatic disconnection for an adequately selective shunting. We have applied this approach in 71 cases, including 67 cirrhotics. The follow-up ranged from 6 months to 6 years 4 months, averaging 3 years 3 months.

*Operative results (Table 4)* The clinical results were satisfactory; the overall operative mortality and postoperative bleeding rates being 1.4 and 4.2%, respectively. Even in the cirrhotics, the operative mortality remained low, 1.5%, as well as postoperative bleeding, 4.5%. The Eck's syndrome was nil.

TABLE 4   Results of DSRS with splenopancreatic disconnection (71 cases)

|  | Overall (71 cases) | Cirrhosis (67 cases) |
|---|---|---|
| Early death | 1 ( 1.4%) | 1 ( 1.5%) |
| Late death | 14 (19.7%) | 10 (14.9%) |
| Survivors | 56 (78.9%) | 56 (83.6%) |
| Postop. bleeding | 3 ( 4.2%) | 3 ( 4.5%) |
| Eck syndrome | 0 ( 0%) | 0 ( 0%) |

TABLE 5   Portal hemodynamics after conventional DSRS and DSRS with splenopancreatic disconnection

|  | DSRS (conventional) | DSRS with S-P disconnection |
|---|---|---|
| Postop. portal malcirculation | 4/20 (20.0%) | 0/33 (0%) |
| Thrombosis | 2 | 0 |
| Stenosis | 2 | 0 |
| PV flow (ml/min) | 169 ± 90/7 cases | 674 ± 189/19 cases |
| Shunt patency rate | 17/20 (85.0%) | 64/68 (94.1%) |

*Portal hemodynamics* Table 5 shows the comparative data of portal hemo-dynamics after conventional DSRS and our procedure. Although there was a 20% incidence of portal malcirculation in the DSRS group, we found no such disadvantage in any case after our procedure. The portal blood flow was well maintained at about 670 ml/min, and the shunt patency was proved in 94.1% of our procedures. Fig. 5 shows the venograms and the pulsed Doppler flowmetry at a remote follow-up after our procedure. The portal vein was well open in Fig. 5A. Pulsed Doppler flowmetry revealed a sufficient portal flow of 896 ml/min (Fig. 5C). The patent shunt was well visualized (Fig. 5B), with a blood flow of 384 ml/min shown in Fig. 5D. The survival of the patients treated by DSRS with splenopancreatic disconnection as well as LGCS proved to be significantly improved, when compared with that after DSRS (Fig. 6).

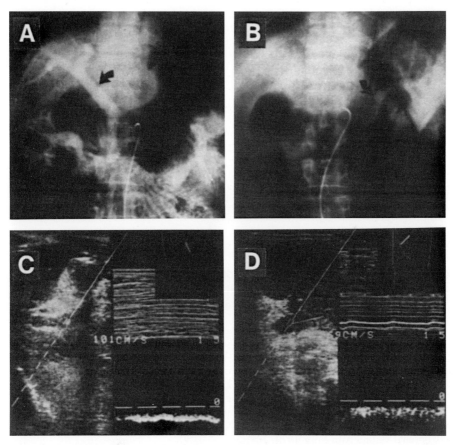

FIG. 5  Angiograms and pulsed Doppler flow meter studies in a cirrhotic patient one month after DSRS with splenopancreatic disconnection. Venous phase (A) of the superior mesentric arteriography indicates a hepatopetal portal flow (arrow). Pulsed Doppler flow meter (C) reveals a sufficient portal blood flow of 896 ml/min. Venous phase (B) of the splenic arteriography indicates a patent shunt (arrow) with a blood flow of 384 ml/min (D).

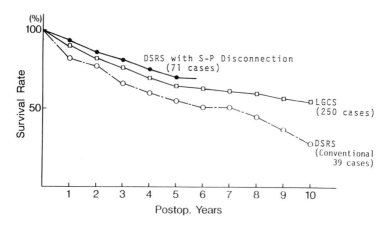

FIG. 6   Survival rate of 360 patients after selective shunts.

## Surgical indications for our procedures

Cirrhosis of the liver and idiopathic portal hypertension are good candidates for these procedures. Regarding liver function, these shunts are applicable to patients with Child's classification A and B, and some of C, and those with less than 40% ICG retention rate as well as more than 0.04/min ICG disappearance rate. Viewed from the hemodynamic standpoint, we perform a left gastric vena caval shunt in patients with predominant left gastric vein and, on the other hand, DSRS with splenopancreatic disconnection in cases of predominant short gastric vein.

## Conclusion

Based on our experience, we recommend not only left gastric vena caval shunt but also an alternative to the Warren shunt, DSRS with splenopancreatic disconnection, for the more selective decompression of esophageal varices.

## References

1   Inokuchi K. A selective portacaval shunt. Lancet 1968; 6: 51 – 52.
2   Warren WD, Zeppa R, Fomon JJ. Selective transsplenic decompression of esophageal varices by distal splenorenal shunt. Ann Surg 1967; 166: 437 – 455.
3   Rikkers LF, Rudman D, Galambos JT. A randomized contolled trial of the distal splenorenal shunt. Ann Surg 1978; 188: 271 – 280.
4   Rostein LE, Makowka L, Langer B, et al. Thrombosis of the portal vein following distal splenorenal shunt. Surg Gynecol Obstet 1979; 149: 847 – 851.
5   Saubier EC, Partensky C, Pinet A, et al. Operation de Warren pour hypertension portale: Appreciation de la methode par controle angiographique precoce de 23 cas. J Chir 1980; 117: 147 – 153.

6  Belghiti J, Grenier P, Nouel O, et al. Long-term loss of Warren's shunt selectivity: Angiographic demonstration. Arch Surg 1981; 116: 1121 – 1124.

7  Henderson JM, Millikan WJ, Chipponi J, et al. The incidence and natural history of thrombus in the portal vein following distal splenorenal shunt. Ann Surg 1982; 196: 1 – 7.

8  Inokuchi K, Beppu K, Koyanagi N, Nagamine K, Hashizume M, Sugimachi K. Exclusion of nonisolated splenic vein in distal splenorenal shunt for prevention of portal malcirculation. Ann Surg 1984; 200: 711 – 717.

9  Warren WD, Millikan WJ Jr, Henderson JM, et al. Splenopancreatic disconnection. Improved selectivity of distal splenorenal shunt. Ann Surg 1986; 204: 346 – 355.

© 1988 Elsevier Science Publishers B.V. (Biomedical Division)
*Treatment of esophageal varices*
*Y. Idezuki, editor*

Chapter 26

# Indication and results of distal splenorenal shunt

Toshio Isomatsu

*Sapporo Teishin Hospital, Sapporo, Japan*

## Introduction

The ideal treatment of bleeding oesophageal varices should permanently eliminate the serious complications of portal hypertension and have no adverse effect on hepatic function. The distal splenorenal shunt would provide both of these advantages, but there are a lot of data available to show that it eventually becomes a total shunt.

In this chapter, we analyse the results of and indications for distal splenorenal shunt. Also, the technical problems involved in improving selectivity of this shunt are examined.

## Materials and Methods

In the past 15 years, we performed distal splenorenal shunts in 70 patients. Two were emergencies, 58 were elective and 10 were prophylactic. The ages of the two

TABLE 1 Distal splenorenal shunt cases

| | No. of cases | Sex | | Age (mean) (years) |
|---|---|---|---|---|
| | | male | female | |
| Emergency | 2 | 1 | 1 | 31 – 50 (40) |
| Elective | 58 | 41 | 17 | 3 – 70 (44) |
| Prophylactic | 10 | 6 | 4 | 43 – 59 (51) |

emergency cases (one male, one female) were 31 and 50. The ages of the 58 elective cases (41 male, 17 female) were from 3 to 70 years (mean of 44) and the ages of the 10 prophylactic cases (6 male, 4 female) were from 43 to 59 (mean of 51) (Table 1).

## Results

*Effect of distal splenorenal shunt on hypersplenism*

*Leucopenia*
Forty patients who had leucopenia prior to distal splenorenal shunt were evaluated. The mean preoperative leucocyte count was 4000 ± 400/cmm. The mean post shunt leucocyte count in these patients was 5000 ± 300/cmm. This improvement in leucocyte counts was statistically significant (p < 0.001) (Fig. 1).

*Thrombocytopenia*
Forty patients with preoperative thrombocytopenia were also evaluated. The mean preoperative platelet count in these patients was 95 000 ± 6000/cmm. Mean postoperative platelet count increased to 120 000 ± 6000/cmm. This change was statistically significant (p < 0.05) (Fig. 2).

*Clinical results*

Immediate and late clinical results following distal splenorenal shunt are given in

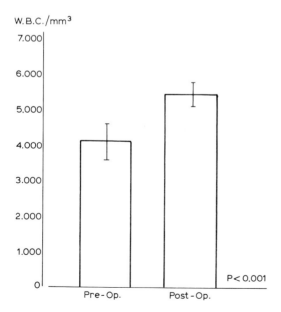

FIG. 1   Late response of leucopenia following distal splenorenal shunt.

Table 2. There were three patients with extra-hepatic portal obstruction, 14 with idiopathic portal hypertension and 53 with liver cirrhosis.

Operative death occurred in none of three with extra-hepatic portal obstruction, in one of 14 with idiopathic portal hypertension and in three of 53 with liver cirrhosis.

Variceal bleeding after distal splenorenal shunt occurred in two of three with extra-hepatic portal obstruction, in none of 13 with idiopathic portal hypertension and in four of 50 cirrhotics. There was bleeding from acute gastromucosal lesions

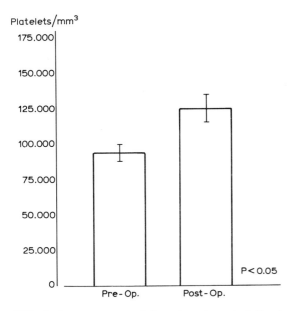

FIG. 2   Late response of thrombocytopenia following distal splenorenal shunt.

TABLE 2   Immediate and late results following distal splenorenal shunt

| | Op. death | Bleeding | | | Cause of late death | | | |
|---|---|---|---|---|---|---|---|---|
| | | varices | AGML | ulcer | hepatic failure | hepatoma | bleeding | others |
| EPO 3 | 0 | 2 | 1 | 0 | 0 | 0 | 0 | 0 |
| IPH 14 | 1 | 0 | 0 | 0 | 0 | 0 | 0 | 2 |
| LC 53 | 3 | 4 | 4 | 6 | 11 | 7 | 2 | 2 |

EPO, extra-hepatic portal obstruction; IPH, idiopathic portal hypertension; LC, liver cirrhosis.

or gastric ulceration in one of three with extra-hepatic portal obstruction and in 10 of 50 cirrhotics who tolerated the operation.

Late death occurred in two of 13 with idiopathic portal hypertension and in 22 cirrhotics. All of the three patients with extra-hepatic portal obstruction hemorrhaged again after operation (two from oesophageal varices, one from an acute gastromucosal lesion), but all patients are still living after a 15 year follow-up period. None of the 13 patients with idiopathic portal hypertension hemorrhaged, but two died from other causes. One 2 years and the other 7 years, respectively, after distal splenorenal shunt.

In cirrhotics, 14 patients hemorrhaged in this follow up period: four from oesophageal varices; four from acute gastromucosal lesions and six from gastric ulcers. During the 15 years of the postoperative period, 22 of 50 cirrhotics who tolerated the operation died. Eleven died from hepatic failure, seven from hepatoma, two from gastrointestinal bleeding and two from miscellaneous causes.

### Survival rate after distal splenorenal shunt
The cumulative survival rate of patients having distal splenorenal shunt are shown in Fig. 3.

In patients with idiopathic portal hypertension, the survival rate at one year after distal splenorenal shunt was 100%, at 3 years it was 92%, at 5 years 92%, at 7 years 84% and at 10 years it was 84%.

In patients with liver cirrhosis, the survival rate at one year was 90%, at 3 years it was 60%, at 5 years 54%, at 7 years 49% and at 10 years it was 45%.

### Indication for distal splenorenal shunt
For 20 patients who survived for more than 10 years after the standard distal splenorenal shunt, the preoperative and 1, 5 and 10 year postoperative shunt biochemical data are summarized in Table 3. There were no statistically significant changes in the patients who survived more than 10 years after distal splenorenal shunt and the portal blood flow in these patients continued to perfuse the liver.

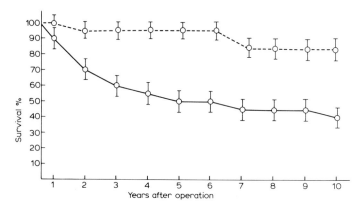

FIG. 3 Cumulative survival curve after distal splenorenal shunt. (− − −) idiopathic portal hypertension; (——) liver cirrhosis.

Therefore, distal splenorenal shunt appears to be the best procedure to obtain long-term survival in these patients.

To select the most favorable candidates for the distal splenorenal shunt, discriminative analysis was designed by use of variables based on hematological, biochemical and hemodynamical data (Table 4).

Discriminative analysis on operative mortality was performed in 50 patients. Thirty-nine of 42 patients were correctly classified in the group actually tolerating the operation and seven of eight patients were correctly classified in the fatality group. The percentage of correctly classified grouped cases was 92% (Fig. 4; Table 5).

Discriminative analysis on survival was performed in 24 patients having distal splenorenal shunt. Actual survivors were classified into: short-term survivors (less than 2 years after distal splenorenal shunt); middle-term survivors (from 2 to 5 years); and long-term survivors (more than 5 years). All of these subgroups were predicted correctly and the percentage of correctly classified grouped cases was 100% (Fig. 5; Table 6).

In the variables used in this series, statistically significant factors influencing operative mortality were; preoperative grade of splenic enlargement, marked

TABLE 3   Biochemical data preoperatively and at 1, 5 and 10 years after distal splenorenal shunt (n = 20)

|  | Pre | 1 year | 5 years | 10 years |
|---|---|---|---|---|
| Total bilirubin (mg/dl) | 1.3 ± 0.4 | 1.2 ± 0.4 | 1.5 ± 0.2 | 2.1 ± 1.1 |
| Direct bilirubin (mg/dl) | 0.5 ± 0.3 | 0.5 ± 0.2 | 0.5 ± 0.2 | 0.6 ± 0.2 |
| Serum albumin (g/dl) | 3.5 ± 0.2 | 3.1 ± 0.2 | 3.1 ± 0.2 | 3.3 ± 0.2 |
| Serum $\gamma$-globulin g/dl) | 1.7 ± 0.4 | 1.6 ± 0.4 | 1.6 ± 0.4 | 2.3 ± 1.2 |
| Hepaplastin test (%) | 61  ± 5.1 | 62  ± 4.9 | 65  ± 8.7 | 69  ± 11 |

TABLE 4   Variables

**I. Clinical**
1) Age
2) Hepatomegaly
3) Splenomegaly
4) OP-time
5) OP-blood loss

**II. Laboratory**
6) K-ICG
7) Insulinogenic Index

8) Blood-$NH_3$
9) T.P
10) $\gamma$-Globulin
11) S-Albumin
12) GOT
13) GPT
14) ALP
15) LDH
16) S-Bilirubin
17) Cho-E

18) WBC
19) RBC
20) PLT

**III. Hemodynamic**
21) PVP
22) Δ-PVP
23) PGX-G[a]
24) W H V P

[a] Portographical grading.

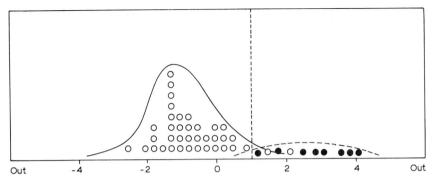

FIG. 4  Discriminative analysis of operative death. Classification groups: 0, alive after surgery ($Z = -0.57249$); ●, operative death ($Z = 5.00558$).

TABLE 5  Classification results on operative death

| Actual group | No. of cases | Predicted group membership | |
|---|---|---|---|
| | | 1 | 2 |
| Group 1 Subfile alive | 42 | 39 92.9% | 3 7.1% |
| Group 2 Subfile death | 8 | 1 12.5% | 7 87.5% |

Percent of 'grouped' cases correctly classified: 92.00%.

TABLE 6  Classification results on survival

| Actual group | No. of cases | Predicted group membership | | |
|---|---|---|---|---|
| | | 1 | 2 | 3 |
| Group 1 Subfile | 10 | 10 100.0% | 0 0.0% | 0 0.0% |
| Group 2 Subfile | 7 | 0 0.0% | 7 100.0% | 0 0.0% |
| Group 3 Subfile | 7 | 0 0.0% | 0 0.0% | 7 100.0% |

Percent of 'grouped' cases correctly classified: 100.00%.

changes of portal pressure before and after operation, serum-ALP, serum-LDH, age, $\gamma$-globulin, anemia, thrombocytopenia, $K_{ICG}$ and serum albumin (Table 7).

The statistically significant factors influencing long-term survival were: $\gamma$-globulin, serum GOT, $K_{ICG}$, serum albumin, thrombocytopenia, grade of pre-

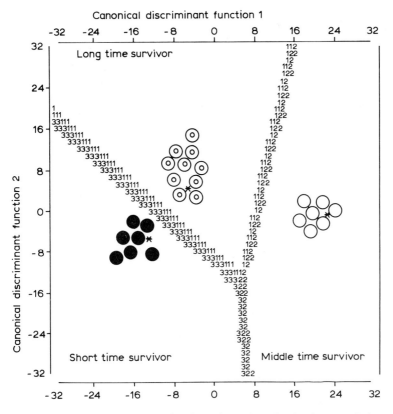

FIG. 5   Discriminative analysis of survival after distal splenorenal shunt.

TABLE 7   Prognostic factors on operative mortality

|  |  |  |
|---|---|---|
| 1. | Grade of splenic enlargement | $P < 0.01$ |
| 2. | Marked changes of portal pressure before and after operation | $P < 0.01$ |
| 3. | Serum ALP | $P < 0.05$ |
| 4. | Serum LDH | $P < 0.05$ |
| 5. | Age | $P < 0.05$ |
| 6. | $\gamma$-Globulin | $P < 0.05$ |
| 7. | Anemia | $P < 0.05$ |
| 8. | Thombocytopenia | $P < 0.05$ |
| 9. | $K_{ICG}$ | $P < 0.05$ |
| 10. | Serum albumin | $P < 0.05$ |

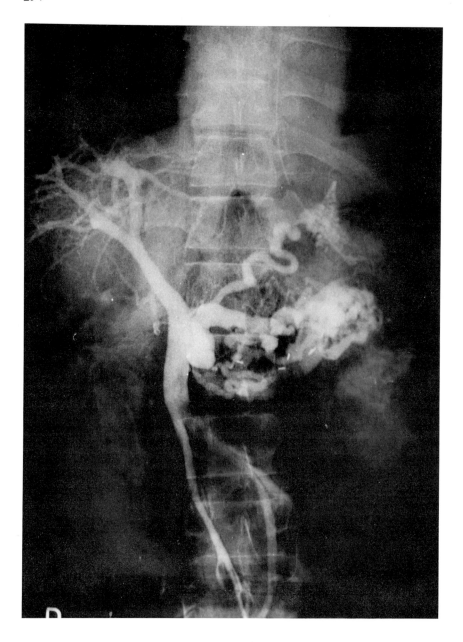

FIG. 6  Narrowing of portal vein (numerous collateral channels to the shunt).

TABLE 8   Prognostic factors on long-term survival

| | | |
|---|---|---|
| **1.** | $\gamma$-Globulin | $P < 0.01$ |
| **2.** | Serum GOT | $P < 0.01$ |
| **3.** | $K_{ICG}$ | $P < 0.01$ |
| **4.** | Serum albumin | $P < 0.01$ |
| **5.** | Thombocytopenia | $P < 0.05$ |
| **6.** | Grade of splenic enlargement | $P < 0.05$ |
| **7.** | Serum ALP | $P < 0.05$ |
| **8.** | Wedged hepatic venous pressure | $P < 0.05$ |
| **9.** | Serum ammonia level | $P < 0.05$ |
| **10.** | Serum LDH | $P < 0.05$ |

operative splenic enlargement, serum ALP, wedged hepatic venous pressure in pre-operative studies, serum ammonia level and serum LDH (Table 8).

In the majority of the patients who underwent standard distal splenorenal shunt, postoperative portography revealed a decrease in diameter of the portal vein compared to preoperative studies and numerous collaterals to distal splenorenal shunt. Postoperative portographical changes in 11 patients who showed considerable change of portal perfusion after standard distal splenorenal shunt are summarized in Table 9.

Figure 6 shows one of the typical patterns of portogram after standard distal splenorenal shunt. This figure shows narrowing of the portal vein, development of large collateral venous channels extending from the porto-mesenteric region and communicating to the shunt.

Therefore, from 1983, our operative technique was improved by including disconnection of the splenic vein from the pancreas to prevent portal malcirculation after the standard distal splenorenal shunt. The patient was positioned with the left side elevated 20° and the left arm adducted across the chest. An upper transverse abdominal incision was made across the right rectus muscle with large extension at the left flank (Fig. 7). This approach facilitated disconnecting the splenic vein from the pancreas at the splenic hilus.

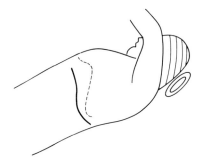

FIG. 7   Patient position and abdominal incision.

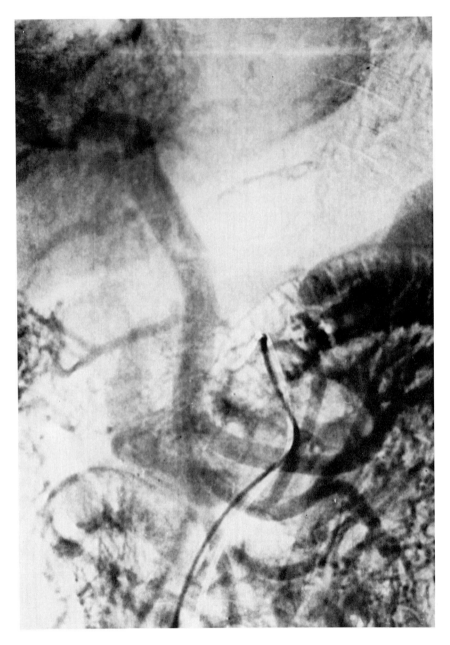

FIG. 8   Portal blood flow continued to perfuse the liver after distal splenorenal shunt with total splenopancreatic disconnection.

TABLE 9  Angiographic changes after conventional distal splenorenal shunt

| Case no. | Sex | Age | Postoperative angiographic changes | Time after operation in which changes occurred | Postoperative encephalopathy | Patient condition (years postop.) |
|---|---|---|---|---|---|---|
| 1 | M | 57 | Portal vein narrowed, numerous collaterals to shunt | 1 year | + | 7, alive |
| 2 | F | 52 | Portal vein narrowed, numerous collaterals | 6 months | + | 5, alive |
| 3 | F | 59 | Portal vein narrowed | 1 month | – | 4, alive |
| 4 | M | 32 | Portal vein narrowed | 4 years | – | 4, alive |
| 5 | M | 55 | Portal vein thrombosed, numerous collaterals | 1 month | – | 2, alive |
| 6 | M | 49 | Portal vein thrombosed, numerous collaterals | 7 years | + | 5, died from hepatoma |
| 7 | F | 58 | Arterio-portal vein fistula, numerous collaterals | 2 years | + | 2, died from hepatic failure |
| 8 | M | 47 | Portal vein narrowed, numerous collaterals | 3 years | + | 3, died from hepatoma |
| 9 | F | 67 | Portal vein narrowed, numerous collaterals | 1 year | + | 1, died from hepatic failure |
| 10 | M | 57 | Portal vein narrowed, numerous collaterals to shunt | 2 months | + | 1, alive |
| 11 | F | 45 | Portal vein narrowed, numerous collaterals to shunt | 1 month | + | 4, alive |

298

After the standard distal splenorenal shunt with total disconnection of the distal splenic vein from the pancreas, portal blood flow continued to perfuse the liver (Fig. 8).

## Discussion

In 1983, we reported that pancreatic veins developed to an enormous size at the area where the non-isolated distal splenic vein was embedded and that such dilated pancreatic veins facilitated flow of mesenteric blood into the distal splenic vein where it was lowered by a distal splenorenal shunt [1]. Since then more data has reinforced the idea that a splenopancreatic disconnection be conceived and implemented as a technical addition to the standard distal splenorenal shunt to preserve portal perfusion and maintain selectivity of the shunt [2, 3]. Rikkers [4] reported that non-alcoholics maintained portal perfusion better than alcoholics after a distal splenorenal shunt and Zeppa [5] observed that survival was also better in non-alcoholics than alcoholics after shunt.

Discriminative analysis based on hematological, biochemical and hemodynamic data in our series showed us that the patients with $-9.85053 < Y_1 < 8.1942$, $1.5363 < Y_2$ of discriminative scores continued portal perfusion and that the survival rate in these patients was better than in the patients with other discriminative scores. It was not ascertained whether the patients with good discriminative analysis scores were non-alcoholics or not, but it was clear that portal malcirculation was linked to decreased survival after the distal splenorenal shunt.

Pancreatic veins communicating to a non-isolated distal splenic vein may play a leading role in the production of malcirculation of the portal system after a distal splenorenal shunt. Here again, I emphasize the necessity of totally disconnecting the splenic vein from the pancreas for improved selectivity of the distal splenorenal shunt.

## References

1   Isomatsu T. Loss of selectivity of Warren shunt in long-time observation. Jpn J Surg 1983; 13: 202 – 206.
2   Inokuchi K, Beppu K, Koyanagi N, et al. Exclusion of nonisolated splenic vein in distal splenorenal shunt for prevention of portal malcirculation. Ann Surg 1984; 200: 711 – 717.
3   Warren MD, Millikan WJ, Henderson JM, et al. Splenopancreatic disconnection improved selectivity of distal splenorenal shunt. Ann Surg 1986; 204: 346 – 355.
4   Rikkers LE, Rudman D, Galambos JT, et al. Randomized controlled trial of the distal splenorenal shunt. Ann Surg 1978; 188: 271 – 282.
5   Zeppa R, Hensley GT, Levi JU, Livingstone AS. Factors influencing survival after distal splenorenal shunt. Ann Surg 1978; 187: 510 – 542.

Chapter 27

# Long-term results of superselective distal splenorenal shunt

Hiroyuki Katoh and Tatsuzo Tanabe

*Second Department of Surgery, Hokkaido University School of Medicine, Kita 14-jyo, Nishi 5-chome, Kita-ku, Sapporo 060, Japan*

Our therapeutic approach to esophageal varices is distal splenorenal shunt. Since 1970 this operative procedure proposed by D. Warren [1] has been applied to 57 cases, 9 of whom died during the early postoperative period, with 5-year and 10-year survival rates of 55 and 30%, respectively.

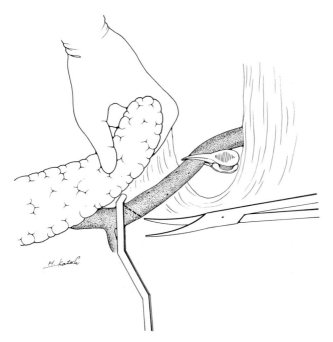

FIG. 1   Complete separation of the pancreatic tail from the splenic vein.

300

The onset of hepatic encephalopathy was observed in 9 cases and death presumably due to hepatic insufficiency involved as many as 18 cases. Then, angiography performed on 12 cases with more than one year postoperative course revealed remarkable decreases in hepatopetal flow. Selectivity loss for shunt via pancreatic veins was confirmed to be responsible for this, which made us improve upon our operative procedure [2 – 4]. The improvement consisted mainly of complete separation of the pancreatic tail from the splenic vein (Fig. 1). However,

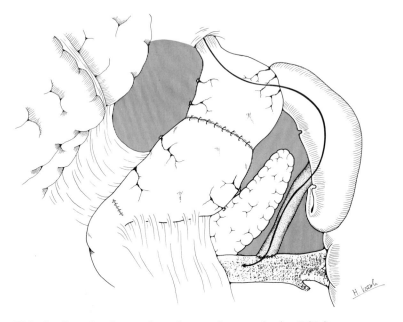

FIG. 2   Completed operative schema of superselective DSRS.

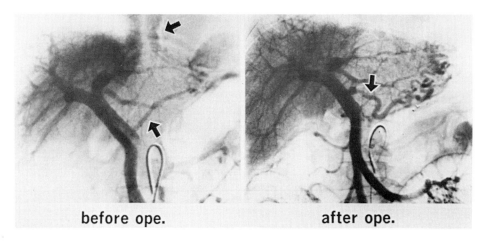

FIG. 3   Longterm angiographic findings of superselective DSRS: early case.

perigastric vascular dissection, which was regarded as unnecessary, was not sufficiently performed. Subsequent examination revealed relapse of esophagogastric varices and selectivity loss for shunt in some cases of insufficient perigastric vascular dissection, so that transection and re-suture of the seromuscular layer of the upper stomach were also added (Fig. 2). We called this procedure superselective distal splenorenal shunt.

With a view to determining postoperative portal circulatory kinetics, angiography was performed on 22 cases with more than one year of postoperative course. Of these 22 cases, 5 received early insufficient perigastric vascular dissection; angiographic findings revealed esophagogastric varix formation, outlining of the shunt and reduction in portal caliber ratio in 3 cases, respectively (Fig. 3). On the other hand, any one of the latter 17 cases showed neither outlining of the shunt nor reduction in portal caliber ratio, presenting ideal angiographic pictures (Fig. 4). These results are shown in Table 1. Also clinically, neither operative mortality nor onset of hepatic encephalopathy was found. Of a total of 31 cases comprising 5 early cases and 26 later cases, 29 have already returned to work. Only one case died of liver cancer postoperatively; 5-year survival rate was 88% (Fig. 5). Superselective

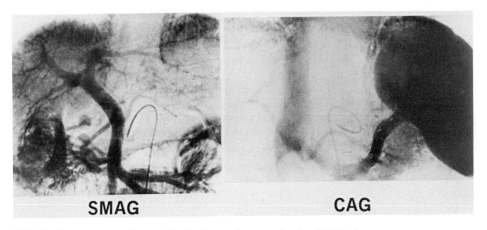

FIG. 4   Longterm angiographic findings of superselective DSRS: late case.

TABLE 1   Angiographic findings after superselective DSRS

|  | Collateral pathway outlined | Esophagogastric varix formation | Shunt outlined |
|---|---|---|---|
| Yes | 14 | 3 | 3 |
| No | 8 | 0 | 0 |

(n = 22)

302

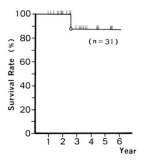

FIG. 5   Cumulative survival rate of superselective distal splenorenal shunt.

distal splenorenal shunt, which we have improved upon Warren's operation, gave excellent postoperative results, which seems to make it a well-established procedure for shunt operation.

## References

1   Warren WD, et al. Selective transsplenic decompression of gastroesophageal varices by a distal splenorenal shunt. Ann Surg 1967; 166: 437 – 444.
2   Behghiti J, et al. Longterm loss of Warren's shunt selectivity. Arch Surg 1981; 166: 1121 – 1130.
3   Warren WD, et al. Splenopancreatic disconnection: improved selectivity of distal splenorenal shunt. Ann Surg 1986; 204: 346 – 355.
4   Katoh H, et al. Superselective distal splenorenal shunt. Gastroenterolog Surg 1985; 8: 246 – 256.

© 1988 Elsevier Science Publishers B.V. (Biomedical Division)
*Treatment of esophageal varices*
*Y. Idezuki, editor*

Chapter 28

# Experimental and clinical effects of vasopressin

KENNETH G. SWAN, JOHN J. FLANAGAN AND DEBORAH M. ROSA

*Department of Surgery, UMDNJ-NJMS, Newark, NJ 07103-2757, USA*

Vasopressin remains one of the three most useful techniques available to the clinician in the nonoperative, emergent care of the patient with bleeding esophageal varices. The other two techniques are the Sengstaken-Blakemore tube for esophagogastric balloon tamponade of the gastric or esophageal varices and endoscopic injection, or sclerotherapy. Of these three techniques the one most readily available and the simplest one to initiate is vasopressin and through an already present and functioning intravenous line. The initial dose is $5 \times 10^{-3}$ units $kg^{-1} min^{-1}$ and can be doubled. The evolution of vasopressin as a clinical modality for control of variceal hemorrhage spans three decades.

Vasopressin was first recommended for treatment of variceal hemorrhage in the 1950s [1, 2] but did not gain popularity until Sherlock [3] advocated its use in the form of an intravenous bolus injection at intervals necessary to control hemorrhage. Reports of toxic side effects [4], including myocardial ischemia, caused others to recommend more selective use of vasopressin.

Nusbaum and Baum [5] popularized the administration of vasopressin directly into the superior mesenteric artery at reduced concentrations than those given systemically to achieve the same degree of relative portal venous hypotension. These authors incorrectly attributed a perceived lessening of systemic side effects of vasopressin, administered intraarterially, to its assumed rapid metabolic breakdown by the liver [6].

It is now known that vasopressin, unlike other vasoactive agents such as the catecholamines, has a relatively long biological half life. Baumann has determined this to be in excess of 24 min in man [7]. This observation led to the hypothesis that vasopressin should exert equal effects upon regional circulations, such as splanchnic vasculature, regardless of route of administration.

We tested this hypothesis in anesthetized Rhesus monkeys [8]. Blood flow through the superior mesenteric artery was measured with an electromagnetic blood flowmeter and effects upon flow in response to intravenous and intraarterial bolus injections of vasopressin were compared (Fig. 1). Vasopressin caused a dose-dependent decrease in superior mesenteric blood flow. Route of injection was an independent variable. We concluded from these studies that, assuming man's response would be similar to that in the monkey, vasopressin could be expected to be equally

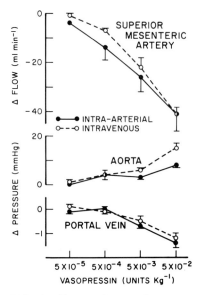

FIG. 1  Changes in superior mesenteric arterial flow, mean arterial pressure, and portal venous pressure. Changes are plotted on the ordinate against doses of injected vasopressin on the abscissa. Values are expressed as the mean ± S.E. of six experiments in six monkeys (intravenous data, ○– – –○; intraarterial data, ●———●).

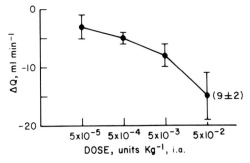

FIG. 2  The effects of intraarterial injections of vasopressin on blood flow through the inferior mesenteric artery of the monkey. Change in flow is expressed on the ordinate in ml/min. Zero indicates control flow; negative values indicate a vasoconstrictor response. The log dose is expressed on the abscissa. Each point represents the mean ± S.E. of five experiments in five animals. The parenthetical figure indicates change in mean arterial pressure at this dose of vasopressin (Gastroenterology, 1977).

effective whether given intraarterially or intravenously. A comparable reduction in superior mesenteric blood flow would be anticipated with either route of administration. Since approximately two thirds of portal venous blood flow comes from the superior mesenteric artery any significant reduction in flow through this vessel should be accompanied by a significant reduction in portal venous pressure. The effects of vasopressin upon blood flow to the large intestine (Fig. 2) are similar to the drug's effects on blood flow to the small intestine [9]. Obviously the intraarterial administration requires the skills of an angiographer which may not be readily available in an emergency. On the other hand intravenous vasopressin can be given immediately upon need and without special skills. We believe its use is best monitored in the intensive care unit since myocardial ischemia secondary to coronary arterial constriction has been reported [10]. Although most patients bleeding from esophageal varices are relatively young (ca 40 years) the cardiomyopathy of acute and chronic alcoholism may predispose the cirrhotic to a higher incidence of cardiac-related complications of vasopressin [10]. What is the optimal dose or concentration or rate of administration of vasopressin?

To address this question we studied the effects of 10-min intravenous infusions of vasopressin upon mesenteric blood flow in dogs (Fig. 3) [11]. A reduction in flow begins at a rate of administration of $5 \times 10^{-4}$ units of vasopressin $kg^{-1}$ $min^{-1}$. This effect is increased when the rate is increased ten-fold ($5 \times 10^{-3}$ units $kg^{-1}$ $min^{-1}$). Flow is halved by this dose of vasopressin but returns to control values promptly after cessation of the infusion. This dose of vasopressin causes only

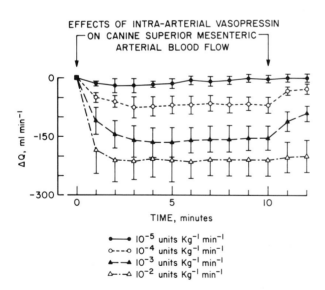

FIG. 3 The effects of intraarterially infused vasopressin upon superior mesenteric arterial blood flow are summarized in five experiments in five animals. The time course of the experiment is presented on the abscissa in minutes, and blood flow, along the ordinate in ml/min. The infusion begins at time 0 and continues through minute 10. Each point on the graph represents the mean ± S.E. error of five experiments in five animals.

a small increase (4 ± 1 mmHg) in mean systemic arterial pressure (126 ± 3 mmHg). A higher dose (5 × 10$^{-2}$ units kg$^{-1}$ min$^{-1}$) of vasopressin reduces blood flow further; the effect persists after cessation of the infusion and the increase in systemic arterial pressure (13 ± 2 mmHg) is significantly ($P < 0.01$) greater. Based upon these canine studies we initially determined the optimal rate for vasopressin clinically to be 5 × 10$^{-3}$ units kg$^{-1}$ min$^{-1}$, intravenously.

Concern for the possible toxic side effects of vasopressin prompted us to evaluate the effects of vasopressin upon other vascular beds. For example if vasopressin exerts its beneficial effects upon bleeding esophageal varices by reducing portal venous pressure, the presumption is that portal venous blood flow is reduced. What if the drug simultaneously constricts the hepatic artery? Would not the combined reduction in hepatic blood flow risk ischemic injury to the liver?

To address this question we measured the effects of intraarterial (superior mesenteric artery) vasopressin upon hepatic and superior mesenteric arterial blood flows in dogs (Fig. 4) [11]. At a relatively high dose (10$^{-2}$ units kg$^{-1}$ min$^{-1}$) of vasopressin, which produced a 75%, sustained reduction in superior mesenteric blood flow, hepatic arterial blood flow was not significantly changed. When vasopressin was infused directly into the canine hepatic artery at the rate we currently recommend for clinical use in man (5 × 10$^{-3}$ units kg$^{-1}$ min$^{-1}$), hepatic arterial blood flow showed a prompt and significant fall to 67% of the control value [12]. This vasoconstrictor response was not sustained, however, and hepatic arterial flow gradually returned to control flow despite continued infusion of vasopressin.

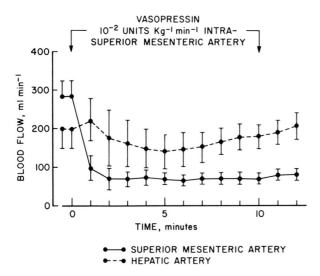

FIG. 4   The effects of intrasuperior mesenteric arterial infusion of vasopressin (10$^{-2}$ units kg$^{-1}$ min$^{-1}$) upon blood flow through the superior mesenteric and hepatic arteries are summarized in five experiments in five animals. The time course of the experiment is presented on the abscissa in minutes. The infusion begins at time 0 and continues through minute 10. Flows along the ordinate are expressed in ml/min. Each point on the graph represents the mean ± S.E.

The value at the fifth minute was not significantly different ($P > 0.05$) from control flow. Following cessation of vasopressin infusion, at 10 min, flow increased beyond the control value (Fig. 5). These phenomena, autoregulatory escape and the overshoot, characterize vasoconstrictor responses to catecholamines, such as norepinephrine, but have not previously been associated with the vasoconstrictor effects of vasopressin. The fact that they are observed only in the hepatic arterial circulation suggests an organ-specific response. In this case the resultant effect is a protective one which appears to maintain some hepatic blood flow despite a significant reduction in portal venous flow. The latter results from a reduction in flow through all splanchnic viscera which are drained by the portal vein, and as a result of vasopressin administration. The major contributor to this circulation (portal venous flow) is the superior mesenteric artery. The reduction in flow through the superior mesenteric artery in response to vasopressin is the same whether vasopressin is given directly into the superior mesenteric artery or into the inferior vena cava or the portal vein [13]. These observations are not peculiar to the canine splanchnic circulation.

In experiments designed to further explore this relationship between portal venous blood flow and hepatic arterial blood flow in response to vasopressin, we studied the subhuman primate. Using the radioactive microsphere technique we measured cardiac output distribution of blood flow to all of the splanchnic viscera of the Rhesus monkey before and at the end of a 10-min infusion of vasopressin [14]. The dose was $5 \times 10^{-3}$ units $kg^{-1}$ $min^{-1}$ (Fig. 6). Blood flow to stomach, small in-

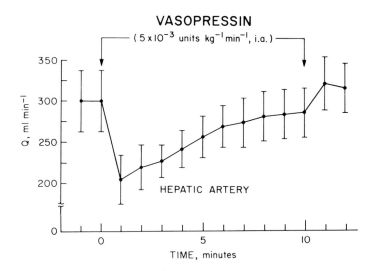

FIG. 5   The effects of intraarterial infusion of vasopressin upon canine hepatic arterial blood flow. The time course of the experiment, in minutes, is depicted along the abscissa; the infusion of vasopressin ($5 \times 10^{-3}$ units $kg^{-1}$ $min^{-1}$) begins at 0 min and ends at 10 min. On the ordinate, flow is expressed in ml/min. Each point on the graph is the mean $\pm$ S.E. of eight experiments in eight animals.

308

testine, large intestine, spleen and pancreas were all significantly decreased by vasopressin. In the case of small intestine, which had the highest absolute flow value of the organs enumerated, its control flow was halved by the ninth minute of vasopressin infusion. Of interest was the observation that vasopressin did not change the rate of blood flow to the kidneys. Hepatic arterial blood flow was increased significantly by vasopressin under the circumstances of these experiments. This observation in monkeys supports previous observations described in dogs indicating that vasopressin appears to spare hepatic arterial flow.

We might speculate from these findings that the dual blood supply to the liver, the portal vein and the hepatic artery have a reciprocal relationship in that a reduction in flow through one is compensated by an increase in flow through the other. This would have teleological merit as many have speculated. In this case a dual circulation to a solitary, vital organ offers protection akin to the pairing of vital organs (e.g., kidneys) with single circulations. In the case of the hepatic circulation these observations in dogs and monkeys indicate that a threat of hepatic ischemia, as a

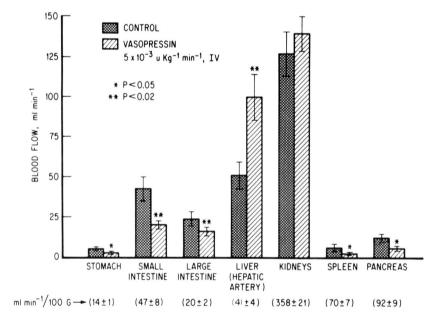

FIG. 6  Effects of intravenous vasopressin infusion at rate of $5 \times 10^{-3}$ units kg$^{-1}$ min$^{-1}$ on distribution of cardiac output to splanchnic viscera as determined by radioactive microspheres. Vertical bars represent blood flow in ml/min during control period (cross-hatched) and at the ninth minute of a 10-min infusion (striped) of vasopressin to various splanchnic organs. Each bar on graph represents mean ± S.E.M. of six experiments in six animals. Parenthetical values along bottom of figure represent blood flow in terms of ml/min per 100 g of tissue during control period. Asterisks represent statistically significant differences between control values and during vasopressin infusion (* $P < 0.05$; ** $P < 0.02$) (J. Vasc. Surg., 1985).

result of systemically administered vasopressin, at recommended clinical doses, is unlikely. The presumption is that man's hepatic circulation would behave similarly to that of these experimental animals.

Perhaps of even greater concern are the effects of vasopressin on the coronary arterial circulation. We studied these effects in Rhesus monkeys (Fig. 7) in which we measured cardiac output with an electromagnetic flowmeter transducer on the ascending aorta [14]. We also recorded systemic arterial pressure. Exponentially increasing bolus injections of vasopressin in doses ranging from $5 \times 10^{-5}$ to $5 \times 10^{-1}$ units $kg^{-1}$ were given intravenously. Cardiac output was 114 ml $min^{-1}$ $kg^{-1}$ or 624 ml $min^{-1}$ in six monkeys whose mean weight was 5.6 kg. Slight decreases in output were observed only at the two highest doses ($5 \times 10^{-2}$, $5 \times 10^{-1}$ units $kg^{-1}$) of vasopressin and these decreases were less than 10% of control output. Mean arterial pressure increased significantly by 16 and 22 mmHg above a control value of 111 mmHg in response to these two highest doses of vasopressin. Thus, vasopressin, at doses which exert significant hypertensive responses in the systemic arterial circulation, have almost negligible effects on cardiac output therefore presumably the coronary arterial circulation in man. Additional studies of vasopressin infusions, intravenously at rates of $5 \times 10^{-3}$ and $5 \times 10^{-2}$ units $kg^{-1}$ $min^{-1}$, confirm these observations with bolus injections in monkeys (Figs. 8 and 9). Only at the higher concentration does vasopressin significantly increase arterial pressure. Concurrent effects on cardiac output are almost negligible.

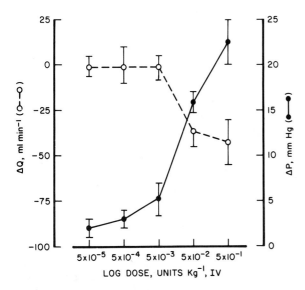

FIG. 7   Effects of intravenous bolus injections of vasopressin on cardiac output and arterial pressure in subhuman primates. Log dose is expressed along abscissa in units $kg^{-1}$, and the resultant changes in cardiac output (open circles) in ml/min and arterial pressure (closed circles) in mmHg are expressed along ordinates. Each point on graph represents mean ± S.E.M. of six experiments in six rhesus monkeys (J. Vasc. Surg., 1985).

310

The real question is man's response to vasopressin. Precise organ-specific blood flows are not easily measured in man; however, inferences can be drawn from several parameters. These include portal pressure determinations. We have measured these effects directly, in the operating room, among patients who have undergone mesocaval shunting for control of exsanguinating hemorrhage secondary to bleeding esophageal varices [15]. All of our patients developed their varices from portal hypertension secondary to cirrhosis of the liver caused by chronic alcoholism. At the end of the operative procedure we measured portal pressure (in cm $H_2O$) with a 21 gauge needle attached to a saline manometer. We then infused vasopressin intravenously at a rate of $10^{-2}$ units $kg^{-1}$ $min^{-1}$ over a 10-min period (Fig. 10). Portal venous pressure was reduced by about 25% from a control value of almost 40 cm $H_2O$ by the tenth minute of the infusion. During the same time systolic arterial pressure (recorded by the anesthesiologist) rose significantly by about 15% and heart rate decreased by a similar order of magnitude. This bradycardia was highly significant ($P < 0.001$).

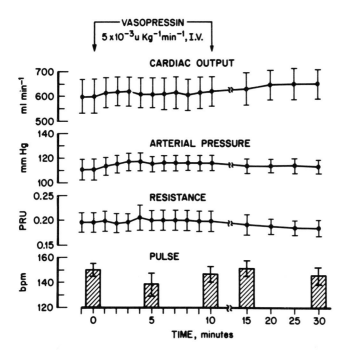

FIG. 8   Effects of 10-min intravenous infusions of vasopressin on subhuman primate hemodynamics. Time course of experiment is presented along the abscissa in minutes. Infusion of vasopressin at rate of $5 \times 10^{-3}$ units $kg^{-1}$ $min^{-1}$ was begun at time zero and continued for 10 min. On the ordinate, cardiac output is expressed in ml/min, arterial pressure in mmHg, total peripheral resistance in peripheral resistance units (PRU) and heart rate in beats $min^{-1}$ (bpm). Each point on graph represents mean ± S.E.M. of six experiments in six rhesus monkeys.

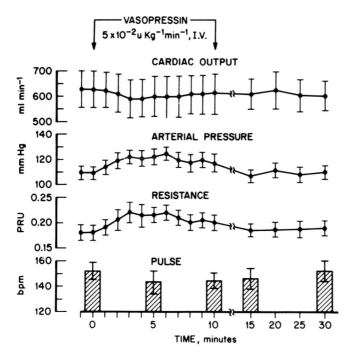

FIG. 9  Effects of 10-min intravenous infusions of vasopressin on subhuman primate hemodynamics. Time course of experiment is presented along the abscissa in minutes. Infusion of vasopressin at rate of $5 \times 10^{-2}$ units $kg^{-1}$ $min^{-1}$ was begun at time zero and continued for 10 min. On the ordinate, cardiac output is expressed in ml/min, arterial pressure in mmHg, total peripheral resistance in peripheral resistance units (PRU) and heart rate in beats $min^{-1}$ (bpm). Each point on the graph represents mean $\pm$ S.E.M. of six experiments in six rhesus monkeys.

These observations in man and experimental animals indicate that vasopressin is a potent splanchnic vasoconstrictor. It exerts its effects through splanchnic arterial constriction, which in turn reduces portal venous blood flow and, hence, portal venous pressure. The reduction in portal venous pressure is modest but presumably (since the precise mechanism remains unknown) sufficient to arrest hemorrhage from bleeding esophageal varices. Despite concerns to the contrary doses of vasopressin which produce this desired effect pose no real threat to liver, kidneys or myocardium. Renal blood flow is unchanged; hepatic arterial blood flow is increased and cardiac output is resistant to change at clinically recommended rates of vasopressin.

Vasopressin can be given intravenously with safety thus it is readily available as a first line of defence against exsanguinating hemorrhage from esophageal varices. The complications associated with intraarterial administration can be eliminated and no special expertise is required for its administration. Thus vasopressin contrasts the other two modalities for emergent control of such hemorrhage, namely esophagogastric balloon tamponade (Sengstaken-Blakemore tube) and endoscopic sclerotherapy. These techniques, especially the latter, require the expertise of those experienced with their use.

Of additional interest, vasopressin has special use in the operating room during emergency and even elective surgery for bleeding from esophageal varices. Operative blood loss should be minimized for two specific reasons other than the obvious benefits associated with careful surgery. These are increased visibility and reduced hepatic injury. Almost all operative procedures for amelioration of bleeding varices will require dissection that produces less or greater amounts of ascites. Even a small amount of bleeding, mixing with ascites, obscures the operative field and hinders visibility. Cross clamping the major venous structures for

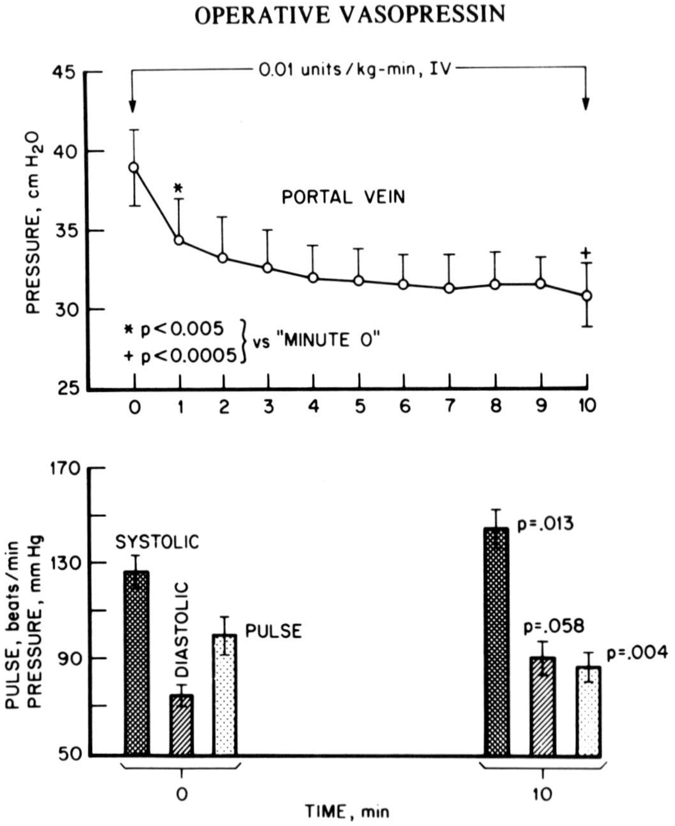

**OPERATIVE VASOPRESSIN**

FIG. 10  The effects of vasopressin upon portal venous pressure, systemic arterial pressure and pulse. The time course of the experiment is presented along the abscissa in minutes. Portal venous pressure is measured in cm $H_2O$. Each point on the graph represents the mean $\pm$ S.E. of 25 observations in 25 patients. The bar graph represents pulse in beats $min^{-1}$ and pressure in mmHg. The statistical significance of apparent differences between values at time 0 and at 10 min is presented (Surgery, 1980).

anastomoses augments portosystemic pressures and blood loss. Concurrent use of vasopressin can minimize this blood loss and hence facilitate the operative procedure. Secondly, the reduction in blood loss equates a reduced volume of homologous blood administration, assuming no autotransfusion. Banked blood carries a definite risk to the cirrhotic's already damaged liver.

Analogues of vasopressin, such as glypressin, have had periodic popularity. Alterations in the aminoacid composition of the molecule can narrow the biological activity or alter the duration of action of the nonapeptide. The vasoconstrictor activity is associated with the terminal amino group and aromatic amino acids in positions two and three [10]. Arginine vasopressin is the naturally occurring mammalian peptide; lysine vasopressin is peculiar to the pig [10]. Triglycyl-lysine vasopressin (glypressin or terlipressin) is a synthetic, slow release hormonogen which has been reported beneficial in the control of variceal hemorrhage [16]. Evidence supporting significant additional benefits of this vasoconstrictor, beyond those of the parent molecule, vasopressin, is conflicting [17, 18].

Some favor the addition of a vasodilator to reduce the threat of myocardial ischemia resulting from coronary vasoconstriction and myocardial failure resulting from increased afterload. Nitroglycerin analogues have been used in conjunction with vasopressin toward this end. Here, again, results are contradictory [19]. Currently we favor vasopressin, alone and in the route and concentration presented.

## References

1   Kehne JH, Hughes FA, Gompertz ML. Use of surgical pituitrin in control of esophageal varix bleeding: experimental study and report of 2 cases. Surgery 1956; 39: 917 – 925.
2   Schwartz SI, Bales HW, Emerson GL, et al. Use of intravenous pituitrin in treatment of bleeding esophageal varices. Surgery 1959; 45: 72 – 80.
3   Shaldon, S, Sherlock S. Use of vasopressin (pitressin) in control of bleeding from esophageal varices. Lancet 1960; ii: 222 – 225.
4   Drapanas T, Crowe CP, Shim WKT, et al. The effect of pitressin on cardiac output and coronary, hepatic and intestinal blood flow. Surg Gynecol Obstet 1961; 113: 484.
5   Nusbaum M, Baum S, Sakiyalak P, et al. Pharmacologic control of portal hypertension. Surgery 1967; 62: 299 – 310.
6   Nusbaum M. Arterial vasopressin infusions: Science or seance? Gastroenterology 1975; 69: 263 – 267.
7   Baumann G, Dingman JF. Distribution, blood transport and degradation of antidiuretic hormone in man. J Clin Invest 1976; 57: 1109 – 1116.
8   Freedman AR, Kerr JC, Swan KG, et al. Primate mesenteric blood flow: effects of vasopressin and its route of delivery. Gastroenterology 1978; 74: 875 – 879.
9   Kerr JC, Hobson RW, Seelig RF, et al. Influence of vasopressin on colon blood flow in monkeys. Gastroenterology 1977; 72: 474 – 478.
10  Blei AT. Vasopressin analogs in portal hypertension: different molecules but similar questions. Hepatology 1986; 6: 146 – 147.
11  Kerr JC, Reynolds DG, Swan KG. Vasopressin and blood flow through the canine small intestine. J Surg Res 1978; 25: 35 – 41.
12  Kerr JC, Reynolds DG, Swan KG. Vasopressin and canine hepatic arterial blood flow. J Surg Res 1977; 23: 166 – 171.

13   Kerr JC, Hobson RW, Seelig RF, et al. Vasopressin: Route of administration and effects on canine hepatic and superior mesenteric arterial blood flows. Ann Surg 1978; 187: 137 – 142.

14   Kerr JC, Jain KM, Swan KG, et al. Effects of vasopressin on cardiac output and its distribution in the subhuman primate. J Vasc Surg 1985; 2: 443 – 449.

15   Swan KG, Howard MM, Rocko JM, et al. Operative vasopressin and mesocaval shunting for portal hypertension. Surgery 1980; 8: 46 – 51.

16   Walker S, Stiehl, A, Raedsch R, et al. Terlipressin in bleeding esophageal varices: a placebo-controlled double blind study. Hepatology 1986; 6: 112 – 115.

17   Fogel MR, Knauer CM, Andres CC, et al. Continuous intravenous vasopressin in active upper gastrointestinal bleeding: a placebo-controlled trial. Ann Int Med 1982; 97: 560 – 565.

18   Freeman JG, Lishman AH, Cobden I, et al. Controlled trial of terlipressin (glypressin) versus vasopressin in the early treatment of oesophageal varices. 1982; Lancet ii: 66 – 68.

19   Way CW. Portal hypertension. In: Way LW, ed. Current Surgical Diagnosis and Treatment, 8th Edn., Appleton & Lange, Norwalk CN, 1988; 471 – 486.

© 1988 Elsevier Science Publishers B.V. (Biomedical Division)
*Treatment of esophageal varices*
*Y. Idezuki, editor*

Chapter 29

# The hemodynamics of esophago-gastric varices: significance of esophago-gastric arterial inflow in their formation

HARUO AOKI, AKITAKE HASUMI AND MOTOHIDE SHIMAZU

*Department of Surgery, Fujita-Gakuen Health University School of Medicine, 1-98, Dengakugakubo, Kutsukake-cho, Toyoake-City, Aichi Pref. 470-11 Japan*

Esophago-gastric varices in patients with portal hypertension are generally thought to develop due to hepatofugal blood flow from the portal system into the collateral vessels. Our clinical and experimental studies revealed, however, that a hyperdynamic state of the lower esophagus and the upper part of the stomach, where varices are usually formed, causes the formation of varices directly.

Since 1978, we have insisted on the significance of esophago-gastric arterial inflow in the development of an abnormal hemodynamic state in the portal area and especially in the formation of esophago-gastric varices [1 – 3].

## Hemodynamics of the left gastric vein

In 66 patients with liver cirrhosis with marked esophageal varices, we studied the hemodynamics of the left gastric vein and the short gastric veins by angiography.

In an intra-operative portogram via splenic puncture and the superior mesenteric vein, a markedly enlarged and meandering left gastric vein was found in the direction of the esophageal varices (Figure 1). This means that the left gastric vein acts as a hepatofugal collateral vessel. We called these cases of reverse flow in the left gastric vein the hepatofugal type (Type I).

In another case, however, hepatofugal blood flow from the portal area through the left gastric and the short gastric veins was not found, although this was a case with marked esophageal varices (Fig. 2a). Figure 2b shows the venography of the stomach wall via the gastro-epiploic vein in the same case. The contrast medium has flowed into the esophageal varices through the vascular net of the stomach wall, and at the same time, is found in the left gastric vein which is not so enlarged nor meandering in the direction of the portal trunk. This indicates that blood flow in

316

the left gastric vein is not hepatofugal. We called these cases without reverse flow in the left gastric vein the non-hepatofugal type (Type II).

The non-hepatofugal type included two subtypes. One was the hepatopetal type (Type IIb), in which blood flow in the left gastric vein was definitely hepatopetal as shown in Fig. 2.

In portograms of the other subtype, the left gastric vein was visualized slightly in portography, but the esophageal varices were not opacified (Fig. 3a). The venous phase of the left gastric arteriography, however, showed the esophageal varices manifestly and slight hepatopetal flow in the left gastric vein (Fig. 3b). Since blood flow in the left gastric vein in these cases is thought to be to and fro, we named this the to and fro type (Type IIa).

In our 66 cases of liver cirrhosis with marked esophageal varices, the frequency of these types was: hepatofugal type (Type I), 21 cases (31.8%) and non-hepatofugal type (Type II), 42 cases (63.6%). Among Type II, 30 cases were of the to and fro type (Type IIa) and 12 of the hepatopetal type (Type IIb). Three cases were unclassifiable due to inconsistent findings (Table 1).

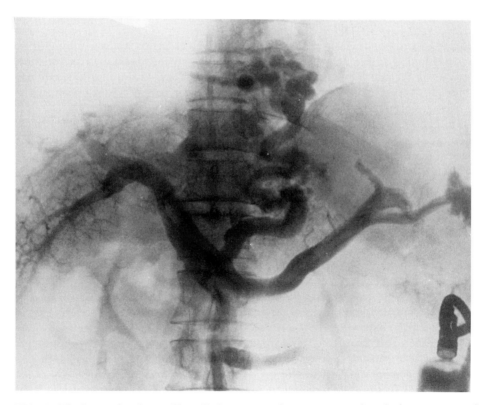

FIG. 1  The hepatofugal type (Type I). Intra-operative portogram via splenic puncture and superior mesenteric vein in patient with liver cirrhosis and esophageal varices. A markedly enlarged and meandering left gastric vein is found in the direction of the esophageal varices.

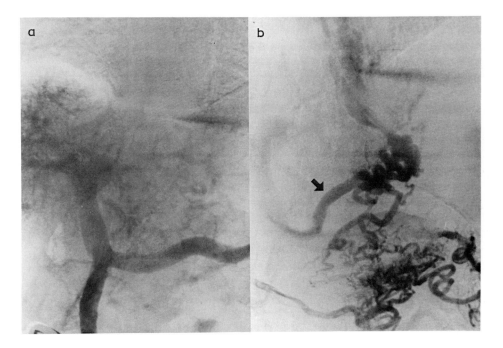

FIG. 2    The hepatopetal subtype (Type IIb) of the non-hepatofugal type (Type II). (a) Intra-operative portogram via splenic puncture and the superior mesenteric vein in patient with liver cirrhosis and esophageal varices. No hepatofugal blood flow from the portal area through the left gastric and short gastric veins is found. (b) Intra-operative venography of the stomach wall via gastro-epiploic vein in the same case. The contrast medium is found in the esophageal varices through the vascular net of the stomach wall and, at the same time, in the left gastric vein which is not so enlarged nor meandering in the direction of the portal trunk.

TABLE 1    Hemodynamics of the left gastric vein in 66 cases of liver cirrhosis with esophageal varices

| Type of hemodynamics | Number of cases |
| --- | --- |
| Type I<br>　Hepatofugal | 21 (31.8%) |
| Type II<br>　Non-hepatofugal<br>　　IIa, to and fro<br>　　IIb, hepatopetal | 30 ⎰ 42 (63.6)<br>12 ⎱ |
| Others | 3 (4.5) |
| Total | 66 |

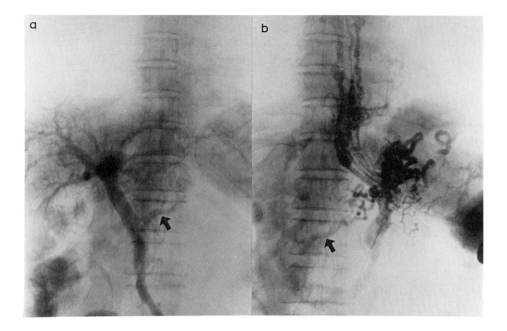

FIG. 3   The to and fro subtype (Type IIa). (a) Intra-operative portography in patient with liver cirrhosis and esophageal varices. The left gastric vein is visualized slightly (arrow), and no esophageal varices are seen. (b) Intra-operative left gastric angiography in the same case. The esophageal varices are demonstrated manifestly, and slight hepatopetal flow in the left gastric vein is seen.

### Evaluation of the blood flow in the left gastric vein by other hemodynamic studies

*(a)* In 42 of the 66 cases, previous judgement of the hemodynamics of the left gastric vein was confirmed by continuous observation using pre-operative cine-angiography or intra-operative video-imaging.

*(b)* In 16 cases, direction and volume of the blood flow in the left gastric vein were measured directly by ultrasonic transit time flowmeter during the operation.

In the hepatofugal type (Type I), blood flow in the left gastric vein was $-90$ to $-120$ ml/min, namely hepatofugal (Fig. 4a). In the to and fro type (Type IIa), blood flow in left gastric vein was hepatofugal and -petal by turns. Its changes were related to both slow respiratory movement and rapid heart beat (Fig. 4b). Therefore, direct measurement of the hemodynamics confirmed our hypothesis that blood flow in the left gastric vein is to and fro.

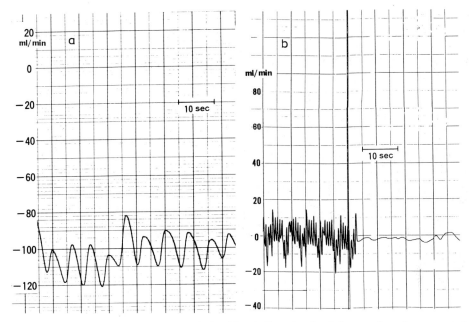

FIG. 4   Direction and volume of the blood flow in the left gastric vein measured by ultrasonic transit time flowmeter. (a) Hepatofugal type (Type I). (b) To and fro type (Type II).

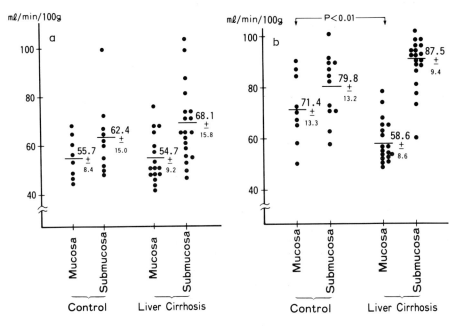

FIG. 5   Tissue blood flow volume in mucosal and submucosal layers of the stomach measured by hydrogen gas clearance technique. (a) Antral portion. (b) Upper part.

**Comparison of the characteristics of each group with respect to the hemodynamics of the left gastric vein**

The clinical features were compared among the cases of each type of blood flow in the left gastric vein.

There was no significant difference among the types, as to frequency of previous variceal hemorrhage, endoscopic findings of the varices, wedged hepatic venous pressure (WHVP) and portal pressure. The diameter of the left gastric vein was significantly enlarged in Type I in comparison with Type II. Also, meandering of the vein was more marked in Type I (Table 2).

Comparing the $Po_2$ of the blood of the portal, superior mesenteric and gastro-epiploic veins collected simultaneously during the operation, that of the gastro-epiploic vein showed the highest value in each group and in Type IIb it was significantly higher. Venous pressure was higher in the gastro-epiploic vein than in the portal trunk in each group. The decrease in pressure in the gastro-epiploic vein during temporary clamping of the splenic artery or the left gastric artery was measured during the operation. The rate of decrease in gastro-epiploic venous pressure was marked in Type I after splenic arterial clamping, and marked in Type II after left gastric arterial clamping (Table 3).

These results revealed that arterial blood flow into the stomach wall through the left gastric artery is a significant factor in the development of venous hypertension in the gastric area especially in Type II patients.

TABLE 2   Clinical features of the cases of each type of blood flow in the left gastric vein

| | Type I (hepatofugal) | Type II (non-hepatofugal) | |
| --- | --- | --- | --- |
| | | IIa (to and fro) | IIb (hepatopetal) |
| Previous variceal hemorrhage | 14/21 (66.7%) | 22/30 (73.3%) | 8/12 (66.7%) |
| Risky varices[c] | 18/20 (90.0%) | 26/30 (86.7%) | 10/12 (83.3%) |
| WHVP[d] (mmH$_2$O) | 324.7 ± 69.4 ($n$ = 21) | 340.4 ± 63.4 ($n$ = 30) | 341.0 ± 50.8 ($n$ = 12) |
| Portal venous pressure (mmH$_2$O) | 347.3 ± 39.0 ($n$ = 21) | 357.5 ± 62.4 ($n$ = 30) | 347.4 ± 79.6 ($n$ = 12) |
| Diameter of left gastric vein (mm) | 9.0 ± 2.0 ($n$ = 20) | 6.7 ± 1.4[b] ($n$ = 23) | 6.1 ± 1.3[b] ($n$ = 11) |
| Meandering of left gastric vein | 15/20 (75.0%) | 7/23[a] (30.4%) | 0/11[a] (0.0%) |

Mean ± SD; [a] $P < 0.05$ vs Type I; [b] $P < 0.01$ vs Type I. [c] According to Beppu and Inokuchi's score [4, 5]. [d] Wedged hepatic venous pressure.

TABLE 3 Comparison of the characteristics of each type of blood flow in the left gastric vein

| | Type I (hepatofugal) | Type II (non-hepatofugal) | |
| --- | --- | --- | --- |
| | | IIa (to and fro) | IIb (hepatopetal) |
| **$Pvo_2/Pao_2$ (× 100)** | | | |
| Portal trunk | 46.9 ± 14.0 ($n$ = 12) | 55.0 ± 17.2 ($n$ = 18) | 53.8 ± 11.8[a] ($n$ = 7) |
| SMV | 50.3 ± 13.8 ($n$ = 11) | 52.0 ± 15.0 ($n$ = 19) | 50.1 ± 12.5 ($n$ = 7) |
| GEV | 57.1 ± 15.4 ($n$ = 12) | 58.4 ± 12.6[b] ($n$ = 19) | 70.6 ± 9.2[c] ($n$ = 7) |
| **GEV pressure ($mmH_2O$)** | 396.4 ± 53.3 ($n$ = 20) | 401.0 ± 72.5 ($n$ = 26) | 380.2 ± 68.0 ($n$ = 11) |
| **Decrease in GEV pressure (%)** | | | |
| after clamping of splenic artery | 6.3 ± 2.5 ($n$ = 7) | 3.5 ± 1.6 ($n$ = 12) | 2.7 ± 1.6 ($n$ = 3) |
| after clamping of left gastric artery | 1.8 ± 0.7[d] ($n$ = 6) | 5.8 ± 4.0[e] ($n$ = 13) | 6.5 ± 3.8 ($n$ = 5) |

Mean ± SD: a vs c, b vs c, d vs e, $P < 0.05$. SMV, superior mesenteric vein; GEV, gastro-epiploic vein.

## Tissue blood flow volume in the mucosal and submucosal layers of the stomach

The tissue blood flow volume in the mucosal and submucosal layers of the stomach was measured by hydrogen gas clearance technique at pre-operative endoscopy. In the antral portion, submucosal blood flow increased slightly in the patients with liver cirrhosis compared with the control. In the upper part of the stomach, however, mucosal blood flow decreased significantly, while submucosal blood flow increased in the patients with liver cirrhosis compared with the control (Fig. 5).

These results indicate that, in liver cirrhosis, a hyperdynamic circulatory state develops in the upper part of the stomach caused by an increase in submucosal A-V anastomoses, and that the arterial blood flow into this area is a significant factor for the higher venous pressure of this area than of the portal trunk.

## The source of blood flow in the submucosal varices of the esophagus

Reuter [6] reported in 1972 that esophageal varices were clearly demonstrated in the venous phase of super-selective angiography of the left gastric artery. This method has since been considered valuable for the diagnosis of varices [7]. It has never been used, however, for evaluating the source of blood flow into the varices.

In our study we estimated the source of blood flow into the submucosal varices of the esophagus from the findings of collateral vessels in portography and of the venous phase of arteriography of the left gastric and proper esophageal arteries.

In some cases of Type I, findings of the varices by portography were the same as those by arteriography (Fig. 6), which means that, in these cases, the source of blood flow into the varices was both portal blood through the hepatofugal collaterals (P) and arterial blood from the esophago-gastric area (A).

In some other cases of Type I, the findings of the collaterals in portography were different from those of the esophageal varices in arteriography (Fig. 7). We propose that the main source of blood flow into the submucosal varices is not portal, but arterial blood.

In Type II, on the other hand, the esophageal varices were demonstrated neither through the left gastric nor the short gastric veins, but were clearly demonstrated

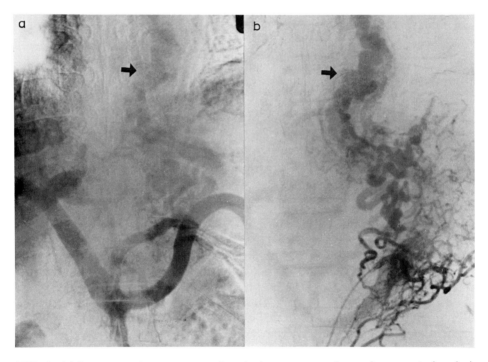

FIG. 6 (a) Intra-operative portogram via splenic puncture and superior mesenteric vein in a case of Type I. (b) Venous phase of intra-operative left gastric angiography. The findings of the varices by portography are the same as those of arteriography (P and A, see text).

by left gastric arteriography (Fig. 3). This indicates that the source of blood flow of the varices is not portal but arterial blood.

As to the source of blood flow of the varices in 12 of 21 cases of Type I, the varices were supplied with both portal blood through the collateral veins and arterial blood from the left gastric artery, proper esophageal artery, etc. In the remaining nine cases the local arteries mainly supplied blood to the varices. On the other hand, in the 42 cases of the non-hepatofugal type (Type II), the sole source of blood was the inflowing artery (Table 4). In other words, arterial inflow (A) plays some role

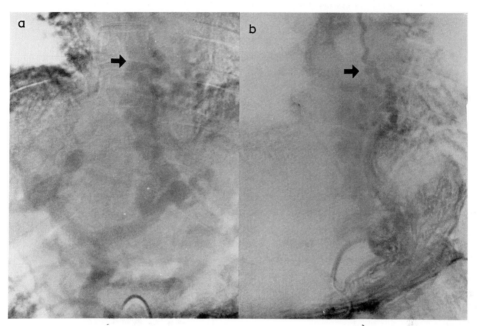

FIG. 7   (a) Venous phase of pre-operative selective superior mesenteric angiography in a case of Type I. (b) Venous phase of pre-operative super-selective left gastric angiography. The findings of the collaterals in the portogram are different from those of the esophageal varices in arteriography (mainly A, see text).

TABLE 4   Source of blood flow in the submucosal varices of the esophagus

| Hemodynamics of left gastric vein | Source of blood flow in varices | Number of cases (%) |
| --- | --- | --- |
| Type I, hepatofugal (n = 21) | both P and A | 12 (19.0) |
| | mainly A | 9 (14.3) |
| Type II, non-hepatofugal (n = 42) | A only | 42 (66.7) |

P, portal blood through hepatofugal collateral vessels; A, arterial blood from the esophago-gastric area.

324

TABLE 5 Experimental study on changes in microcirculation of stomach wall in liver cirrhosis, and influence of estrogen

| Material: | male wistar rats (150 – 200 g) |
|---|---|
| Groups: | **a)** control |
| | **b)** estrogen administration; intramuscular administration of estradiol 5 mg × 2/week, 8 weeks |
| | **c)** liver cirrhosis; induced by wrapping the residual liver for 8 weeks after 60% hepatectomy according to Iwata et al. [8] |
| | **d)** Liver cirrhosis plug estrogen administration (b + c) |
| Procedure: | animals were examined 2 weeks after completion of experimental preparation |

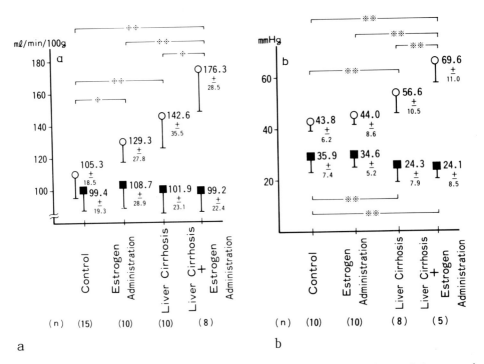

FIG. 8   Tissue blood flow volume and tissue $Po_2$ of the submucosal layer of the stomach wall ($\bigcirc$, upper part of stomach; $\blacksquare$, antral portion; * $P < 0.05$, ** $P < 0.01$). (a) Tissue blood flow volume by hydrogen gas clearance technique. (b) Tissue $Po_2$ by microelectrode technique.

in the development of varices in all cases, while contrariwise portal blood (P) through hepatofugal collaterals plays a role in only half of the Type I cases, a mere fifth of all cases.

## Experimental study of the micro-circulation in the stomach wall

Experimentally we studied the changes in micro-circulation of the stomach wall in rats with liver cirrhosis, and the influence of estrogen (Table 5).

The tissue blood flow volume of the submucosal layer in the upper part of the stomach increased in the group with estrogen administration and the group with liver cirrhosis, and increased even more in the group with liver cirrhosis and estrogen administration (Fig. 8a). The tissue $Po_2$ of the submucosal layer in the upper part of the stomach did not change in the estrogen group, but increased in the liver cirrhosis group and further increased in the liver cirrhosis plus estrogen group (Fig. 8b).

Observation of submucosal A-V anastomoses by the dual dye injection method, in which cobalt blue is injected from the artery and light red from the venous system [9], demonstrated $10-15$ $\mu$ A-V anastomoses (Fig. 9). In the liver cirrhosis plus estrogen group the distribution of A-V anastomoses, indicated by red arrows, was much denser than in the control (Fig. 10). The number of A-V anastomoses per square cm increased in the estrogen group, significantly increased in the liver cirrhosis group and even more significantly increased in the liver cirrhosis plus estrogen group (Fig. 11).

The results of this experimental study prove that a hyperdynamic state develops due to an increase in submucosal A-V anastomoses and that hyper-estrogenemia is one of its causes in patients with liver cirrhosis.

## Discussion

It has already been reported that a systemic hyperdynamic state with an increase in cardiac output, left ventricular stroke work, cardiac index and pulmonary A-V anastomoses, develops in patients with liver cirrhosis. And it has been suggested that this systemic hyperdynamic state is related to abnormally high levels of hormones, such as estrogen, glucagon, etc. However, a hyperdynamic state in the portal area is not known except for intra-hepatic and intra-splenic A-V anastomoses.

A hyperdynamic state in the portal area was first described by Inokuchi et al. [10] in 1977.

We investigated the hemodynamics of the portal area in cirrhotic patients with marked esophageal varices by angiography and found that the cases in which the left gastric and the short gastric veins acted as hepatofugal collaterals (Type I) occupied only about one third of all, while the cases in which these veins were not hepatofugal collaterals (Type II) were in the majority. This Type II includes two subtypes with to and fro (Type IIa), and hepatopetal (Type IIb) blood flow in these veins.

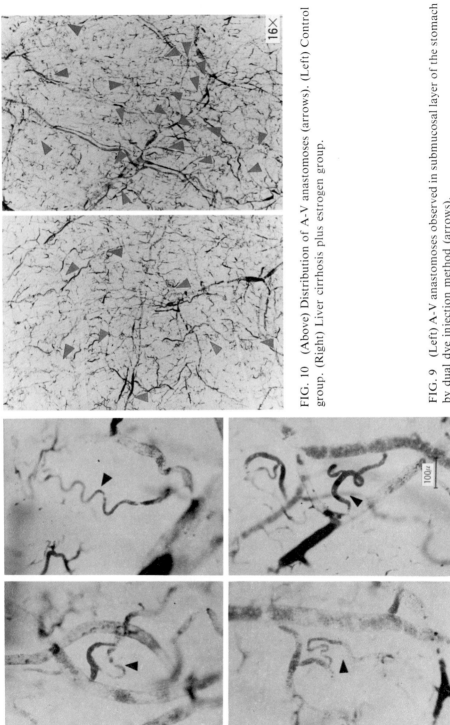

FIG. 10 (Above) Distribution of A-V anastomoses (arrows). (Left) Control group. (Right) Liver cirrhosis plus estrogen group.

FIG. 9 (Left) A-V anastomoses observed in submucosal layer of the stomach by dual dye injection method (arrows).

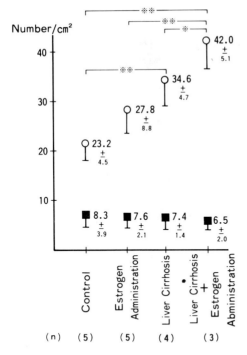

FIG. 11 Number of A-V anastomoses per square cm in submucosal layer of the stomach (○, upper part of stomach; ■, antral portion; * $P < 0.05$, ** $P < 0.01$).

As to the source of blood flow in the submucosal varices of the esophagus, the cases in which portal blood was a source occupied only 19%. On the other hand, in all cases one source was arterial inflow into the lower esophagus and the upper part of the stomach through the left gastric artery, proper esophageal artery, etc.

These results show that esophago-gastric varices not only form due to hepatofugal blood flow from the portal area, but also due to hypertension of the local venous system due to a hyperdynamic state caused by an increase in A-V anastomoses in the submucosal layer of the esophagus and stomach. Therefore, the interruption of the arterial inflow into the esophago-gastric area is important in the treatment of esophageal varices.

We further demonstrated experimentally that hyperestrogenemia, which occurs due to disturbance of liver function, is one of the causes of the increase in submucosal A-V anastomoses.

**References**

1   Aoki H, Funabiki T, Sasaki T, et al. Significance of left gastric arterial inflow in the formation of the esophageal varices. Nihon Geka Gakkaisi (J Jpn Surg Soc) 1978; 79: 353 (in Japanese).

2   Aoki H. An inflow arterial embolization therapy for esophago-gastric varices based on

the new concept of formation of varices. Shoukakigeka Semina (Seminar on Gastroenterological Surgery) 1985; 18: 178 – 186 (in Japanese).

3  Aoki H, Hasumi A, Shimazu M. Pathogenesis of the portal hypertension. In: Kimoto S, Wada T, Idezuki Y, et al. eds. Shin Gekagaku Taikei (New Encyclopedia of Surgical Science) Tokyo: Nakayama Shoten, 1986; 89 – 134 (in Japanese).

4  Japanese Research Society for Portal Hypertension. The general rules for recording endoscopic findings on esophageal varices. Jpn J Surg 1980; 10: 84 – 87.

5  Beppu K, Inokuchi K, Nakayama S, et al. Endoscopic study of esophageal varices especially its diagnostic values for variceal bleeding. Kanzou (Acta Hepatol Jpn) 1981; 22: 102 – 109 (in Japanese).

6  Reuter SR, Atkin TW. High-dose left gastric angiography for demonstration of esophageal varices. Radiology 1972; 105: 573 – 578.

7  Lunderquist A. Pharmacoangiography of the left gastric artery in oesophageal varices. Acta Radiol Diagn 1974; 15: 157 – 160.

8  Iwata M, Akiyama K, Sugawara T, Tatebe T, Ishii K. A new technique on inducing experimental liver cirrhosis. Nihon Syoukakibyou Gakkaishi (Jpn J Gastroenterol) 1981; 78 (Suppl): 461 (in Japanese).

9  Kobayashi K. An experimental study of arterio-venous anastomoses in the stomach. Nihon Syoukakibyou Gakkaishi (Jpn J Gastroenterol) 1973; 70: 442 – 453 (in Japanese).

10  Inokuchi K, Kobayashi M, Saku M, Nagasue N, Iwaki A, Nakayama S. Characteristics of splanchnic circulation in portal hypertension as analysed by pressure study in clinical cases. Kanzou (Acta Hepatol Jpn) 1977; 12: 891 – 898 (in Japanese).

© 1988 Elsevier Science Publishers B.V. (Biomedical Division)
Treatment of esophageal varices
Y. Idezuki, editor

Chapter 30

# Continuous intravenous infusion of pitressin for esophageal variceal bleeding and combined therapy for esophageal varices

JIROICHI ONO AND TAKETO KATSUKI

*First Department of Surgery, Miyazaki Medical College, 5200 Kihara, Kiyotake-cho, Miyazaki 889-16, Japan*

While sclerotherapy is currently an acceptable means of halting esophageal variceal bleeding, it can be performed only in a limited number of institutes. Classical procedures employing pitressin and the Sengstaken-Blakemore (S-B) tube are still widely used for initial management. This report presents the clinical results of pitressin in control of hemorrhage and combined therapy for the treatment of esophageal varices.

## I. Continuous intravenous infusion of pitressin for esophageal variceal bleeding

*(A) Historical note on pitressin therapy (Table 1)*
The usefulness of pitressin was described by Trimble and Wood [1] in 1950 for the control of pulmonary hemorrhage. In experimental animals, Bainbridge and Trevor (1917) [2], Clark (1928) [3], McMichael (1932) [4] and Katz and Rodbard (1939) [5] had demonstrated that intravenous pitressin caused an elevation of hepatic arterial pressure and an abrupt fall in portal pressure. With knowledge of these reports, Kehne and his colleagues (1956) [6] first used pitressin clinically for control of bleeding from esophageal varices. The portal hypotensive effect of pitressin in patients with and without cirrhosis was published soon after. The use of pitressin in the control of esophageal bleeding was suggested as a form of adjunct emergency therapy and not as a substitute for tamponade. Since then, pitressin has become a popular drug in the management of massive esophageal variceal hemorrhage. The original technique of administration consisted of an intravenous infusion of 20 units of pitressin repeated at hourly intervals. To avoid its systemic effects and related complications, Nusbaum and Baum (1967) [7] employed selective infusion into the superior mesenteric artery, and their success rate in controlling variceal bleeding exceeded that obtained by the original technique. Conn and colleagues (1975) [8]

reported in the first prospective randomized controlled trial of pitressin that it was significantly more effective in controlling hemorrhage. Barr (1975) [9] showed in his experiments that there was no statistically significant difference between the degree of changes in portal flow, portal and systemic blood pressure and cardiac output among those treated with selective arterial and intravenous infusions. Recently, Athanasoulis (1976) [10] and Chojkier (1979) [11] reported that a continuous intravenous pitressin infusion was as effective as intraarterial infusions in the treatment of hemorrhage from varices, and recommended that a brief, low-dose therapeutic trial of intravenous pitressin be used early in the treatment of variceal bleeding.

Pitressin has been known to reduce splanchnic blood flow by its effect of vasoconstriction, thus resulting in lowered portal venous pressure. However, reports on its effect on portal venous pressure in man have been somewhat conflicting [12, 13]. Ohnishi (1987) [14] reported that pitressin significantly decreased portal venous pressure ($-36\%$) and flow ($-54.3\%$), investigating in cases of portal hypertension by catheterization of the portal vein using an echo-Doppler flowmetry. Estimated hepatic blood flow was also lowered as previously described by several reports. With the fear that this effect may result in hepatic ischemia, the magnitude of hepatic arterial flow has been of great concern. According to Barr (1975) [15], the hepatic arterial flow showed a biphasic response with an initial decrease followed by a substantial increase in spite of a continued pitressin infusion. A compensatory increase in hepatic arterial blood flow after transient pitressin-induced vasoconstriction protects against hepatic ischemia. This has also been confirmed with direct hepatic artery infusions [16]. The efficacy of pitressin in controlling variceal

TABLE 1   A review of literature in experimental and clinical studies of pitressin

| Author | Year | Achievement |
| --- | --- | --- |
| **Experimental** | | |
| Bainbridge and Trevor | 1917 | Decrease in portal pressure and elevation of hepatic arterial pressure |
| Clark | 1928 | Action in the capillaries of splanchnic region |
| McMichael | 1932 | Presinusoidal A-V shunt |
| Katz and Rodbard | 1939 | Splanchnic vasospasm |
| Barr | 1975 | Comparison of intraarterial and intravenous infusion |
| **Clinical** | | |
| Trimble and Wood | 1950 | Use for pulmonary hemorrhage |
| Kehne | 1956 | First use for esophageal varices |
| Nusbaum | 1967 | Selective intraarterial use |
| Conn | 1975 | Controlled trial |
| Athanasoulis | 1976 | Continuous IV infusion |
| Chojkier | 1979 | Controlled trial of IA and IV infusion |
| Ohnishi | 1987 | Direct measurement of portal hemodynamics |

bleeding may not be explained, since the response to pitressin is somewhat variable that portal venous pressure is not lowered in all patients. The suggestion has been made that constriction of esophageal smooth muscle may shut off the blood flow in the penetrating vessels connecting the para-esophageal coronary vein with the submucosal varices. The pitressin effect is actually on the smooth muscle of the lower one-third of the esophageal wall [17] (Fig. 1).

### (B) Clinical results

During 1978 and 1982, a comparison of a continuous intravenous infusion of pitressin (IVP) and Sengstaken-Blakemore (S-B) tube tamponade in control of esophageal variceal bleeding was carried out. The technique of IVP was to give 200 units in 500 ml of normal saline and then 0.4 units/min continuously for 3 – 4 hours. After bleeding had been controlled, the dosage was slowly tapered off over 24 to 48 hours. Of a total of 34 patients, 22 patients were treated with IVP and 12 patients with S-B tube tamponade. These patients were divided into two groups according to the treatment given. Table 2 compares the two groups with respect to demographic and clinical data. There were no significant differences in liver function between the two groups. In the IVP group, there were 14 men and 7 women with a mean age of 46.8 ± 19.2 and a 9-year-old child with extrahepatic portal obstruction. The causes of esophageal varices were cirrhosis of the liver in 17 patients, idiopathic portal hypertension in 3 patients and extrahepatic portal obstruction in 2 patients. There were 12 patients in Child's A, five in Child's B and five in Child's C classes. The majority of patients had two or three episodes of hematemeses prior to admission except for five patients with initial bleeding from esophageal varices.

The success in control of bleeding was 82% in the IVP group compared with 44% in the S-B tube tamponade group (Fig. 2). The average requirements of blood transfusion were 2700 ml in the IVP group and 5100 ml in the S-B tube tamponade group. The duration of the treatment of IVP ranged from 32 to 80 hours, with an average of 56 hours. The total amount of pitressin dosage was 520 ± 40 units (Table 3). Recurrent bleeding occurred in 36% of the patients. As a major complication,

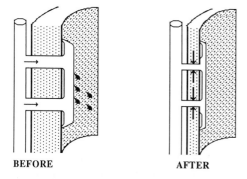

BEFORE                    AFTER

FIG. 1   Mechanism of action of pitressin in esophageal variceal bleeding.

TABLE 2    Clinical data on liver function

|  | Pitressin infusion (n = 22) | S-B tube tamponade (n = 12) |
|---|---|---|
| Sex (M:F) | 15:7 | 10:1 |
| Age (yr) | 46.8 ± 19.2[a] | 48.5 ± 12.2 |
| Liver disease |  |  |
|   Cirrhosis | 17 | 9 |
|   IPH[b] | 3 | 2 |
|   EHPO[c] | 2 | 1 |
| Liver function |  |  |
|   Bilirubin (mg/dl) | 1.5 ± 1.3 | 1.8 ± 1.2 |
|   Total protein (gm/dl) | 6.2 ± 1.4 | 6.0 ± 1.0 |
|   A/G ratio | 1.2 ± 0.4 | 1.2 ± 0.5 |
|   SGOT (IU/l) | 51.8 ± 41.0 | 73.6 ± 35.2 |
|   Alkaline phosphatase (K.A.) | 10.4 ± 9.9 | 10.4 ± 9.2 |
| Child's criteria | A:12, B:5, C:5 | A:5, B:4, C:3 |

[a] Except for one 9-yr-old child.
[b] Idiopathic portal hypertension.
[c] Extrahepatic portal obstruction.

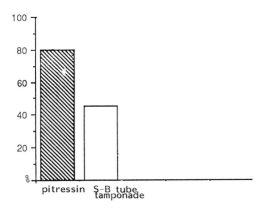

FIG. 2    The success in control of bleeding.

acute pulmonary edema was observed in two patients, but it resolved following cessation of pitressin. No other serious complications were observed.

*(C) Discussion and conclusion*
A continuous intravenous infusion of pitressin (IVP) was reported to seem as effective as an intraarterial infusion [18]. By its simplicity and practical convenience, we have routinely used IVP as well as sclerotherapy for esophageal variceal bleeding. However, the efficacy of pitressin infusion in controlling bleeding is controversial

TABLE 3    Treatments with pitressin and S-B tube tamponade

|  | Episodes of bleeding | Duration of therapy (days) | Requirement of blood transfusion (ml) |
|---|---|---|---|
| Pitressin | 2.5 ± 1.6 | 3.8 ± 2.2 | 2720 ± 2400 |
| S-B tube tamponade | 2.8 ± 2.1 | 1.8 ± 0.6 | 5116 ± 3450 |

[11]. The overall efficacy depends on the patient's clinical status and the severity of the underlying liver disease. Although the numbers of patients in our data were too small to speculate, patients nonresponsive to IVP were one in Child's A, one in Child's B and two in Child's B classes. According to Athanasoulis [10], a 90 – 95% success rate for bleeding control should be expected among patients of Child's A, 75% for Child's B and 55% for Child's C classes. Following mesenteric vasoconstriction and decrease of portal flow induced by pitressin, the lack of hepatic arterial response for compensation is observed in some patients. They may have a poor prognosis and would not tolerate portocaval shunt.

With regard to the dosage of pitressin, Chojkier [11] started to use 0.3 U/min for at least 30 min and, if ineffective, progressively increased the dose at approximately 30 to 60 min intervals to 0.6, 0.9, 1.2 and 1.5 U/min. It is possible that the systemic side-effects and complications of pitressin may contribute to the high mortality rate. To avoid such potential risks, he recommends that a brief (2 – 4 h), low dose (0.3 to 0.9 U/min) be used early in the treatment of variceal bleeding. Athanasoulis [10] successfully treated 10 patients with intravenous infusion of pitressin at a rate of 0.3 U/min for 12 hours, followed by 0.2 U/min for 24 hours and 0.1 U/min for an additional 24 hours. It would make much better sense to administer pitressin in weight-related dosages, and the proper dose should be $5 \times 10^{-3}$ units/kg [19]. Bleeding recurred within 5 days of initial control in 33 – 45% of patients [8]. This must be considered a disappointing result. Moreover, Conn and associates failed to demonstrate improved survival in the pitressin treated group.

In conclusion, IVP is recommended to be used in a brief therapeutic trial for the initial management of esophageal variceal bleeding. Then, sclerotherapy and/or surgery should be performed.

## II. Combined therapy for esophageal varices

### (A) Theoretical possibilities

Sclerotherapy is currently the most popular form of therapy for esophageal variceal bleeding, although recurrence is common. According to one report [20], sclerotherapy reduced the recurrence of varices in patients who developed new and/or enlarged collaterals, and was accompanied by a decrease in portal pressure. Thus, any additional shunting may improve the efficacy of sclerotherapy, but the surgical procedures must be technically simple and safe since the majority of these patients are cirrhotic. On the basis of our experience [21 – 23], portopulmonary shunt by

334

splenopneumopexy is a reasonable shunt procedure which facilitates natural collateral formation. A concept of combined therapy was established. This consists of sclerotherapy, splenopneumopexy and transcatheter arterial embolization (TAE) of the splenic and left gastric arteries (Fig. 3). Thus the theoretical possibilities of this combined therapeutic approach can be explained as follows. (1) Intravariceal sclerotherapy will lead to endoscopic devascularization. (2) Portopulmonary shunt by means of splenopneumopexy facilitates effective collateral formation. (3) Transcatheter arterial embolization of the splenic artery and of the left gastric artery aids in the safe performance of splenopneumopexy and helps to eliminate those factors that contribute to portal hypertension and esophageal varices, as well as hypersplenism.

*(B) Clinical results*

The technique of combined therapy was previously described in detail [24, 25]. In patients with actual variceal bleeding, sclerotherapy was the first treatment choice. One week later, endoscopic examination was carried out and sclerotherapy was performed if any unthrombosed varices were present. One to two weeks after the initial sclerotherapy, TAE of the splenic and left gastric arteries was carried out along with angiographic evaluation of the portal system. When platelet counts increased after splenic artery embolization, splenopneumopexy was performed. Usually a period of 2 – 3 weeks was required for platelet counts to increase to the maximum level. However, thrombocytopenia may not be a counterindication for elective splenopneumopexy.

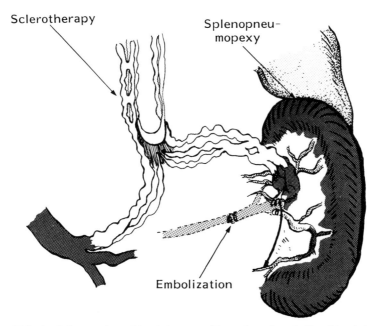

FIG. 3   Schema of combined therapy. (From Ono J et al: Combined therapy for esophageal varices. Surgery 1987; 101: 535 – 543. Used by permission of the C. V. Mosby Company.)

Thirty-eight patients were consecutively treated for esophageal varices. The patients were divided into two groups according to the treatment given. Group A was treated with sclerotherapy and TAE of the splenic and left gastric arteries. Group B was treated with sclerotherapy, TAE of the splenic and left gastric arteries, and splenopneumopexy. There were no significant differences in liver function between the two groups (Table 4). The follow-up period has been 20 months, and there has been a high rate of recurrence in group A (63%) as compared with group B (5%) (Table 5). The majority of recurrences in group A were within 6 months after treatment. There was recurrent bleeding in three of 19 patients in group A and none in group B. Three patients died, two of recurrent bleeding and one of hepatic failure

TABLE 4    Clinical data on liver function in groups A and B

|  | Group A (n = 19) | Group B (n = 19) |
|---|---|---|
| Sex (M:F) | 17 : 2 | 11 : 8 |
| Age (years) | 56.9 ± 10.1 | 57.3 ± 6.6 |
| Liver disease |  |  |
| Cirrhosis | 19 | 16 |
| IPH | 0 | 3 |
| Liver function |  |  |
| Bilirubin (mg/dl) | 1.1 ± 0.6 | 0.8 ± 0.3 |
| Albumin (g/dl) | 3.2 ± 0.6 | 3.4 ± 0.5 |
| SGOT (IU/l) | 52.0 ± 33.0 | 41.8 ± 12.9 |
| Alkaline phosphatase (K.A.) | 12.2 ± 5.4 | 10.7 ± 2.9 |
| ICG $R_{15}$ (%) | 32.5 ± 17.2 | 30.8 ± 19.1 |
| Ascites moderate | 5/19 (26.3%) | 4/19 (21.1%) |
| Encephalopathy moderate | 3/19 (15.8%) | 1/19 (5.3%) |
| Child's criteria | A:4, B:8, C:7 | A:8, B:8, C:3 |

TABLE 5    Postoperative results in groups A and B

|  | Group A (n = 19) | Group B (n = 19) |  |
|---|---|---|---|
| Follow-up (months) | 14 – 36 | 10 – 35 |  |
| (mean ± SD) | (22.1 ± 6.8) | (19.6 ± 7.2) |  |
| Disappearance of varices | 2 (10.5%) | 7 (36.8%) |  |
| Recurrence of varices |  |  |  |
| F factor | 12 (63.2%)[a] | 1 (5.3%)[a] |  |
| R-C sign | 15 (78.9%)[a] | 2 (10.5%)[a] |  |
| Recurrent bleeding | 4 (21.1%) | 1 (5.3%) | gastric varices |
| Late death | 3 (15.8%) | 2 (10.5%) |  |

[a] $p < 0.05$.

in group A. Two patients died of hepatic failure in group B over four months after surgery. Esophageal varices with 'red color sign' disappeared in most patients in group B. Significant improvements in the esophageal varices were observed at periodic endoscopic examinations of the other subjects.

### (C) Discussion and conclusion

In our experience, 77 splenopneumopexies were performed in patients with portal hypertension. The reductions of postoperative splenic pulp pressure and wedged hepatic venous pressure were previously reported [24]. Thus this procedure effects a low grade of portal hypertension with well-controlled esophageal variceal bleeding, and an adequate hepatic blood flow is maintained to prevent hepatic impairment. Furthermore, in this shunt the spleen plays an important role in controlling blood flow through the shunt, as well as in portal flow, similar to Warren-Zeppa's distal splenorenal shunt. The patency of the portopulmonary shunt is well-maintained without thrombosis formation. The long-time survival data were also similar to those for distal splenorenal shunt, being 68% at 5 years and 54% at 10 years, compared with 59% at 5 years and 50% at 10 years in distal splenorenal shunt [26] (Fig. 4).

Complications have been observed in each of the procedures (sclerotherapy, TAE and splenopneumopexy). Although they occur frequently, minor complications, such as ulcerations in sclerotherapy and fever with abdominal pain in splenic embolization, are resolved by the use of conservative measures.

In conclusion, splenopneumopexy is an additional procedure which may resolve some of the problems associated with sclerotherapy. It is safe, simple and effective.

**References**

1   Trimble HG, Wood HR. Pulmonary hemorrhage: its control by the intravenous use of pituitrin. Dis Chest 1950; 18: 345 – 351.
2   Bainbridge FA, Trevor JW. Some action of adrenalin upon the liver. J Physiol 1917; 50: 460 – 468.
3   Clark GA. Comparison of the effects of adrenalin and pituitrin on the portal circulation. J Physiol 1928; 66: 274 – 279.
4   McMichael J. The portal circulation: the action of adrenalin and pituitary pressor extract. J Physiol 1932; 75: 241 – 263.
5   Katz LN, Rodbard S. The integration of the vasomotor responses in the liver with those in other systemic vessels. J Pharmacol Exp Ther 1939; 67: 407 – 421.
6   Kehne JH, Hughes FA, Gompertz ML. The use of surgical pituitrin in the control of esophageal varix bleeding: an experimental study and report of two cases. Surgery 1956; 39: 917 – 925.
7   Nusbaum M, Baum S, Kuroda K, et al. Control of portal hypertension by selective mesenteric arterial drug infusion. Arch Surg 1968; 97: 1005 – 1012.
8   Conn HO, Ramsby GR, Storer EH, et al. Intraarterial vasopressin in the treatment of upper gastrointestinal hemorrhage: a prospective, controlled clinical trial. Gastroenterology 1975; 68: 211 – 221.
9   Barr JW, Lakin RC, Rosch J. Vasopressin and hepatic artery: effect of selective celiac infusion of vasopressin on the hepatic artery flow. Invest Radiol 1975; 10: 200 – 205.
10  Athanasoulis CA, Waltman AC, Novelline RA, et al. Angiography: its contribution to

the emergency management of gastrointestinal hemorrhage. Ther Rad Clin N Am 1976; 15: 265 – 280.

11　Chojkier M, Groszmann RJ, Atterbury CE, et al. A controlled comparison of continuous intraarterial and intravenous infusions of vasopressin in hemorrhage from esophageal varices. Gastroenterology 1979; 77: 540 – 546.

12　Ranek L, Vilstrup H, Iversen J, et al. The effect of continuous vasopressin infusion on splanchnic blood flow, liver function, and portal and central venous pressures in patients with cirrhosis. Scand J Clin Lab Invest 1984; 44: 251 – 256.

13　Mols P, Hallemans R, Kuyk MV, et al. Hemodynamic effects of vasopressin, alone and in combination with nitroprusside, in patients with liver cirrhosis and portal hypertension. Ann Surg 1984; 199: 176 – 181.

14　Ohnishi K, Saito M, Nakayama T, et al. Effects of vasopressin on portal hemodynamics in patients with portal hypertension. Am J Gastroenterol 1987; 82: 135 – 138.

15　Barr JW, Lakin RC, Rosch J. Similarity of arterial and intravenous vasopressin on portal and systemic hemodynamics. Gastroenterology 1975; 69: 13 – 19.

16　Kerr JC, Reynolds DG, Swan KG. Vasopressin and canine hepatic arterial blood flow. J Surg Res 1977; 23: 166 – 171.

17　Cort JH, Schwartz IL. An early look at the therapeutic uses of some new vasopressin analogs in gastroenterology. Yale J Biol Med 1978; 51: 605 – 614.

18　Johnson WC, Widrich WC, Ansell JE, et al. Control of bleeding varices by vasopressin: a prospective randomized study. Ann Surg 1977; 186: 369 – 376.

19　Chandler JG. Vasopressin and splanchnic shunting. Ann Surg 1982; 195: 543 – 553.

20　Toyonaga A, Eguchi S. Prognostic study on 205 patients with endoscopic injection sclerotherapy (EIS) for esophageal varices. Gastroenterol Endosc 1985; 27: 2361 – 2362 (in Japanese with English abstract).

21　Akita H, Sakoda K. Portopulmonary shunt by splenopneumopexy as a surgical treatment of Budd-Chiari syndrome. Surgery 1980; 1: 85 – 94.

22　Ono J, Sakoda K, Kawada T. Membranous obstruction of the inferior vena cava. Ann Surg 1983; 197: 454 – 458.

23　Ono J, Sakoda K, Kawada T, Nishi S, Tabata M, Mizouchi J, Furukawa T, et al. Long-term follow-up result of portopulmonary shunt by splenopneumopexy on membranous obstruction of the inferior vena cava. Surgery 1984; 95: 116 – 119.

24　Ono J, Katsuki T, Kodama Y. Combined therapy for esophageal varices: sclerotherapy, embolization, and splenopneumopexy. Surgery 1987; 101: 535 – 543.

25　Ono J, Katsuki T, Kodama Y. New approach in the management of esophageal varices. Br J Surg 1987; 74: 607 – 609.

26　Warren WD, Millikan WJ, Henderson JM, et al. Ten years portal hypertensive surgery at Emory. Ann Surg 1982; 195: 530 – 542.

Chapter 31

# The effect of an amino acid solution granule-enriched with branched chain amino acids, and arginine, in patients with portal systemic encephalopathy

KENSHO SANJO[1], YASUO IDEZUKI[1] AND HIROSHI OKA[2]

[1] *The Second Department of Surgery and* [2] *The First Department of Medicine, Faculty of Medicine, University of Tokyo, Tokyo, Japan*

## Introduction

Chronic portal-systemic encephalopathy following systemic shunts may be incapacitating and non-responsive to intensive medical management. At our surgical department, 111 shunt procedures were done between 1949 and 1964.

Portal-systemic decompressive operation was done with successful control of hemorrhage, but hepatic encephalopathy was recognized as a serious complication post shunt operation. Eighteen patients died within the first 30 days of the procedure. Thirty-six patients suffered from at least one episode of hepatic encephalopathy during follow up. Six patients are alive at more than 25 years following portal systemic shunts, and are free of recurrence of variceal bleeding in the long-term follow up.

Several hypotheses for the pathogenesis of HE have been presented. Accumulation of toxic products in the brain such as ammonia, mercaptans, short and medium chain fatty acids or deranged metabolism of glutamine, glutamate, GABA and alpha-ketoglutaramate are generally regarded to be of importance for the development of HE [1]. Disturbances in central neurotransmission as a consequence of amino acid imbalance in plasma have also been suggested [2].

An amino acid solution (named THF) enriched with branched chain amino acids and arginine has been established, intending to correct the blood ammonia level, supply nutrition and promote the improvement in symptoms. Basic experiments were performed. In the basic experiments, psychoneurotic symptoms and the electroencephalogram were improved with the lowering of the blood ammonia level [3].

The therapeutic efficacy of orally administered amino acids, granule (THF-G) enriched in branched chain amino acids and arginine, in 108 patients with liver cirrhosis and chronic hepatic encephalopathy was examined in a randomized double-blind cross-over study.

## Methods

### Subjects

One hundred and eight patients with stable cirrhosis of varying etiology were selected from 21 hospitals between April 1983 and March 1984. The following selection criterion was used: evidence of chronic hepatic encephalopathy. Patients were randomly allocated to THF-G group and placebo group. The two randomly assigned groups were comparable with respect to age, sex, history of hepatitis, alcoholic abuse and modified Child's grading (Table 1). The severity of hepatic encephalopathy in their previous history was comparable and at entry there was no difference in severity of hepatic encephalopathy. The two randomly assigned groups were highly comparable in clinical and laboratory characteristics. There were no differences in laboratory features such as albumin, prothrombin time, blood urea nitrogen, blood ammonia, total bilirubin and BCAA/AAA ratio (Table 2).

TABLE 1    Comparison of clinical features in the two patient groups at entry into the trial

|  | THF-G ($n$ = 56) | Placebo ($n$ = 52) | $P$ value |
|---|---|---|---|
| Sex (F:M) | 33:23 | 34:18 | NP |
| Mean age ± SD HBs | 57.7 ± 9.8 | 58.1 ± 9.6 | NP |
| (−) | 45 | 43 | NP |
| (+) | 11 | 9 | NP |
| Hepatitis | 13 | 13 | NP |
| Alcohol abuse | 22 | 24 | NP |
| Modified Child's grading |  |  |  |
| A | 10 | 9 |  |
| B | 15 | 13 | NP |
| C | 30 | 28 |  |

TABLE 2    Laboratory values (mean ± SD)

|  | THF-G | Placebo | $P$ value |
|---|---|---|---|
| Albumin (gm/l) | 3.3 ± 0.6 | 3.3 ± 0.6 | NP |
| Prothrombin activity (%) | 70 ± 22 | 67 ± 24 | NP |
| BUN (mg/dl) | 14.9 ± 5.4 | 15.5 ± 6.7 | NP |
| Blood ammonia (µg/dl) | 110 ± 80 | 106 ± 56 | NP |
| Bilirubin (mg/dl) | 2.3 ± 1.6 | 2.2 ± 1.3 | NP |
| BCAA/AAA | 1.09 ± 0.35 | 1.07 ± 0.35 | NP |
| ICG (15 mm) | 51.0 ± 16.4 | 50.5 ± 16.3 | NP |

## Experimental design

The study was designed to compare, in a double-blind, randomized, cross-over fashion, THF-G or placebo in a dosage of 9 g/day was administered for 8 weeks. Each diet was given in random order. The composition of THF-G is outlined in Table 3.

## Neurologic assessment

Mental status, asterixis and psychomotor function were graded according to the following criteria.

### Mental status
A modified Sherlock criterion was used [17]. Grade I, confused, altered mood or behaviour, slurred speech; grade 2, drowsy, inappropriate behaviour; grade 3, stuporous but speaking and obeying simple commands, inarticulate speech, marked confusion; grade 4, coma; grade 5, deep coma with no response to painful stimuli and no spontaneous movements.

### Trailmarking test
Part A of the Reitan number-connecting test (NCT) was used [18]. Patients were asked to connect a series of 25 numbers as quickly as possible. To avoid the learning effect, four different versions of the NCT were used.

### Asterixis
Presence of asterixis was tested by having the patients hold both arms and forearms extended with the wrists dorsiflexed.

### Medications
All maintenance medications were continued during the clinical trial. But lactulose, neomycin and psychoactive agents were not administered.

TABLE 3   Amino acid (granule enriched in branched chain amino acids and arginine)

Composition of THF-G (g)

| | | | |
|---|---|---|---|
| Ile[a] | 0.131 | His | 0.044 |
| Leu[a] | 0.136 | Ala | 0.120 |
| Lys | 0.056 | Asp | 0.003 |
| Met | 0.009 | Cys | 0.003 |
| Phe | 0.004 | Gly | 0.077 |
| Thr | 0.042 | Pro | 0.076 |
| Trp | 0.010 | Ser | 0.037 |
| Val[a] | 0.127 | Tyr | 0.009 |
| Arg[a] | 0.131 | | |

[a] THF-G, enriched in branched chain amino acids and arginine.

*Plasma aminograms*
Quantitative determination of amino acids was carried out by a column chromatographic technique.

*Blood ammonia concentration*
Fasting blood ammonia levels were measured. Data were subjected to analysis of Chi-square and Wilcoxon.

*Statistical analysis*
Results are reported as the mean ± SD.

## Results

*Mental state*
Sixteen (29%) of the 56 patients receiving oral administration of THF-G had an improved grade of mental state. There was no detectable improvement in six (11%) of the THF-G group. Mental status grades indicated a statistically significant difference on the patients' response of THF-G compared with placebo (Table 4).

*NCT*
The NCT showed improvement after administration of THF-G. Twenty-two (41%) of the 56 patients had an improved NCT. No detectable improvement was observed

TABLE 4   Physician's evaluation (mental status grade)

|  | THF-G (No. of patients) | Placebo (No. of patients) | $P$ value |
|---|---|---|---|
| Excellent | 1 | 1 |  |
| Good | 15 | 7 | < 0.05 |
| No change | 33 | 24 |  |
| Poor | 6 | 14 |  |
| No evaluation | 1 | 6 |  |

TABLE 5   Number connection test

|  | THF-G (No. of patients) | Placebo (No. of patients) | $P$ value |
|---|---|---|---|
| Excellent | 5 | 1 |  |
| Good | 18 | 10 |  |
| No change | 21 | 18 | < 0.05 |
| Poor | 2 | 7 |  |
| No evaluation | 10 | 16 |  |

in only two patients. There was a statistically significant difference between THF-G and placebo (Table 5).

*Plasma aminogram*
The ratio of plasma BCAA to AAA molar concentration greatly increased after administration of THF-G (from $1.09 \pm 0.35$ to $1.25 \pm 0.31$), but no substantial change was seen in the placebo group. The difference between THF-G and placebo was statistically significant for the ratio of plasma BCAA to AAA molar concentration (Table 6).

*Blood ammonia concentration*
The mean value of blood ammonia levels showed a tendency to improve after administration of THF-G. There was a wide range of variation in blood ammonia values. The mean value of blood ammonia levels was aggravated in the placebo group. There was a statistically significant difference between THF-G and placebo (Table 7).

*Liver function tests*
There was no significant improvement in liver function tests on completion of the study. General evaluation of clinical observations indicated a statistically significant difference in the patients' response to THF-G compared with placebo. Fifty-six of the patients who were administered THF-G observed apparent efficacy, but this was only 23% in the placebo group (Table 8). Improvements in asterixis were observed, showing a statistically significant difference between THF-G and placebo.

TABLE 6   Results of laboratory values (BCAA/AAA[a] ratio)

|              | THF-G            | Placebo          |
| ------------ | ---------------- | ---------------- |
| At entry     | $1.09 \pm 0.35$  | $1.07 \pm 0.35$  |
| Post 1 week  | $1.20 \pm 0.37$  | $1.08 \pm 0.52$  |
| Post 6 weeks | $1.25 \pm 0.31$  | $1.02 \pm 0.31$  |

[a] BCAA, branched chain amino acid; AAA, aromatic amino acid.

TABLE 7   Results of laboratory values (blood ammonia ($\mu$g/dl))

|              | THF-G             | Placebo           |
| ------------ | ----------------- | ----------------- |
| At entry     | $109.8 \pm 79.9$  | $106.6 \pm 56.2$  |
| Post 1 week  | $93.6 \pm 54.5$   | $123.8 \pm 63.6$  |
| Post 6 weeks | $96.4 \pm 49.1$   | $114.9 \pm 58.9$  |

TABLE 8   General evaluation of clinical observations

|  | THF-G (No. of patients) | Placebo (No. of patients) | P value |
|---|---|---|---|
| Excellent | 1 | 0 | |
| Good | 25 | 11 | |
| No change | 23 | 18 | < 0.01 |
| Poor | 6 | 17 | |
| No evaluation | 1 | 6 | |

## Discussion

Treatment for hepatic encephalopathy aims principally at reducing the blood ammonia level, and protein-restricted diets, antibiotics, oral lactulose and enema have been commonly employed with fair clinical success.

Since the 19th century when Eck [4] discovered that cerebral symptoms could be induced in dogs with portacaval shunts by feeding them meat, abnormal ammonia metabolism has been regarded to be an important cause in the development of hepatic encephalopathy. The acute administration of ammonium salts to experimental animals will produce convulsions, coma, and death [5, 6]. The concentration of ammonia is usually elevated in the blood and cerebrospinal fluid of patients with hepatic encephalopathy [7].

Hyperammonemia accompanies the comas of Reye's disease [8, 9], inherited disorders caused by a deficiency of one or more of the enzymes of the Krebs-Henseleit cycle. Chronic hyperammonemia in animals, achieved either by the infusion of ammonium salts [10], administration of jack-bean urease [11] or construction of a portacaval shunt [12], leads to the development of Alzheimer astrocytic changes and other neuropathologic abnormalities that are strikingly similar to those found in the brains of patients who die in hepatic coma.

It can readily be presumed from the present investigation that the improvement in ammonemia contributes largely to the development of therapeutic effects of THF-G.

The question of which amino acid among THF-G actually acts and how it promotes the ammonia metabolism is a difficult problem. It is reported that ammonemia in hepatic insufficiency promotes glutamine synthesis in the brain, and when the glutamine flows out from the brain cells, aromatic amino acids flow into the brain cells [13].

Since ammonia metabolism in healthy humans occurs mainly in the liver, the ammonia level in the hepatic venous blood shows a low value compared with that of other sites. In patients with liver cirrhosis, the ammonia level in the hepatic venous blood is not always low, due to effects of an intrahepatic shunt added to that of the ammonia metabolism in the liver. In contrast, the ammonia level in the jugular venous blood exhibits a lower value compared with that of other sites [14]. In cases of hepatic insufficiency accompanying chronic liver diseases, ammonia metabolism occurs in the compensatory phase; metabolism of $\alpha$-ketoglutarate $\rightarrow$ glutamate $\rightarrow$ glutamine has led to a partial compensation of the metabolism in which the urea cycle has been predominant [15].

Of the amino acids that are contained in THF, those which play important roles in ammonia metabolism are considered to be arginine in the urea cycle in the liver, and branched chain amino acids in the glutamine cycle in the brain and muscle. Other amino acids need further study.

Infusion of BCAA reduces the concentrations of aromatic amino acids and the indoles in the brain but does not seem to influence the mental state at 6 h after inducing liver ischemia in the rat.

However, the altered metabolism of the amino acids and serotonin in the brain is probably not the only reason for the development and maintenance of hepatic coma and encephalopathy. Therefore, although the BCAA infusion can be of importance, no apparent influence on the mental state with the present methods could be demonstrated [17].

## Summary

The therapeutic efficacy of orally administered amino acids, granule (THF-G) enriched in branched chain amino acids and arginine, in 108 patients with liver cirrhosis and chronic hepatic encephalopathy was examined in a double-blind randomized cross-over study. The two randomly assigned groups were highly comparable in clinical and labaoratory characteristics. THF-G or placebo at a dosage of 9.0 g/day was administered in a cross-over fashion for 8 weeks. Each diet was given in random order.

Mental status grade ($P < 0.05$), number connection test ($P < 0.05$), venous blood ammonia ($P < 0.05$), BCAA/AA ratio ($P < 0.01$) and clinical observations ($P < 0.01$) indicated a statistically significant difference on the patient's response to THF-G compared with placebo.

It can be concluded that oral administration of THF-G reduces the affection of hepatic encephalopathy.

## Acknowledgements

I am indebted to Drs Toshitugu Oda, Tatsuo Wada, Tatsuo Negishi (controller) and Mr Shunpei Banno, and finally to members of the THF-G study, mainly for their cooperation in clinical investigation.

## References

1  Conn HO, Liebeberthal MM. The Hepatic Coma Syndromes and Lactulose. Baltimore: Williams & Wilkins Co., 1979.
2  Fischer J, Baldessarini R. False neurotransmitters and hepatic failure. Lancet 1971; i: 75 – 80.

346

3 Sanjo K. Effect of an amino acid solution and amino acid granules – enriched with branched-chain amino acids – on the blood ammonia levels. In: Parenteral and Enteral Hyperalimentation. Amsterdam: Elsevier Science Publishers, 1984.

4 Eck NV. Ligature of the portal vein. Med J St Petersburg 1877; 130: 1–2 (translated by Child CG. (1953) in Eck fistula. Surg Gynecol Obstet 96: 375–376).

5 Torda C. Ammonium ion content and electrical activity of the brain during the preconvulsive and convulsive phases induced by various convulsants. J Pharmacol Exp Ther 1953; 107: 197–203.

6 Hindfelt B, Siesjo BK. Cerebral effects of acute ammonia intoxication. I. The influence on intracellular and extracellular acid-base parameters. Scand J Clin Lab Invest 1971; 28: 353–364.

7 Plum F. The CSF in hepatic encephalopathy. Exp Biol Med 1971; 4: 34–41.

8 Huttenlocher PR, Schwartz AD, Klatskin G. Reye's syndrome: ammonia intoxication as a possible factor in the encephalopathy. Pediatrics 1969; 43: 443–454.

9 Glasgow AM, Cotton RB, Dhiensiri K. Reye's syndrome. I. Blood ammonia and consideration of the nonhistologic diagnosis. Am J Dis Child 1972; 124: 827–836.

10 Cole M, Rutherford RB, Smith FO. Experimental ammonia encephalopathy in the primate. Arch Neurol. 1972; 26: 130–136.

11 Gibson GE, Zimber A, Krook L, Richardson EP Jr, Visek WJ. Brain histology and behavior of mice injected with urease. J Neuropathol Exp Neurol 1974; 33: 201–211.

12 Cavanagh JB. Liver bypass and the glia. Res Publ Assoc Nerv Ment Dis 1974; 53: 13–35.

13 James JH, Ziparo V, Jeppsson B. Hyperammonemia, plasma amino acid imbalance, and blood-brain amino acid transport: a unified theory of portal-systemic encephalopathy. Lancet 1979; ii: 772.

14 Sanjo K, Hidai K, Kawasaki S, et al. Basic study of THF. J THF Study Meeting 1981; 4, 174.

15 McMenamy RH, Drapanas T. Amino acid and $\alpha$-keto acid concentrations in plasma and blood of the liver-less dog. Am J Physiol 1965; 209, 1046.

16 Bugge M, Bengtsson F, et al. Amino acids and indoleamines in the brain after infusion of branched-chain amino acids to rats with liver ischemia. JPEN 1985; 10(5): 474–478.

17 Sherlock, S. Diseases of the Liver and Biliary System. Tokyo: Igaku Shoin Ltd, 1973.

18 Conn HO. Trailmarking and number-connection tests in the assessment of mental state in portal systemic encephalopathy. Digest Dis 1977; 22: 541–550.

© 1988 Elsevier Science Publishers B.V. (Biomedical Division)
*Treatment of esophageal varices*
*Y. Idezuki, editor*

Chapter 32

# Emergency control of bleeding esophageal varices using a transparent tamponade tube (Idezuki's tube)

MASARU HAGIWARA, YASUHARU SATO, MASAHIRO SAKAI AND HIROMU WATANABE

*First Department of Surgery, St. Marianna University School of Medicine, Kanagawa, Japan*

Successful control of massive bleeding from ruptured esophageal varices using an esophagogastric balloon tamponade tube is life-saving and also important in preventing further deterioration of the condition of patients with hepatic failure. Among the several kinds of tubes developed for this purpose, the Sengstaken-Blakemore tube [1], which is the most widely used in the world, is shown in the upper part of Fig. 1, in the middle is a new type of tube, made of silicon rubber, and the lower part also shows a new type of esophageal balloon tamponade tube, which is called Idezuki's tube (Fig. 1).

## The instrument

The transparent tamponade tube was designed to control esophageal and gastric bleeding in 1975 by Professor Idezuki [2], who was a president of the Tokyo symposium.

The structure of Idezuki's tube is basically similar to that of the Sengstaken-Blakemore tube. This tube has a triple-lumen core tube, a gastric balloon and an esophageal balloon. The length of the core tube is 55 cm and the inside diameter of the main lumen of the tube is 8 mm. The core tube is made of polyvinyl chloride. The esophageal balloon is cylindrical in shape and is made of a polyurethane membrane, and the gastric balloon is made of latex rubber.

The central tube is large enough to accomodate a standard-diameter bronchofiberscope. One of the unique aspects of this tube is that it is designed to accomodate an endoscope inserted through it and not vice versa. Since the material of the balloon is transparent, the resolution of the visual image is not significantly impaired (Fig. 2).

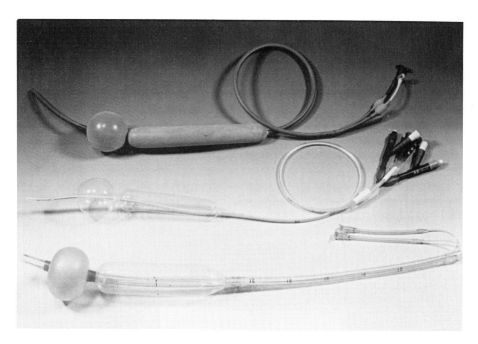

FIG. 1 Esophagogastric balloon tamponade tubes.

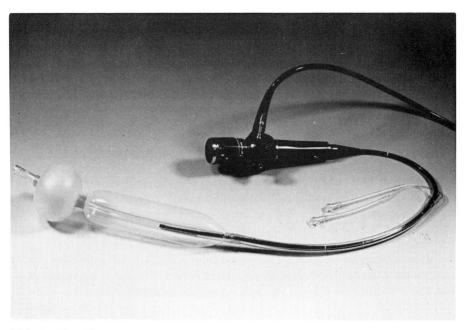

FIG. 2 Idezuki's tube with bronchofiberscope.

## Materials and methods

Between February 1975 and February 1987, 45 patients with esophageal varices were intubated with Idezuki's tube when esophageal varices ruptured at St. Marianna University School of Medicine [3]. The cases of rupture of esophageal varices consisted of 2 Child's A, 11 Child's B, and 32 Child's C cases.

First, the larynx of the patient is anesthetized with xylocaine solution and the patient is placed in the prone or left lateral position. The tube is inserted through the mouth and the tip of the tube is carefully advanced to the esophagus and then into the stomach.

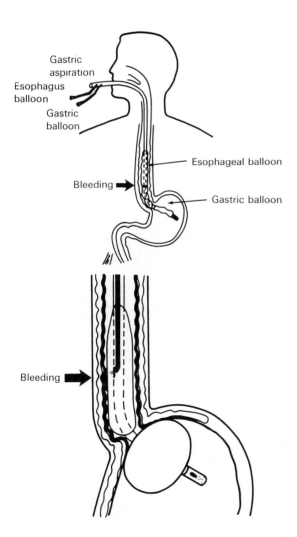

FIG. 3   Close examination of esophageal varices with endoscopic balloon tamponade.

TABLE 1  Endoscopic balloon tamponade for upper gastrointestinal bleeding

| Source of bleeding | Number of cases | Number of trials | Successful hemostasis (%) |
|---|---|---|---|
| Esophageal varices | 45 | 84 | 82/84 (97) |
| Esophageal ulcer | 7 | 13 | 8/13 (62) |
| Gastric varices | 2 | 2 | 1/2 (50) |
| Total | 54 | 99 | 91/99 (92) |

TABLE 2  Relationship between initial time and frequency in Child's classification

| Child's classification | n | Time (hours) | Number of cases and trials | | |
|---|---|---|---|---|---|
| | | | 1 time (%) | 2 times (%) | 3 times (%) |
| A | 2 | 28.5 | 2 (100) | | |
| B | 11 | 26.6 | 10 (90) | 1 (10) | |
| C | 32 | 67.5 | 16 (50) | 5 (16) | 11 (34) |
| Total | 45 | | 28 | 6 | 11 |

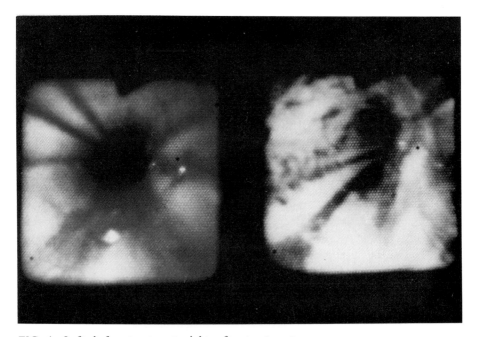

FIG. 4  Left, before treatment; right, after treatment.

The gastric balloon is inflated with 150 – 300 ml of air and the esophageal balloon is inflated slowly with 50 – 80 ml of air to attain a pressure equivalent to 30 mmHg (Fig. 3).

We can thus examine the esophagus endoscopically at will, so that failure to control bleeding can be rectified and also mucosal damage due to overcompression by the balloon can be avoided.

## Results

These are the clinical results using the balloon tamponade for upper G-I bleeding. Treatment with Idezuki's tube was performed on 84 occasions on 45 patients with rupture of esophageal varices. Hemostasis was achieved in 82 times out of 84 (97%) with this tube (Table 1).

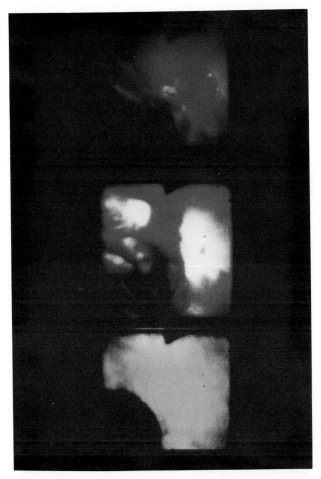

FIG. 5   Top, before treatment; middle, after 1 h treatment; bottom, one day later.

The tube was inserted for an average of 28.5 hours to achieve hemostasis in Child's A, 26.6 hours in Child's B and 67.5 hours in Child's C.

In over 90% of the cases of Child's A and B, hemostasis was achieved with only one session with this tube, but two or more sessions were needed to control bleeding in Child's C cases (Table 2). We have not come across any complications [4].

**Two case reports**

In the left-hand photograph in Fig. 4, there is bleeding from a varix. The tamponade tube was maintained in place for 24 hours, after which fiberscopy revealed that hemostasis had been successfully achieved.

Fig. 5 shows another case. Here massive bleeding is observed and, as can be seen in the middle photograph, even after tamponade treatment for one hour bleeding was still observed. However, the bleeding was brought under control three hours later, and in the lower photograph one can see that hemostasis was achieved, after one day.

**Discussion**

At first Fig. 6 may appear slightly puzzling. One might assume that a higher pressure would yield more effective control of bleeding. However, these results show that in

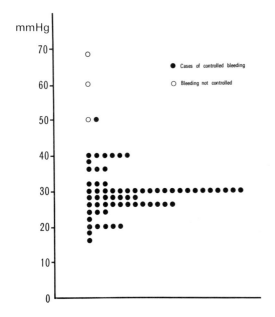

FIG. 6 Pressure of the esophageal balloon at successful control of bleeding (initial pressure).

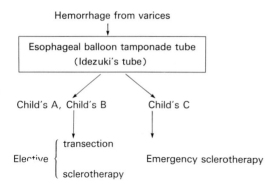

FIG. 7    Treatment of bleeding esophageal varices.

fact cases that respond to this method will respond to relatively low pressure, whereas a few cases of uncontrollable massive bleeding will not respond even at high pressure levels.

Following temporary control of esophageal bleeding of varices with this method, patients with Child's A or Child's B classification are worked up for staged treatment such as esophageal transection or sclerotherapy.

However, recurrent bleeding after the removal of the tube is often noticed in Child's C cases, so it is necessary to perform sclerotherapy soon after the removal of the tube (Fig. 7).

Finally, these are the overall results we have obtained with this method. We use it primarily to control bleeding from esophageal varices, and as you can see here we have obtained a very high rate of hemostasis, close to a hundred percent.

We are very satisfied with our results. We find this instrument very easy to use and consider it to be a convenient clinical instrument.

## References

1    Sengstaken RW, Blakemore AH. Balloon tamponade for the control of hemorrhage from esophageal varices. Ann Surg 1950; 131: 781 – 789.

2    Idezuki Y, Hagiwara M, et al. Endoscopic balloon tamponade for emergency control of bleeding esophageal varices using a new transparent tamponade tube. Trans Am Soc Artif Intern Organs 1977; 23: 646 – 650.

3    Sato Y. Clinical effectiveness of a new type of esophageal balloon tamponade tube (Idezuki's tube) in rupture of esophageal varices. St. Marianna Med J 1988; 15: 624 – 633.

4    Hagiwara M, Ikari J, Kurihara H, et al. Practice of endoscopic sclerotherapy for esophageal varices; its technique and knack. Rinsho Geka 1986; 41: 1403 – 1408.

© 1988 Elsevier Science Publishers B.V. (Biomedical Division)
*Treatment of esophageal varices*
*Y. Idezuki, editor*

Chapter 33

# Angiographic study of hemodynamics in portal hypertension

SHUNJI FUTAGAWA, RYO NAKANISHI, YASUHIKO HISHIMURA AND MITSUO SUGIURA

*IInd Department of Surgery, Juntendo University, Tokyo, Japan*

I would like to discuss mainly the clinical meaning of blood flow of the left gastric vein (LGV) in cases of esophageal varices.

Left gastric arteriography (LGA), celiac arteriography (CA) and superior mesenteric arteriography (SMA) were performed on cirrhotic patients with esophageal varices; these were classified into four groups according to LGV blood flow; i.e., hepatofugal, hepatopetal, bi-lateral and unknown. In the hepatofugal group, the LGV was recognized by CA or SMA and not recognized by LGA.

In the hepatopetal group, the LGV was recognized by LGA and not recognized by the other series.

In the bi-lateral group, the LGV was recognized by all series.

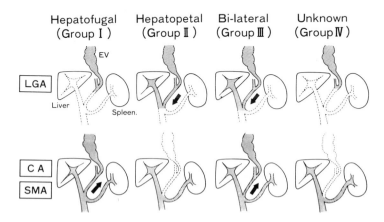

FIG. 1 Blood flow of left gastric vein. LGA, left gastric arteriography; CA, celiac arteriography; SMA, superior mesenteric arteriography.

TABLE 1   Grouping of blood flow of left gastric vein

| Group | Patients | |
|---|---|---|
| | No. | % |
| Hepatofugal (Group I) | 130 | 65 |
| Hepatopetal (Group II) | 18 | 9 |
| Bi-lateral (Group III) | 30 | 15 |
| Unknown (Group IV) | 22 | 11 |
| Total | 200 | 100 |

TABLE 2   Group and liver function (1)

| Group | ICG $R_{15}$ (%) | T-Bil (mg/dl) | Alb (g/dl) |
|---|---|---|---|
| I (Hepatofugal) | 36.8 ± 12.1* ⎤ | 1.4 ± 0.8** ⎤ | 3.6 ± 0.5 |
| II (Hepatopetal) | 25.2 ± 14.7* ⎦ ⎤ | 0.9 ± 0.9** ⎦ | 3.8 ± 0.5 |
| III (Bi-lateral) | 39.8 ± 16.8* ⎦ ⎤ | 1.6 ± 1.2 | 3.7 ± 0.6 |
| IV (Unknown) | 37.1 ± 13.5* ⎦ | 1.5 ± 1.1 | 3.4 ± 0.8 |

$*P < 0.01; **P < 0.05.$

TABLE 3   Group and liver function (2)

| Group | Cholinesterase (IU/l) | PT (%) | | NH$_3$ ($\mu$g/l) |
|---|---|---|---|---|
| I (Hepatofugal) | 540 ± 163 | 60 ± 13* ⎤ | | 124 ± 52** ⎤ |
| II (Hepatopetal) | 610 ± 217 | 75 ± 18* ⎦ | **⎤ | 95 ± 28** ⎦ |
| III (Bi-lateral) | 481 ± 102 | 64 ± 18 | **⎦ | 106 ± 35 |
| IV (Unknown) | 612 ± 189 | 57 ± 13* ⎦ | | 111 ± 41 |

$*P < 0.01; **P < 0.05.$

In the unknown group, the LGV was not recognized by any series (Fig. 1).

Two hundred patients with esophageal varices were studied. Of these, 130 (65%) were in the hepatofugal group, and only 18 (9%) were in the hepatopetal group. Thirty (15%) were bi-lateral and 22 (11%) were in the unknown group (Table 1).

Mean ICG retention rate at 15 min, serum total bilirubin and albumin were studied in all of the four groups.

TABLE 4   Group and clinical findings (1)

| Group | Mean age (years) | Sex: $n$ | Child's group ($n$) |
|---|---|---|---|
| I (Hepatofugal) | 54 ± 9.4* | M:74<br>F: 46 | A (39)<br>B (60*)<br>C (31) |
| II (Hepatopetal) | 48 ± 7.5* | M:13<br>F: 5 | A (14)<br>B (3*)<br>C (1) |
| III (Bi-lateral) | 51 ± 8.6 | M:22<br>F: 8 | A (10)<br>B (10)<br>C (10) |
| IV (Unknown) | 50 ± 10 | M:17<br>F: 5 | A (3)<br>B (10)<br>C (9) |

*$P < 0.05$.

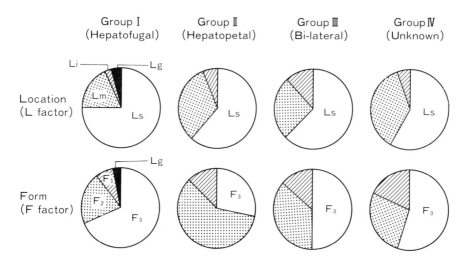

FIG. 2   Group and endoscopic findings of varices.

358

Liver function in the hepatopetal group was well preserved compared with other groups (Table 2).

Other laboratory data were also studied, showing the same tendency: that liver function in the hepatopetal group was well maintained compared with other groups (Table 3).

*Clinical findings*

Fourteen cases (78%) of 18 cases in the hepatopetal group were classified as Child's A. But in the 130 cases of the hepatofugal group, only 39 (30%) were Child's A and

TABLE 5   Group and CA, SMA, LGA

| Group | Dia. of portal vein | Dia. of splenic vein | Dia. of I. gastric vein |
|---|---|---|---|
| I (Hepatofugal) | 14.8 ± 2.5*⌉ | 11.7 ± 2.9 | 7.8 ± 2.2**⌉ |
| II (Hepatopetal) | 16.2 ± 2.3*⌋ | 10.7 ± 2.1 | 5.1 ± 0.7** |
| III (Bi-lateral) | 15.6 ± 1.8 | 10.5 ± 2.6 | 6.0 ± 1.3**⌋ |
| IV (Unknown) | 15.9 ± 2.0 | 11.8 ± 3.1 | 5.5 ± 0.8 |

*$P < 0.05$; **$P < 0.01$.

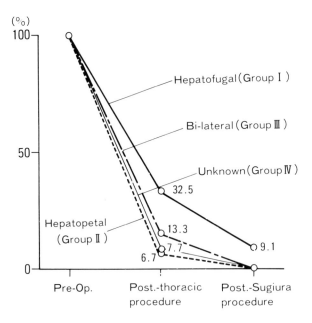

FIG. 3   Residual rate of varices after the Sugiura procedure.

91 (70%) were Child's B or C. There was a significant difference between these two groups (Table 4).

*Endoscopic findings*
The hepatofugal group showed severe endoscopic findings compared with the hepatopetal group, i.e., the varices of the hepatofugal group were more often recognized from the upper part of the esophagus and were larger than those of the hepatopetal group (Fig. 2).

*Mean diameters*
The left gastric vein of the hepatofugal group was larger than that of the hepatopetal group (Table 5). Table 5 shows the residual rate of the esophageal varices after two-staged Sugiura procedure in four groups.

After the transthoracic procedure, varices did not completely disappear in all groups. But when the Sugiura procedure was completed by a transabdominal procedure, the varices disappeared completely in three groups, but not in the hepatofugal group (Fig. 3).

To prevent recurrent or residual varices, it is important to perform complete devascularization right up to the inferior pulmonary vein. During this procedure, we often observed the proper esophageal artery; it is important to identify and cut these arteries.

**Summary**

1. The blood flow of the left gastric vein was shown to be hepatofugal in 65% of the cases with esophageal varices.
2. The hepatofugal group showed poor liver function compared with the hepatopetal group.
3. The hepatofugal group showed severe endoscopic findings of varices compared with the hepatopetal group.
4. Residual varices after the Sugiura procedure were seen only in the hepatofugal group.

© 1988 Elsevier Science Publishers B.V. (Biomedical Division)
*Treatment of esophageal varices*
*Y. Idezuki, editor*

Chapter 34

# Study on portal hypertension in Japan: activities of the Japanese Research Society for Portal Hypertension during a period of 20 years

Kiyoshi Inokuchi

*Saga Prefectural Hospital Koseikan, Saga, Japan*

During the War, our teacher Professors in Japan could not help closing their eyes to the brilliant advances in the study of portal hypertension, when Whipple and his associates established a historic concept of 'portal hypertension' around 1940. After the War we were apparently behind the progress of medical science. There were three or four major institution families in Japan which were devotedly engaged in the study of portal hypertension: Dr. H. Imanaga of Ngoya University, teacher Professor of Prof. Yamamoto; Dr. S. Kimoto of University of Tokyo, teacher Professor of Prof. Sugiura; and Dr. M. Tomoda of Kyushu University, my own teacher. They accumulated a certain number of experiences with portal hypertension in about 1955 (Table 1).

To our regret, however, we were disappointed with the clinical results, showing a high rate of Eck's syndrome [1]. We also realized that the survival of patients with portacaval shunt has not been significantly different from that of those without shunt. This was because the preventive effect of bleeding from esophageal varices rendered by the shunt was cancelled by the enhancement of hepatic deterioration due to decreased hepatic perfusion after the shunt.

Such a situation prompted us to search for a better method of operation for controlling esophageal variceal bleeding. In 1967, the experts organized the Japanese Research Society for Portal Hypertension. Twelve institutions were gathered at the 1st Meeting. Unanimous agreement was reached to search for a pertinent method of operation, in which portal pressure is not lowered after surgery. 'Portal non-decompression surgery' was a testimony to surgical therapy for controlling esophageal variceal bleeding.

The major works this Society collaborated in were:
(1) Devices of portal non-decompression procedures;
(2) Determination of the general rules for recording the endoscopic findings of esophageal varices;

(3) Appraisal of prophylactic operations for esophageal varices;

(4) Approach to new trends of multidisciplinary treatment of esophageal bleeding.

## (1) Devices of portal non-decompression procedures

At the same time that Prof. Warren and associates [2] reported their ingenious approach to selective shunting through the trans-splenic route, i.e. distal splenorenal shunt, in 1967, I myself [3] reported an alternative selective shunting through a left gastric vein in 1968. Most Japanese surgeons dealt with non-shunting direct interruption procedures. Prof. Sugiura and others [4] developed the transthoracic-abdominal approach for esophageal transection with adequate devascularization in

TABLE 1   Clinical results of portacaval shunt in Japan around 1960

|  | Operative mortality (%) | Late survival (%) | | Eck's syndrome (%) |
|---|---|---|---|---|
|  |  | 5 yr | 4 yr |  |
| Kimoto |  |  |  |  |
| End-to-side | 29.5 | 37.5 | 25.0 | 45.4 |
| Side-to-side | 11.8 | 47.4 | 26.3 | 41.0 |
| Imanaga |  |  |  |  |
| Cirrhosis | 28.0 |  | 13.3 | 77.8 |
| Non-cirrhosis | 21.5 |  | 48.1 | 72.6 |

TABLE 2   Results of portal non-decompression vs. portal decompression surgery (3588 collected cases; 1982)

|  | Cases | Operative mortality (%) | Survivors (%) | Variceal bleeding (%) | Eck's syndrome (%) |
|---|---|---|---|---|---|
| Non-decompression |  |  |  |  |  |
| Direct interruption | 3136 | 8.8 | 69.7 | 6.8 | 4.8 |
| Selective shunt | 452 | 5.1 | 61.1 | 7.5 | 4.2 |
| Total | 3588 | 8.3 | 68.6 | 6.9 | 4.8 |
| Decompression* |  |  |  |  |  |
| Portacaval shunt | 312 | 20.8 | 57.4 | 8.0 | 48.5 |
| Splenorenal shunt | 166 | 13.2 | 66.7 | 16.8 | 13.2 |
| Total | 476 | 18.2 | 60.7 | 11.1 | 36.4 |

* Mostly before 1970.

1967, which is well-known as Sugiura's procedure. Prof. Yamamoto [5] also proposed proximal gastric resection in 1967. The late 1960s was really the time of the efflorescence of portal non-decompression procedures. Details of clinical results of individual procedures will be omitted from my talk, since they are already mentioned in this meeting.

In 1982, a national survey was carried out in 3588 patients with portal hypertension who underwent non-decompression surgery, and this was published in 1985 [6]. Operative mortality overall was 8.3%, variceal bleeding 6.9% and Eck's syndrome 4.8%. Long-term survival was seen in 68.6%. These figures were found far superior to those obtained with decompression surgery before 1970 (Table 2).

Regarding the cumulative bleeding rate postoperatively in the long term, an interesting trend was found (Fig. 1). In cases of selective shunt, the cumulative bleeding rate became less after 5 years postoperatively, tending to be about 12% at

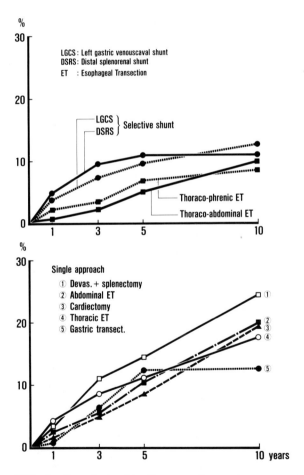

FIG. 1  Cumulative bleeding rate for various operations in non-decompression surgery (Japan, 1982; from Ref. 6).

10 years postoperatively. In cases of direct interruption procedures, the cumulative bleeding rate was generally proportional to the time elapsed postoperatively, and the figures were less in dual approaches, tending to be about 10% at 10 years postoperatively. It may be suggested that more adequate devascularization lessens the rate of postoperative bleeding accordingly.

Regarding the selective shunting, I should like to add some comments. Prof. Warren reported his pioneering work on what is known as the Warren shunt in 1967. At the time I myself was developing my own left gastric venacaval shunt. I was, of course, fascinated and impressed by his work. I myself have later been engaged in studies to prevent the portal malcirculation occasionally occurring after distal splenorenal shunt and came to the conclusion that complete isolation of the splenic vein from the pancreas is mandatory for this type of operation.

I reported this in the Annals of Surgery in 1984 [7]. Later I realized that our view was essentially identical to Prof. Warren's concept of splenopancreatic disconnection, which was reported soon after with relevant evidence [8].

From the evidence of Warren's and our group, I believe that occasional occurrence of portal malcirculation will be prevented by complete splenopancreatic disconnection, and hope that this mode of thinking will be widely understood and that establishment of a true distal splenorenal shunt will become prevalent. I would like to express my deep appreciation to Prof. Warren for his contribution to this field of surgery.

## (2) Determination of the general rules for recording the endoscopic findings of esophageal varices

The ability to accurately predict variceal bleeders prior to acute bleeding episodes would have important therapeutic implications. The Japanese Research Society for Portal Hypertension in 1979 [9] unified the description of endoscopic findings of esophageal varices observed by the naked eye.

Findings consist of four main categories: fundamental color, red color signs on varices, form and location. Using these criteria, Beppu et al. [10] reviewed endoscopic findings observed in our series of patients with esophageal varices and analysed the relationship of the bleeding history to the respective findings retrospectively to determine which findings are most likely to be associated with future bleeding.

It was concluded that red color signs such as red wale marking, cherry red spot or hematocystic spot as well as blue varices in fundamental color category are valuable in predicting bleeding. Other factors such as the form and location were of minor significance in prediction of bleeding. Multivariate analysis makes it possible to quantify the risks of each of these factors.

Some authors described the correlation of the form and size or location, but these are merely the factors which appear to be associated with red color signs, the leading potential factors.

Such a way of predicting the risk of variceal bleeding has been well accepted among the experts, but as far as the blue varices are concerned the problems remained. Small straight varices usually located in the upper esophagus are non-risky and often observed as bluish colored varices. These varices have been included in the blue varices category, thus making the definition of blue varices controversial.

After studying this problem intensely, our Research Society defined specific blue varices really associated with bleeding as large-sized and fully expanded blue varices with a glossy surface like an over-inflated balloon, and proposed a term 'prognostic blue varices (p-Cb)' to discriminate them from general bluish colored varices [11]. It may be supposed that a p-Cb has a thin variceal wall and a high intravariceal pressure. The occurrence of p-Cb accounted for about 25% of all bluish colored varices in our series.

These high-risk bluish varices should thus be specified as p-Cb.

## (3) Appraisal of prophylactic operations for esophageal varices

It is the general opinion in western countries that prophylactic operations for esophageal varices are not warranted. The reasons may be that (1) the varices do not always bleed, and (2) the risks of elective operations are not low. However, the results achieved in our Research Society have changed the situation as mentioned above. The patient at risk of variceal bleeding can be predicted by endoscopic findings. Elective surgery using portal non-decompression procedures can be safely performed with an acceptably low risk. Based on such situations, we carried out a prospective controlled randomized study in 1980 to evaluate prophylactic surgery [12].

Methods of operation included selected shunts and non-shunting interruption procedures. 112 Japanese patients who had risky varices based on endoscopic findings, but no bleeding episode, were allocated to the 'operated group' of 60 patients or the 'non-operated group' of 52 patients. Variceal bleeding, endoscopically confirmed or controlled by Sengstaken-Blakemore tube tamponade, was significantly less frequent in the operated group (6.7%) than in the non-operated group (34.6%). Long-term follow-up of patients showed a total 25% death rate, including 2 operative deaths in the operated group, while there was a 48.1% death rate in the non-operated group, which is a statistically significant difference. Cumulative survival rate at 5 years in the operated group was 71.6%, and was significantly higher than the 37.4% in the non-operated group. It was concluded that prophylactic portal non-decompression surgery satisfactorily prevented variceal bleeding and led to an improvement of the patient's survival (Table 3).

TABLE 3   Prospective randomized controlled study of prophylactic portal non-decompression surgery for esophageal varices (Japanese Research Society for Portal Hypertension, Oct. 1980 – Jan. 1983)

| Groups | Variceal bleeding | Late deaths | 5-yr survival |
|---|---|---|---|
| Operated (n = 62) | 6.7% | 25% | 71.6% |
| Non-operated (n = 52) | 34.6% | 48% | 37.4% |
| $P <$ | 0.001 | 0.01 | 0.05 |

366

## (4) Approach to new trends of multidisciplinary treatment of esophageal bleeding

While such development in the surgical treatment of esophageal varices was steadily achieved during these two decades, endoscopic sclerosing palliative therapy has recently become prevalent. We recall the situation similarly seen in the treatment of gastroduodenal ulcer, in which surgical treatment has mostly been replaced by the medical therapy. However, whatever the advancement of palliative treatment, there will remain a small but significant number of patients incurable with palliative treatment, necessitating standard surgical therapy. I seriously hope that the correct and pertinent knowledge of the surgical treatment for esophageal varices which our colleagues have achieved with great effort should be well understood and utilized for improvement in treatment through a multidisciplinary approach.

## References

1  Inokuchi K. Current status of surgical treatment of portal hypertension in Japan. Jpn J Surg 1972; 2: 171 – 181.
2  Warren WD, Zeppa R, Fomon JJ. Selective trans-splenic decompression of gastroesophageal varices by distal splenorenal shunt, Ann Surg 1967; 166: 437 – 455.
3  Inokuchi K. A selective portacaval shunt. Lancet 1968; 6: 51 – 52.
4  Idezuki Y, Sugiura M, Sakamoto K, Abe H, Miura T, Hatano S, Kimoto S. Rationale for transthoracic esophageal transection for bleeding varices. Dis Chest 1967; 52: 621 – 631.
5  Yamamoto S. Proximal gastrectomy for the treatment of portal hypertension. Geka Shinryo 1967; 9: 1357 – 1358 (in Japanese).
6  Inokuchi K. Jpn Res Soc Portal Hypertension: Present status of surgical treatment of esophageal varices in Japan: A nationwide survey of 3,588 patients. World J Surg 1985; 9: 171 – 180.
7  Inokuchi K, Beppu K, Koyanagi N, Nagamine K, Hashizume M, Sugimachi K. Exclusion of non-isolated splenic vein in distal splenorenal shunt for prevention of portal malcirculation. Ann Surg 1984; 200: 711 – 717.
8  Warren WD, Millikan WJ, Henderson JM, Abu-Elmagd KM, Galloway JR, Shires GT, Richards WO, Salam AA, Kutner MH. Splenopancreatic disconnection – Improved selectivity of distal splenorenal shunt. Ann Surg 1986; 204: 346 – 355.
9  Japanese Research Society for Portal Hypertension. The general rules for recording endoscopic findings on esophageal varices. Jpn J Surg 1980; 10: 84 – 87.
10  Beppu K, Inokuchi K, Koyanagi N, Nakayama S, Sakata H, Kitano S, Kobayashi M. Prediction of variceal hemorrhage by esophageal endoscopy. Gastrointest Endosc 1981; 27: 213 – 218.
11  Koyanagi N and Cooperative study group of portal hypertension in Japan. Prognostic blue varices as a discriminant factor of findings of esophageal varices. Jpn J Surg, 1988; 18: 142 – 145.
12  Inokuchi K and Cooperative study group of portal hypertension in Japan. Prophylactic portal non-decompression surgery in patients with esophageal varices – An interim report. Ann Surg 1984; 200: 61 – 65.

© 1988 Elsevier Science Publishers B.V. (Biomedical Division)
*Treatment of esophageal varices*
*Y. Idezuki, editor*

Chapter 35

# Current status of treatment of esophageal varices in Japan: endoscopic sclerotherapy in Japan

YASUO IDEZUKI

*The Second Department of Surgery, University of Tokyo, Faculty of Medicine, Tokyo, Japan*

The recent development of endoscopic sclerotherapy using the flexible fiberoptic endoscope and new sclerosants is remarkable. During the last several years, the number of operations for esophageal varices in Japan has decreased considerably. This is mainly because endoscopic sclerotherapy has become increasingly popular and many of the patients are now being treated by this method rather than surgery. This trend is continuing and more and more of the patients with esophageal varices are being treated by endoscopists rather than by surgeons.

We established the Japanese Research Society for Sclerotherapy of Esophageal Varices in 1886 (Executive Office: Second Department of Surgery, University of Tokyo, Faculty of Medicine, Hongo, Bunkyo-ku, Tokyo, Japan), and at present 167 surgical and medical institutions are the members of the Society.

As one of the activities of this Society, a nationwide survey on endoscopic sclerotherapy was performed at the end of 1986 in order to summarize the up-to-date status of sclerotherapy in Japan. Questionnaires were sent to 151 institutions and 98 institutions (30 medical and 68 surgical institutions) responded. Results obtained from these 98 institutions are summarized and reported here.

## Chronological number of institutions performing sclerotherapy

Endoscopic sclerotherapy using the flexible fiberscope in Japan started in 1967, and the number of institutions using this method of treatment for esophageal varices has been increasing very rapidly; 98 institutions had started to use this treatment by the end of 1986 (Fig. 1).

### Number of patients treated by endoscopic sclerotherapy

The total number of patients treated by this method is listed in Fig. 2. Seven thousand two hundred and seven patients were treated by sclerotherapy by November 1986. Sclerotherapy was performed in 1870 patients at the time of bleeding to control active bleeding from varices, electively in 2231 patients and prophylactically in 3106.

It is interesting to note that this treatment was performed prophylactically in more than 40% of patients. The effect of slcerotherapy in these patients without previous history of bleeding should be carefully followed and evaluated.

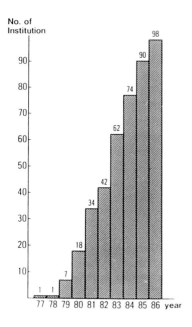

FIG. 1   Development of endoscopic sclerotherapy in Japan.

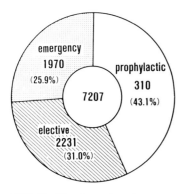

FIG. 2   Number of patients treated by sclerotherapy.

The total number of sclerotherapies in these patients was 18 762, of which 72.4% was for intravariceal injection, 20.8% for paravariceal injection and 6.8% for combination of both (Fig. 3).

## Number of sclerotherapies per patient

The average number of sclerotherapies per patient was 2.8, ranging from a single injection to as many as 18. This therapy usually requires hospitalization of the patient, and the average number of hospital days for a series of sclerotherapy treatment was 32.8 days (6–80 days).

## Sclerosants

Sclerosing agents used for sclerotherapy in Japan are ethanolamine oleate, polydocanol, sodium tetradecylsulfate, sodium morrhuate, ethyl alcohol, 50%

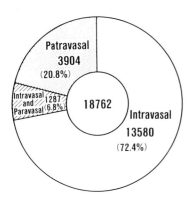

FIG. 3   Number of injection sclerotherapies in patients.

TABLE 1   Sclerosing agents used for sclerotherapy

| Sclerosing agents | No. institutions | Average vol. (range) |
|---|---|---|
| Ethanolamine oleate (EO) | 55 | 20 ml (7–80 ml) |
| Polydocanol (AS) | 25 | 18 ml (6–50 ml) |
| EO + AS | 6 | |
| Sodium tetradecylsulfate | 6 | 11 ml (7–15 ml) |
| Others (ethyl alcohol, thrombin, 50% glucose) | 12 | |
| Sodium morrhuate | 2 | 3 ml (1–5 ml) |
| Total | 106 | |

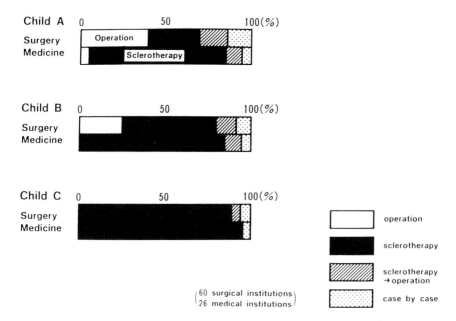

FIG. 4    Strategy for treatment of esophageal varices in emergency cases.

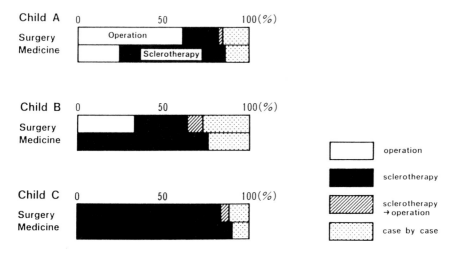

FIG. 5    Strategy for treatment of esophageal varices in elective cases.

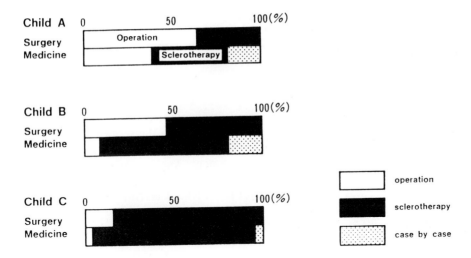

FIG. 6   Strategy for treatment of esophageal varices in prophylactic cases.

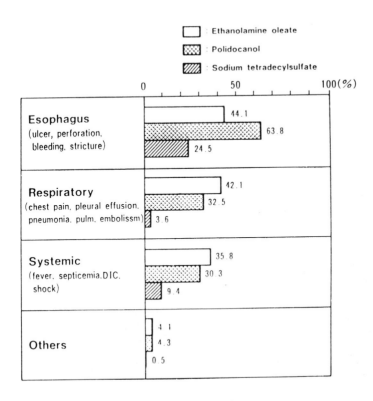

FIG. 7   Sclerosing agents and complications.

glucose, and thrombin. The widely used drugs were ethanolamine oleate and polydocanol (Table 1).

## Indications for sclerotherapy

Since the recent development of sclerotherapy, strategy for treatment of varices has changed considerably. Strategy for treatment of varices in the surgical and medical institutions was surveyed. The method of treatment of varices is usually decided by the severity of the disease and the timing of treatment. Analysis was made according to the Child's classification.

Emergency surgery was the first choice for treatment of bleeding in Child's A patients, in 40% of surgical institutions and 4% of medical institutions, whereas 30% of surgical institutions and 80% of medical institutions selected sclerotherapy. For Child's B patients, 25% of surgical institutions recommended emergency surgery, but 60% preferred sclerotherapy. For Child's C patients, no institutions recommended emergency operation (Fig. 4).

TABLE 2  Mortality and morbidity associated with sclerotherapy

| Complication | No. of cases (%) | No. of fatalities |
|---|---|---|
| Esophagus | | |
| Ulceration | 2972 (34.8) | 8 |
| Bleeding from ulcer | 207 (2.4) | 24 |
| Perforation | 27 (0.5) | 12 |
| Stricture | 108 (1.3) | 2 |
| Bleeding from varices | 34 (0.4) | 5 |
| Bleeding from peptic ulcers | 99 (1.2) | 9 |
| Respiratory | | |
| Pleural effusion | 330 (3.9) | 5 |
| Pulmonary embolism | 31 (0.4) | 7 |
| Pneumonia | 34 (0.4) | 4 |
| Chest pain | 1941 (22.4) | 8 |
| Shock | 145 (1.7) | 9 |
| DIC | 16 (0.2) | 12 |
| Fever | 1760 (20.6) | 8 |
| Septicemia | 15 (0.2) | 2 |
| Portal vein thrombosis | 6 (0.1) | 5 |
| Hepatic failure | 196 (2.3) | 42 |
| Renal failure | 28 (0.4) | 8 |
| Cerebral vascular compl. | 13 (0.2) | 3 |
| Others | 572 (6.7) | 34 |
| Total | 8535 | 207 |

For elective treatment in Child A patients, 52% of surgical institutions and 24% of medical institutions recommended surgical treatment. Approximately 20% of surgical institutions and 60% of medical institutions selected sclerotherapy for Child's A patients. In Child's B patients, 34% of surgical institutions selected surgery, however, 30% of surgical institutions and 76% of medical institutions recommended sclerotherapy. In Child's C patients, almost all institutions recommended sclerotherapy for treatment of varices (Fig. 5).

For prophylactic treatment, of Child's A patients, 64% of surgical institutions and 38% of medical institutions recommended surgery. In Child's B patients, more than half of surgical institutions and 10% of medical institutions selected sclerotherapy as the treatment of choice. In Child's C patients, sclerotherapy was the most common method of treatment in both surgical and medical institutions (Fig. 6). It is no wonder that the number of operative cases is decreasing and that sclerotherapy is rapidly increasing.

**Mortality and morbidity associated with sclerotherapy**

As many as 207 patients died because of complications of some kind associated with sclerotherapy. Complications were observed in many patients and a vast variety of complications have been reported. Ulcerations of the esophagus and bleeding from ulcers, perforations of the esophagus, chest pain, pleural effusion, fever and dyspnea were not uncommon, although most of these complications were transient.

TABLE 3   Problems in endoscopic sclerotherapy

**Sclerosants**
   Toxicity, mechanism, absorption
   volume, production, distribution

**Intravasal? Paravasal?**
   How far should be thrombosed?
   Should afferent vessels be thrombosed?
   Is arterial embolisation necessary?

**Morbidity and mortality** associated
   with sclerotherapy

**Effects on gastric circulation**

**Long-term results?**
   Recurrent bleeding
   Survival rate

**Rehabilitation of patients**

**Indication of sclerotherapy**

Obstruction of esophagus, bleeding from peptic ulcers, shock, hepatic failure and renal failure have been reported sporadically (Table 2).

Most of these complications were due to the toxicity of sclerosants and to the inadequate techniques. Complications were more frequently seen when ethanolamine oleate or polydocanol was used. When tetradecylsulfate was used as sclerosant, occurrence of complications was less frequent compared to the other sclerosants (Fig. 7; Table 3).

Almost ten years have elapsed since the revival of this therapy in Japan, and remarkable developments have been made, yet many of the problems remain unsolved. Further critical analysis and careful evaluation of the long-term results of endoscopic sclerotherapy is necessary and important to decide the ultimate fate of endoscopic sclerotherapy in the treatment of esophageal varices.

# Summary of general discussion on the treatment of esophageal varices

**Chairpersons:** W.D. WARREN AND YASUO IDEZUKI

## 1. Treatment of portal hypertensive gastropathy

**W.D. Warren:** Shunt operations will control gastric bleeding whether they are selective-type shunts or total portacaval shunts.

**K. Inokuchi:** One third of the cases treated by shunt operations were bleeding from the stomach. I think selective shunt is not always effective for portal hypertensive gastropathy.

**R.A.J. Spence:** I know one report that $\beta$-blocker has been effective in portal hypertensive gastropathy.

**M. Sugiura:** We have used $\beta$-blocker for 30 patients and obtained improvement in endoscopic findings of portal hypertensive gastropathy.

**K. Tanikawa:** We have used $\beta$-blocker for 400 patients and only one died of bleeding from portal hypertensive gastropathy.

**F.E. Eckhauser:** From several reports, shunt procedure seems to be more effective than non-shunting procedure in portal hypertensive gastropathy.

## 2. Strategy for control of active bleeding from ruptured varices

**K.G. Swan:** At first, we use vasopressin and balloon tamponade and then carry out sclerotherapy. And if bleeding continues, we perform mesocaval shunt. We think Child C patients are not contraindicative in emergency.

**K. Tanikawa:** Hemostasis is obtained in almost 100% of cases by sclerotherapy. So we don't recommend emergency operations.

**Y. Takase:** After hemostasis by balloon tamponade and vasopressin, we carry out sclerotherapy.

**E.P. DiMagno:** We obtain hemostasis by sclerotherapy using overtube while bleeding.

**W.D. Warren:** The final therapy is operation when hemostasis cannot be obtained by any other conservative therapy. And a surgeon must do it.

**K.-J. Paquet:** We carry out sclerotherapy while bleeding. When hemostasis is not obtained (about 10%), we use Linton's tube. From direct measurement of esophageal variceal pressure, we found that vasopressin was not effective for decreasing portal pressure and so we don't use vasopressin.

**R.A.J. Spence:** At first, we try to obtain hemostasis by vasopressin and balloon tamponade and then carry out sclerotherapy. When these methods are ineffective, we do a non-shunting operation.

**Huang Yan-Ting:** We obtain hemostasis by vasopressin, balloon tamponade and sclerotherapy and then carry out operation for good liver function patients within 2 weeks.

**K. Inokuchi:** At first, we carry out balloon tamponade and then sclerotherapy.

**M. Sugiura:** After hemostasis by balloon tamponade, we perform non-shunting operation for Child A and B patient. Even among Child C patients there are some in whom operation is possible.

**S. Yamamoto:** In emergency, patients without previous history of bleeding are often difficult to estimate for liver function. So we obtain hemostasis conservatively and then carry out operation electively.

### 3. Problems in shunt operations

**W.D. Warren:** Splenopancreatic disconnection contributes to the maintenance of hepatic perfusion and selectivity of the Warren shunt.

**K. Inokuchi:** Splenopancreatic disconnection seems to be essential to maintain selectivity of the Warren shunt.

**H. Ashida:** Distal splenorenal shunt after sclerotherapy was performed in 17 patients and an excellent result was obtained.

### 4. Problems in non-shunting operations

**Y. Idezuki:** The results of non-shunting operations in Japan are much better than those in European countries and the United States. It has been suggested that this difference in results is mainly due to the difference in liver disease, i.e. alcoholic or non-alcoholic cirrhosis.

**M. Sugiura:** About 40% of our recent operative cases were esophageal varices caused by alcoholic liver cirrhosis, and prognosis of these patients has not been different from that of postnecrotic liver cirrhosis.

**S. Yamamoto:** Liver function in alcoholic liver cirrhosis in Europe and the United States is comparable to that in non-alcoholic cirrhosis in Japan. But operations in alcoholic cirrhosis, either shunt procedures or non-shunting procedures, are more difficult because of its hepatomegaly.

**K. Inokuchi:** From my experience, the prognosis of alcoholic liver cirrhosis has not differed from that of postnecrotic liver cirrhosis when the operation is performed properly.

**R.A.J. Spence:** When Sugiura's procedure was performed in Europe and in the United States, its mortality would be three or four times higher than that in Japan. So alcoholic liver cirrhosis in Europe and the United States seems to be different from that in Japan.

**W.D. Warren:** Technical superiority (?) of Japanese non-shunting operations would be a factor in good prognosis.

## 5. Problems in sclerotherapy

**Y. Idezuki:** Results of sclerotherapy are different among the institutions. What is this difference due to?

**K. Tanikawa:** We have carried out sclerotherapy in 400 cases and the results have been excellent. I think the reason for not-so-good results in Europe and the United States is mainly due to the fact that many patients continue to drink after sclerotherapy. Also, it is important in sclerotherapy to eradicate esophageal varices completely.

**E.P. DiMagno:** With many changeable factors, it is difficult to estimate the results of sclerotherapy accurately. Prospective controlled trials are needed.

**K.-J. Paquet:** The reason for excellent results in Japan seems to be due to pre-selection of patients and not using any other therapy. Sclerosants are poisonous essentially and many complications have been reported. Prospective trials are necessary.

**W.D. Warren:** Quality control of operation or any other treatment is important in controlled trials.

## 6. Rationale of prophylactic treatment

**Y. Idezuki:** One-third of the Japanese cases have been treated prophylactically. On the other hand, most of the doctors in Europe and the United States are reluctant to use prophylactic treatment. Why so much difference?

**K.-J. Paquet:** The pressure over 30 mmHg in direct measurement of esophageal varices is found only in few patients with huge varices. Prophylactic treatment is necessary for these patients but not for many others.

**K. Inokuchi:** It has been clearly shown from our controlled study that prophylactic treatment is effective. The difference between this study and other studies in the past seems to be mainly due to technical improvement of operation.

**R.A.J. Spence:** Considering the results of operations in Europe and the United States, it is difficult to recommend prophylactic operations.

**W.D. Warren:** Even in a controlled study, bleeding patients should be treated in some way. Strict controlled trial is difficult in this situation.

**E.P. DiMagno:** We don't carry out sclerotherapy or operation prophylactically.

**K.G. Swan:** There are many medical lawsuits in the United States. They are also obstacles to prophylactic treatment.

**K.-J. Paquet:** Judgement of the risk of bleeding from the varices is important. The diagnosis criteria for this in Japan are too complicated.

**S. Yamamoto:** Even if varices bleed after prophylactic sclerotherapy, we can repeat sclerotherapy again.

**Y. Takase:** We think that rebleeding after sclerotherapy is failure. The evaluation of success or failure is controversial among doctors who do sclerotherapy.

## 7. Strategy for rebleeding after sclerotherapy

**Y. Takase:** If we cannot stop bleeding from varices after three or four episodes of sclerotherapy, we do a non-shunting operation.

**K. Tanikawa:** We repeat sclerotherapy again. It is an advantage that we can always repeat it again.

**S. Yamamoto:** We can control rebleeding easily by repeating sclerotherapy.

**M. Sugiura:** We prefer operative devascularization.

**Huang Yan-Ting:** If the patient's condition is suitable to undergo operations, we try to do some operations.

**E.P. DiMagno:** We carry out sclerotherapy at first. If it fails, we do shunt operations.

**K.G. Swan:** If bleeding occurs after sclerotherapy, we would repeat sclerotherapy again. But I think an alternative shunt is one solution too.

**W.D. Warren:** If rebleeding occurs because of shunt thrombosis, we would struggle with sclerotherapy. If that failed, we then do the devascularization procedure including taking out the spleen or, if the patient has massive ascites, we do H-graft interposition.

**R.A.J. Spence:** Most of our patients get additional acute sclerotherapy. And if we failed (probably less than 10% of cases) after two or three episodes of sclerotherapy, we then consider going on to an emergency operation (transection and devascularization procedure).

**K.-J. Paquet:** When sclerotherapy fails, patients are treated in urgent or emergency situations by devascularization procedure, sometimes combined with Nissen's fundplication.

**F.E. Eckhauser:** If a patient experiences an early or late rebleeding, I can't emphasize strongly enough the importance of interventional radiography. It provides us with valuable information about persistent large collaterals, thrombosis of shunt and therefore choice of treatment.

(The editor of the volume is responsible for any inaccuracies or errors in this summary.)

# Closing remarks

YASUO IDEZUKI

We are now closing the two-day symposium on the treatment of esophageal varices. As an organizer of this symposium, I would like to take this opportunity to thank all of the participants for your beautiful presentation and active participation in the discussion. I believe that this has been a very productive symposium, and will become an important step for the future development of treatment of varices. Although it seems that controversy over many issues still continues, many aspects have been clarified through the discussion and which were very helpful for the mutual understanding among the participants.

I would like to thank again especially the guests from abroad who came a very long way to participate in the symposium and gave us the up-to-date data and information which could not have been obtained from reading the literature.

I have been deeply impressed and am very much grateful to Dr. W. Dean Warren because I have been aware that he had been ill and did not feel well during the symposium, he had to retire from all of the social events; however, he did attend the whole session through the symposium and gave us so much important information and suggestions. I found in him the good conscience of the American surgeons and the real frontier or pioneering spirit of the United States of America. Because of that I respect him and salute him.

I should like to thank the members of the committees of this symposium and the staff of our department of surgery for helping me in every step of the planning and through the symposium. I would also like to express my sincere gratitude to the sponsors who gave us generous financial support which made this international symposium possible. I am also grateful to the staff of the Jeff Corporation, who helped us in preparing the symposium.

I hope we will be able to get together again in the near future. Thank you very much again and *SAYONARA* for now.

# Author index

Aoki, H., 315
Arakawa, M., 111

DiMagno, E.P., 23

Eckhauser, F.E., 239

Flanagan, J.J., 257, 303
Fukasawa, M., 149
Futagawa, S., 149, 355

Hagiwara, M., 347
Hashizume, M., 85
Hasumi, A., 315
Henderson, J.M., 205
Hishimura, Y., 355

Idezuki, Y., 175, 339, 367
Inokuchi, K., 277, 361
Ishikawa, T., 167
Isomatsu, T., 287

Kage, M., 111
Kasukawa, R., 75
Katoh, H., 299
Katsuki, T., 329
Kinoshita, E., 149
Kitano, S., 85
Kobayashi, M., 277
Kobayashi, S., 161
Kobayashi, Y., 95
Kohyama, M., 45
Kokudo, N., 175
Koyama, H., 175
Koyama, K., 187
Kumagai, Y., 105

Maguchi, H., 53
Makuuchi, H., 105
Masaki, M., 75
Masuda, K., 45
Miho, O., 45
Millikan, Jr, W.J., 205
Mitsuhashi, H., 75
Mizuno, M., 53
Muto, T., 195

Nakanishi, R., 149, 355
Namiki, M., 53
Nishimura, Y., 149

Obara, K., 75
Ohmasa, R., 45
Oka, H., 339
Okamoto, E., 37
Okano, S., 53
Ono, J., 329
Ouchi, K., 187

Paquet, K.-J., 1, 271

Rocko, J.M., 257
Rosa, D.M., 303

Sakai, M., 347
Sakamoto, H., 175
Sanjo, K., 175, 339
Sate, T., 187
Sato, Y., 347
Sekiya, C., 53
Shibuya, S., 95
Shimazu, M., 315
Spence, R.A.J., 123

Sugimachi, K., 85, 277
Sugiura, M., 149, 355
Suzuki, H., 45
Suzuki, T., 53
Swan, K.G., 257, 303

Takasaki, K., 161
Takase, Y., 95
Tanabe, T., 299
Tanikawa, K., 67
Tominaga, Y., 53
Toyonaga, A., 67
Tsukada, K., 195
Turcotte, J.G., 239

Uehara, A., 53
Umeyama, K., 167

Warren, W.D., 205
Watanabe, H., 347
Watanabe, Y., 45

Yamaga, H., 85
Yamamoto, S., 141
Yamashita, T., 167
Yan-Ting Huang, 247
Yazaki, Y., 53
Yoshida, K., 195
Yoshikawa, K., 167

Zuidema, G.D., 239

# Subject index

**Prepared by H. Kettner, M.D.,**
**Middelburg, The Netherlands**

Aethoxysklerol
  *see* polidocanol
Alcoholism
  Rebleeding, liver cirrhosis, 257
  survival, sclero- vs.
    non-sclerotherapy, 29
Angiography
  esophageal varices, 322
Arginine
  hepatic encephalopathy, 339
Autosuture proximal gastrectomy, 141

Bleeding recurrence
  elective sclerotherapy, 14, 100
  esophagus transection, 129
  non-shunting surgery vs.
    sclerotherapy, 199
  prophylactic sclerotherapy, 61
Sengstaken tube vs. paravariceal
    sclerotherapy, 11
Blood flow pattern
  esophagus varices, 124
  portal hypertension, 119
Boerema button
  esophagus stricture, 125
Bradycardia
  vasopressin i.v., 310
Branched-chain amino acids
  hepatic encephalopathy, 339

Cardia varices
  sclerotherapy indications, 105
Cardiac output
  vasopressin, 309

Chest pain
  sclerotherapy complication, 80
Child classification, 24
  emergy sclerotherapy results, 58
  post-decompression prognosis, 239
  varices sclerotherapy, 3
China
  portal hypertension epidemiology,
    247
Cine-angiography
  left gastric vein hemodynamics, 318
Combined injection technique
  polidocanol 1%, 45
Complications
  endoscopic sclerotherapy, 56, 80, 99
Coronary blood flow
  vasopressin, 309
Coronary venous caval shunt
  portal hypertension, China, 248

Death cause
  Elective sclerotherapy follow-up, 100
Distal splenorenal shunt, 205, 271, 287
  China, portal hypertension, 248
  hemodynamics, 212, 229, 280
  hepatic encephalopathy, 219
  hypersplenism, 288
  indications, 290
  vs. left gastric vena caval shunt, 277
  liver function, 231
  vs. mesocaval shunt, 260
  portal flow, 218
  portal vein thrombosis, 225
  prognosis, 273

vs. sclerotherapy, 91, 222
splenopancreatic disconnection, 282
superselective, long-term results, 299
technique, 207, 272
vs. total shunts, 219
Drapana's shunt
*see* mesocaval shunt
Dysphagia
post-esophagus transection, 129

Eck fistula
*see* portocaval shunt
Elective sclerotherapy, 14, 55, 95
death cause, follow-up, 100
vs. emergency, 12
ethanolamine oleate, 95
indications, 1
long-term results, 37, 39, 58, 72, 98
vs. non-shunting surgery, 199
Emergency sclerotherapy, 11, 55, 69
combined injections, polidocanol
1%, 47
flexible vs. rigid endoscope, 9
histopathology, 111
indications, 1
long-term results, 37, 38, 58
vs. non-sclerotherapy, 27
vs. non-shunting surgery, 198
results, 57, 91
series results, 7
Endoscopic sclerotherapy
see sclerotherapy
Endoscopy
findings recording, 364
Idezuki's tube, 347
surgery assistance, 141, 145
Endothelium damage
*see* vein damage
Epidemiology
sclerotherapy, Japan, 367
Esophagoscopy
*see* endoscopy
Esophagus mucosa removal
varices recurrence prevention, 88
Esophagus perforation

sclerotherapy complication, 56, 80
Esophagus stricture
Boerema button, 125
post-esophagus transection, 129
sclerosants comparison, 90
sclerotherapy complication, 56, 80,
99
Esophagus transection, 123, 161, 167,
175, 187
complications, 129
efficacy, 169
follow-up, 161
immediate residual varices, 157
indications, 127, 151, 161
results, 127, 153
vs. sclerotherapy, 42, 91
technique, 125, 176
Esophagus ulcer
sclerosants comparison, 90
sclerotherapy induced, 39, 46, 56, 80,
99
Esophagus varices
anatomy, 1
blood flow source, 322
etiology, 24
obliteration time, survival, 30
Esophagus wall
histology after sclerotherapy, 114
Estrogen
gastric wall circulation, cirrhotic rat,
325
Ethanolamine oleate
elective sclerotherapy, 95
esophagus wall histopathology, 111
indications, 77
injection volume, 86, 90
other sclerosants comparison, 90
sclerotherapy, 26, 67
vein damage, dog, 76, 82
Ethanolamine oleate + polidocanol
long-term results, 75

Fever
sclerotherapy complication, 80
Flexible endoscope

emergency sclerotherapy, 9

Gastric varices
    classification, 108
    ethanolamine oleate, 77
    sclerotherapy, 107
Gastric wall
    histology after sclerotherapy, 114
    microcirculation, 325
Gastric wall blood flow, 321
Gastrointestinal bleeding
    esophageal varices, bleeding source,
        1
Glypressin
    esophagus varices bleeding, 313


Hassab operation, 152, 177
Hemodynamics
    angiographic evaluation, 355
    distal splenorenal shunt, 212, 229,
        290
    esophago-gastric varices, 315
    left gastric vena caval shunt, 278
    mesocaval shunt, 265
    superselective distal splenorenal
        shunt, 301
Hemorrhagic gastritis
    histopathology, after sclerotherapy,
        114
    sclerotherapy complication, 80
Hepatic artery flow
    vasopressin, 307
Hepatic coma
    sclerotherapy complication, 80
Hepatic encephalopathy
    branched-chain amino acids +
        arginine, 39
    distal splenorenal shunt, 273
    distal splenorenal vs. total shunt, 219
    elective portacaval shunt, 1
    porto-azygos disconnection surgery,
        249
    post-esophagus transection, 129
    shunt surgery contra-indication, 258
    shunt type, 250, 254, 259

superselective distal splenorenal
    shunt, 300
Hepatic reserve
    see also child classification
    distal splenorenal shunt, prognosis,
        295
    endoscopic sclerotherapy, survival,
        23, 48
    patient selection, portal
        decompression, 241
    post-decompression prognosis, 239
    survival, sclero- vs.
        non-sclerotherapy, 27
Hepatoma
    non-shunting surgery, 153
Histopathology
    see pathohistology
History
    distal splenorenal shunt, 205
Hypersplenism
    distal splenorenal shunt, 288
Hypotension
    sclerotherapy complication, 99

Idezuki tube
    emergency bleeding control, 347
Immediate endoscopic injection
        sclerotherapy
    see emergency sclerotherapy
Injection sclerotherapy
    see sclerotherapy
Intestinal necrosis
    sclerotherapy complication, 80
Intravarix thrombus
    histopathology after sclerotherapy,
        116

Japan
    portal hypertension, 361
    sclerotherapy, 367

Leakage
    esophagus transection, 129
Left gastric artery flow
    gastric venous hypertension, 320

Left gastric vein
  cine-angiography, 318
  hemodynamics, varices, 315, 355
Left gastric vena caval shunt, 277
Leukopenia
  hypersplenism, distal splenorenal
    shunt, 288
Life expectancy
  elective sclerotherapy, 14
Linton shunt
  see proximal splenorenal shunt
Linton-Nachlas tube
  bleeding varices, 12
Liver cancer
  see hepatoma
Liver cirrhosis
  bleeding source, gastro-intestinal
    bleeding, 1
  elective sclerotherapy, life
    expectancy, 14
  natural history, esophageal bleeding,
    14, 239
Liver disease severity
  see hepatic reserve
Liver function
  branched-chain amino acid diet +
    arginine, 343
  distal splenorenal shunt, 231
  distal splenorenal shunt vs.
    sclerotherapy, 223
  hemodynamics, portal hypertension,
    358
  surgical mortality, 250

Mental status
  branched-chain amino acids +
    arginine, 342
Mesenteric artery flow
  vasopressin, 303
Mesocaval shunt, 257
  China, portal hypertension, 248
  vs. distal splenorenal shunt, 219, 260
  emergency vs. elective, mortality, 265
  encephalopathy, 253
  technique, 262

Mesorenal shunt
  vs. distal splenorenal shunt, 219
Mortality
  see also life expectancy and survival
  absominal esophagus transection,
    162
  distal splenorenal shunt, 273
  elective sclerotherapy, 14, 100
  emergency portocaval shunt, 258
  emergency sclerotherapy, 9
  esophagus transection, 178, 188
  porto-azygos disconnection surgery,
    249
  prophylactic sclerotherapy, 16
  sclerotherapy, Japan, 373
  shunt type, 250, 259
  surgery timing, 243
  transabdominal esophagus
    transection, 168
  varices bleeding, natural history, 14,
    240

Natural history
  esophageal bleeding, liver cirrhosis,
    14, 240
Nephrotoxicity
  sclerotherapy complication, 80, 99
Non-alcoholic varices
  survival, sclero- vs.
    non-sclerotherapy, 29
Non-shunting surgery, 141, 149, 167,
    175, 187, 195
  indications, 150, 175, 187
  results, 156
  + sclerotherapy, 154
  vs. sclerotherapy, 195
Number-connecting test
  branched-chain amino acids,
    encephalopathy, 342

Overtubes
  field of vision, 86

Paravariceal sclerotherapy
  schedule, 6

vs. Sengstaken tube, emergency, 9
Pathohistology
  esophagus wall, 111
  ethanolamine oleate, vein damage,
    dog, 76, 81
  polidocanol, vein damage, dog, 76,
    81
Patient selection
  distal splenorenal shunt, 271
  portal decompression results, 241
Pitpressin
  *see* vasopressin
Plasma amino acids
  branched-chain amino acid diet +
    arginine, 343
Plasma ammonia
  branched-chain amino acid diet +
    arginine, 343
Pleura effusion
  sclerotherapy complication, 56, 80
Polidocanol 1%
  cardia varices, 105
  indications, 77
  other sclerosants comparison, 90
  sclerotherapy, 45
  vein damage, dog, 76, 82
Portal azygos disconnection surgery,
    141, 248
  China, epidemiology, 248
  indications, 142
  portal pressure rise, 255
Portal flow
  distal splenorenal shunt, 218, 230
Portal hypertension
  blood flow pattern, 119
  China, epidemiology, 247
  hemodynamics, angiography, 355
  Japan, research society, 361
  natural history, 239
  portosystemic shunt, evaluation, 252
  propranolol, 123
  vasopressin, administration route,
    306
Portal pressure
  pre- vs. post-sclerotherapy, 69

varices bleeding, 240
  vasopressin, 310, 329
Portal-systemic encephalopathy
  *see* hepatic encephalopathy
Portal vein thrombosis
  distal splenorenal shunt, 225
  sclerotherapy complication, 80
Portocaval shunt
  vs. distal splenorenal shunt, 206
  emergency, mortality, 1
  emergency procedure, 258
  encephalopathy, 253
Portography
  sclerotherapy-resistant varices, 70
Portosystemic shunt
  China, epidemiology, 248
  contra-indications, 258
  Japan, epidemiology, 363
  mortality, 252
  shunt type, encephalopathy, 251
Preventive surgery
  esophagus varices, 365
Prophylactic sclerotherapy, 16, 55
  bleeding prevention, 63
  complications, 72
  indications, 1
  long-term results, 37, 39, 59, 91
Propranolol
  portal hypertension, 123
Proximal gastric transection, 141
Proximal splenorenal shunt, 258
Pulmonary edema
  vasopressin complication, 332
Pulmonary embolism
  sclerotherapy complication, 80

Recurrent bleeding
  *see* bleeding recurrence
Red color sign
  abdominal esophagus transection,
    172
Renal blood flow
  vasopressin, 311
Renal damage
  *see* nephrotoxicity

Residual varices
    esophagus transection (Sugiura), 157
Revarication
    see varices recurrence
Rigid endoscope
    emergency sclerotherapy, 9

SBI
    see Sengstaken-Blakemore tube
Sclerosants
    comparison, 90
    mechanism, 3
Sclerotherapy
    cardia varices, indications, 105
    complications 56, 72, 80, 258, 373
    vs. distal splenorenal shunt, 222
    elective, see elective sclerotherapy
    vs. esophagus transection, 42
    histopathology, 112
    immediate, see emergency
        sclerotherapy
    indications, 3, 85, 372
    Japan, 367
    long-term results, 37
    + non-shunting surgery, 154
    vs. non-shunting surgery, 195
    polidocanol 1%, 45
    portal pressure decrease/increase, 69
    postoperative rebleeding, 164
    prophylactic, see prophylactic
        sclerotherapy
    + splenopneumopexy + splenic
        artery embolization, 334
    techniques, 3, 85, 96
    transparent over-tube, 87
Sclerotherapy results
    hepatic reserve, 23
    varices cause, 23
Sengstaken-Blakemore tube
    vs. endoscopic sclerotherapy, 9
    vs. vasopressin, 331
Serum
    see plasma
Shock
    sclerotherapy complication, 80

Shunt patency
    distal splenorenal shunt, 211
    mesocaval shunt, 266
Side-effects
    vasopressin, 303
Sodium tetradecyl sulfate
    other sclerosants comparison, 90
Splanchnic blood flow
    vasopressin, 311, 330
Splanchnic circulation
    vasopressin, administration route,
        303
Splenectomy
    Schistosomal portal hypertension,
        247
Splenectomy + coronary vein
    embolization, 254
Splenocaval shunt
    China, portal hypertension, 248
    indications, 212
Splenopancreatic disconnection
    distal splenorenal shunt, 282
Splenopneumopexy, 259
    + sclerotherapy + splenic artery
        embolization, 334
Splenorenal shunt
    China, portal hypertension, 248
    distal, see distal splenorenal shunt
    encephalopathy, 253
Stapler gun
    transabdominal esophagus
        transection, 161
Sugiura procedure
    see esophagus transection
Superior mesenteric artery
    hemodynamics, portal hypertension,
        355
    intra-arterial vasopressin, 303
Superior mesenteric artery flow
    vasopressin, administration route,
        303
Surgery
    blood loss, vasopressin, 312
    endoscopic assistance, 141, 145
    non-shunting, see non-shunting

surgery
  timing after bleeding, 243
Survival
  abdominal esophagus transection,
    170
  bleeding etiology, 29
  combined injection sclerotherapy,
    polidocanol 1%, 48
  distal splenorenal shunt, 215, 290
  distal splenorenal shunt vs.
    sclerotherapy, 222
  elective sclerotherapy, 58, 72, 98
  emergency sclerotherapy, 58
  esophagus transection, 127, 131, 133,
    182, 190
  non-shunting surgery vs.
    sclerotherapy, 200
  prophylactic sclerotherapy, 59, 72
  sclero- vs. non-sclerotherapy, 27
  shunt type, 259
Suture material
  mesocaval shunt, 263

Terminal esophago-proximal
    gastrectomy, 141
  blind vs. endoscopic assistance, 145
THF
  *see* branched-chain amino acids
Thrombocytopenia
  hypersplenism, distal splenorenal
    shunt, 288
  splenic artery embolization, 334
[201]Tl-chloride
  varices recurrence, 55
Total portosystemic shunt
  portal hypertension, 252
Trailmarking test
  Branched-chain amino acids,
    encephalopathy, 342
Transabdominal esophagus
    transection, 161, 167
  follow-up, 161
  technique, 167

Varices
  angioarchitecture, 119, 124
  endoscopic findings recording, 364
  hemodynamics, 315
  non-shunting surgery, 149
Varices bleeding
  bleeding localization, 124
  Idezuki tube, 347
  natural history, 14, 240
  sclero- vs. non-sclerotherapy, 24
  vasopressin, 303, 329
  vasopressin vs. Sengstaken tube, 331
Varices eradication
  combined injection therapy,
    polidocanol 1%, 48
  ethanolamine oleate + polidocanol,
    78
Varices rebleeding
  abdominal esophagus transection,
    170
  distal splenorenal shunt, 211, 217
  distal splenorenal shunt vs.
    sclerotherapy, 223
  emergency sclerotherapy, 38, 56
  portal-azygos disconnection surgery,
    144
  sclero- vs. non-sclerotherapy, 31, 258
  shunting surgery, 250, 252
Varices recurrence
  elective sclerotherapy, 100
  esophagus mucosa removal, 88
  esophagus transection (Sugiura), 158
  histopathology, 117
  polidocanol 1%, 77
  portal-azygos disconnection surgery,
    143
  post-sclerotherapy portal pressure,
    69
  prophylactic sclerotherapy, 61
  [201]Tl-chloride scintigraphy, 55
Vasopressin
  administration route, 303
  bradycardia, 310
  continuous i.v. therapy, 329
  coronary artery flow, 309

peroperative blood loss, 312
pulmonary edema, 332
splanchnic hemodynamics, 311
varices bleeding, 303
Vasopressin analog, 313
Vein damage

ethanolamine oleate, dog, 76, 81
polidocanol, dog, 76, 81

Warren shunt
   *see* distal splenorenal shunt